**1993**
**YEAR BOOK OF**
**SURGERY**®

# Statement of Purpose

## The YEAR BOOK Service

The YEAR BOOK series was devised in 1901 by practicing health professionals who observed that the literature of medicine and related disciplines had become so voluminous that no one individual could read and place in perspective every potential advance in a major specialty. In the final decade of the 20th century, this recognition is more acutely true than it was in 1901.

More than merely a series of books, YEAR BOOK volumes are the tangible results of a unique service designed to accomplish the following:

- *survey* a wide range of journals of proven value
- *select* from those journals papers representing significant advances and statements of important clinical principles
- provide *abstracts* of those articles that are readable, convenient summaries of their key points
- provide *commentary* about those articles to place them in perspective

These publications grow out of a unique process that calls on the talents of outstanding authorities in clinical and fundamental disciplines, trained literature specialists, and professional writers, all supported by the resources of Mosby, the world's preeminent publisher for the health professions.

## The Literature Base

Mosby subscribes to nearly 1,000 journals published worldwide, covering the full range of the health professions. On an annual basis, the publisher examines usage patterns and polls its expert authorities to add new journals to the literature base and to delete journals that are no longer useful as potential YEAR BOOK sources.

## The Literature Survey

The publisher's team of literature specialists, all of whom are trained and experienced health professionals, examines every original, peer-reviewed article in each journal issue. More than 250,000 articles per year are scanned systematically, including title, text, illustrations, tables, and references. Each scan is compared, article by article, to the search strategies that the publisher has developed in consultation with the 270 outside experts who form the pool of YEAR BOOK editors. A given article may be reviewed by any number of editors, from one to a dozen or more, regardless of the discipline for which the paper was originally published. In turn, each editor who receives the article reviews it to determine whether or not the article should be included in the YEAR BOOK. This decision is based on the article's inherent quality, its probable usefulness to readers of that YEAR BOOK, and the editor's goal to represent a balanced picture of a given field in each volume of the YEAR BOOK. In addition, the editor indicates when to include figures and tables from the article to help the YEAR BOOK reader better understand the information.

Of the quarter million articles scanned each year, only 5% are selected for detailed analysis within the YEAR BOOK series, thereby assuring readers of the high value of every selection.

## The Abstract

The publisher's abstracting staff is headed by a physician-writer and includes individuals with training in the life sciences, medicine, and other areas, plus extensive experience in writing for the health professions and related industries. Each selected article is assigned to a specific writer on this abstracting staff. The abstracter, guided in many cases by notations supplied by the expert editor, writes a structured, condensed summary designed so that the reader can rapidly acquire the essential information contained in the article.

## The Commentary

The YEAR BOOK editorial boards, sometimes assisted by guest commentators, write comments that place each article in perspective for the reader. This provides the reader with the equivalent of a personal consultation with a leading international authority—an opportunity to better understand the value of the article and to benefit from the authority's thought processes in assessing the article.

## Additional Editorial Features

The editorial boards of each YEAR BOOK organize the abstracts and comments to provide a logical and satisfying sequence of information. To enhance the organization, editors also provide introductions to sections or individual chapters, comments linking a number of abstracts, citations to additional literature, and other features.

The published YEAR BOOK contains enhanced bibliographic citations for each selected article, including extended listings of multiple authors and identification of author affiliations. Each YEAR BOOK contains a Table of Contents specific to that year's volume. From year to year, the Table of Contents for a given YEAR BOOK will vary depending on developments within the field.

Every YEAR BOOK contains a list of the journals from which papers have been selected. This list represents a subset of the nearly 1,000 journals surveyed by the publisher, and occasionally reflects a particularly pertinent article from a journal that is not surveyed on a routine basis.

Finally, each volume contains a comprehensive subject index and an index to authors of each selected paper.

# The 1993 Year Book Series

**Year Book of Anesthesia and Pain Management:** Drs. Miller, Abram, Kirby, Ostheimer, Roizen, and Stoelting

**Year Book of Cardiology®:** Drs. Schlant, Collins, Engle, Gersh, Kaplan, and Waldo

**Year Book of Chiropractic:** Drs. Phillips and Adams

**Year Book of Critical Care Medicine®:** Drs. Rogers and Parrillo

**Year Book of Dentistry®:** Drs. Meskin, Currier, Kennedy, Leinfelder, Berry, Roser, and Zakariasen

**Year Book of Dermatologic Surgery:** Drs. Swanson, Salasche, and Glogau

**Year Book of Dermatology®:** Drs. Sober and Fitzpatrick

**Year Book of Diagnostic Radiology®:** Drs. Federle, Clark, Gross, Madewell, Maynard, Sackett, and Young

**Year Book of Digestive Diseases®:** Drs. Greenberger and Moody

**Year Book of Drug Therapy®:** Drs. Lasagna and Weintraub

**Year Book of Emergency Medicine®:** Drs. Wagner, Burdick, Davidson, Roberts, and Spivey

**Year Book of Endocrinology®:** Drs. Bagdade, Braverman, Horton, Kannan, Landsberg, Molitch, Morley, Odell, Rogol, Ryan, and Sherwin

**Year Book of Family Practice®:** Drs. Berg, Bowman, Davidson, Dietrich, and Scherger

**Year Book of Geriatrics and Gerontology®:** Drs. Beck, Reuben, Burton, Small, Whitehouse, and Goldstein

**Year Book of Hand Surgery®:** Drs. Amadio and Hentz

**Year Book of Health Care Management:** Drs. Heyssel, Brock, Moses, and Steinberg, Ms. Avakian, and Messrs. Berman, Kues, and Rosenberg

**Year Book of Hematology®:** Drs. Spivak, Bell, Ness, Quesenberry, and Wiernik

**Year Book of Infectious Diseases®:** Drs. Wolff, Barza, Keusch, Klempner, and Snydman

**Year Book of Infertility®:** Drs. Mishell, Paulsen, and Lobo

**Year Book of Medicine®:** Drs. Rogers, Bone, Cline, O'Rourke, Greenberger, Utiger, Epstein, and Malawista

**Year Book of Neonatal and Perinatal Medicine®:** Drs. Klaus and Fanaroff

**Year Book of Nephrology:** Drs. Coe, Favus, Henderson, Kashgarian, Luke, Myers, and Curtis

**Year Book of Neurology and Neurosurgery®:** Drs. Bradley and Crowell

# Contributors

The Editors of the YEAR BOOK OF SURGERY gratefully acknowledge the contribution of John M. Porter, M.D., Professor of Surgery and Head, Division of Vascular Surgery, Oregon Health Sciences University School of Medicine, Portland, Oregon, and Editor of the YEAR BOOK OF VASCULAR SURGERY, for his assistance in the selection process for the Vascular chapter. We also thank our contributors to the Vascular chapter:

**James M. Seeger, M.D., F.A.C.S.**

*Professor and Chief, Section of Vascular Surgery, Department of Surgery, University of Florida College of Medicine, Gainesville, Florida*

**Timothy C. Flynn, M.D., F.A.C.S.**

*Associate Professor, Section of Vascular Surgery, Department of Surgery, University of Florida College of Medicine; and Chief of Surgical Services, Veterans Administration Medical Center, Gainesville, Florida*

**Timothy R.S. Harward, M.D.**

*Assistant Professor, Section of Vascular Surgery, Department of Surgery, University of Florida College of Medicine, Gainesville, Florida*

1993

# The Year Book of SURGERY®

Editor-in-Chief
## Edward M. Copeland, III, M.D.
*The Edward R. Woodward Professor and Chairman, Department of Surgery, University of Florida College of Medicine, Gainesville, Florida*

Editorial Board
## Edwin A. Deitch, M.D.
*Professor of Surgery, Louisiana State University School of Medicine in Shreveport; Louisiana State Medical Center, Shreveport, Louisiana*

## Timothy J. Eberlein, M.D.
*Associate Professor of Surgery, Harvard Medical School; Chief, Division of Surgical Oncology, Program Director, Laboratory of Biologic Cancer Therapy, Brigham and Women's Hospital; Surgical Director, Breast Evaluation Clinic, Dana Farber Cancer Institute, Boston, Massachusetts*

## Richard J. Howard, M.D., Ph.D.
*Professor of Surgery, University of Florida College of Medicine, Shands Hospital at the University of Florida, Gainesville, Florida*

## Wallace P. Ritchie, Jr., M.D.
*Professor and Chairman, Department of Surgery, Temple University School of Medicine, Temple University Hospital, Philadelphia, Pennsylvania*

## Martin C. Robson, M.D.
*Professor and Chief, Plastic Surgery, University of Texas Medical School at Galveston, Galveston, Texas*

## Wiley W. Souba, M.D., Sc.D.
*Chief, Division of Surgical Oncology, Massachusetts General Hospital, Harvard Medical School, Boston, Massachusetts*

## David J. Sugarbaker, M.D.
*Associate Professor of Surgery, Harvard Medical School; Chief, Division of Thoracic Surgery, Brigham and Women's Hospital, Boston, Massachusetts*

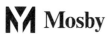 Mosby

St. Louis  Baltimore  Boston  Chicago  London  Madrid  Philadelphia  Sydney  Toronto

*Vice President and Publisher, Continuity Publishing:* Kenneth H. Killion
*Sponsoring Editor:* Diana Dodge
*Manager, Literature Services:* Edith M. Podrazik, R.N.
*Senior Information Specialist:* Terri Santo, R.N.
*Senior Medical Writer:* David A. Cramer, M.D.
*Project Supervisor:* Tamara L. Smith
*Senior Production Assistant:* Sandra Rogers
*Production Assistant:* Rebecca Nordbrock
*Senior Project Manager:* Max F. Perez
*Proofroom Manager:* Barbara M. Kelly

1993 EDITION
Copyright © September 1993 by Mosby-Year Book, Inc.

Printed in the United States of America
Composition by International Computaprint Corporation
Printing/binding by Maple-Vail


Mosby, Inc.
11830 Westline Industrial Drive
St. Louis, MO 63146


Editorial Office:
Mosby, Inc.
200 North LaSalle St.
Chicago, IL 60601

International Standard Serial Number: 0090-3671
International Standard Book Number: 0-8151-7792-5

# Table of Contents

# Journals Represented

Mosby subscribes to and surveys nearly 1,000 U.S. and foreign medical and allied health journals. From these journals, the Editors select the articles to be abstracted. Journals represented in this YEAR BOOK are listed below.

Acta Oto-Laryngologica
American Journal of Gastroenterology
American Journal of Medicine
American Journal of Pathology
American Journal of Psychiatry
American Journal of Surgery
American Surgeon
Annals of Internal Medicine
Annals of Surgery
Annals of Thoracic Surgery
Archives of Internal Medicine
Archives of Otolaryngology–Head and Neck Surgery
Archives of Surgery
British Journal of Cancer
British Journal of Plastic Surgery
British Journal of Surgery
Burns
Canadian Journal of Surgery
Cancer
Cancer Research
Chest
Circulatory Shock
Clinical Pediatrics
Clinical Pharmacology and Therapeutics
Clinical Science
Critical Care Medicine
Der Chirurg
Diseases of the Colon and Rectum
European Journal of Plastic Surgery
European Journal of Surgery
European Journal of Vascular Surgery
Gastroenterology
Gynecologic Oncology
Head and Neck
Hepatology
Human Pathology
International Journal of Cancer
International Journal of Dermatology
International Journal of Radiation, Oncology, Biology, and Physics
Journal of Burn Care and Rehabilitation
Journal of Clinical Endocrinology and Metabolism
Journal of Clinical Oncology
Journal of Clinical Pathology
Journal of Craniofacial Genetics and Developmental Biology
Journal of Heart and Lung Transplantation
Journal of Immunology
Journal of Investigative Dermatology
Journal of Oral and Maxillofacial Surgery
Journal of Pediatric Surgery
Journal of Surgical Research

Journal of Thoracic and Cardiovascular Surgery
Journal of Trauma
Journal of Urology
Journal of Vascular Surgery
Journal of the American Medical Association
Journal of the National Cancer Institute
Journal of the Royal College of Surgeons of Edinburgh
Laboratory Investigation
Lancet
Life Sciences
Medicine
Microsurgery
Nephrology, Dialysis, Transplantation
New England Journal of Medicine
Otolaryngology–Head and Neck Surgery
Plastic and Reconstructive Surgery
Radiology
Respiratory Medicine
Scandinavian Journal of Plastic and Reconstructive Surgery and Hand Surgery
Surgery
Surgery, Gynecology and Obstetrics
Thorax
Transplantation
World Journal of Surgery

### STANDARD ABBREVIATIONS

The following terms are abbreviated in this edition: acquired immunodeficiency syndrome (AIDS), the central nervous system (CNS), cerebrospinal fluid (CSF), computed tomography (CT), electrocardiography (ECG), human immunodeficiency virus (HIV), and magnetic resonance (MR) imaging (MRI).

# Introduction

The new Editorial Board members of the YEAR BOOK OF SURGERY are honored to be asked to carry on the tradition of excellence established by Seymour I. Schwartz and his associate editors, Olga Jonasson, Martin C. Robson, G. Tom Shires, Frank C. Spencer, and James C. Thompson, during the past 22 years.

We have elected to have a slightly different format. Each section is introduced with an overview written by the section editor, and several abstracts may be discussed together when appropriate.

Surgical education and cost containment were bigger issues this past year and are contained in the section on General Considerations. I suspect that in the next few years, the importance of these subjects will dictate the dedication of an entire section to each as we grapple with the new reimbursement system and the training of surgical residents within its framework.

The members of the Editorial Board have enjoyed our inaugural year as YEAR BOOK editors, and we look forward to attaining the same success as our predecessors.

Edward M. Copeland, III, M.D.

# 1 General Considerations

**Guidelines for Surgical Residents' Working Hours: Intent vs Reality**
Schwartz RJ, Dubrow TJ, Rosso RF, Williams RA, Butler JA, Wilson SE (Harbor-UCLA Med Ctr, Torrance, Calif)
*Arch Surg* 127:778–783, 1992                                                 1–1

*Background.*—Legislation in New York State in 1989 provided that residents caring for hospitalized patients work no more than 80 hours in a week, averaged over a 4-week period. Shifts are limited to 24 hours, and the house officer is entitled to a 24-hour work-free period each week. Anticipating similar legislation in California, the general surgical residence program at Harbor-UCLA has scheduled a 72-hour work week by changing in-house call from 1 in 3 nights to 1 in 4 and by providing 1 free day each weekend. There is 1 full weekend without call each month.

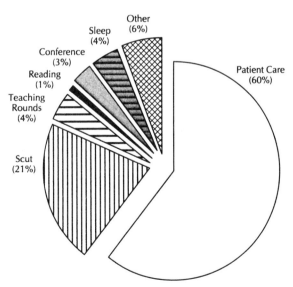

**Fig 1–1.**—Analysis of house staff hours. (Courtesy of Schwartz RJ, Dubrow TJ, Rosso RF, et al: *Arch Surg* 127:778–783, 1992.)

*Methods.*—The results of these changes were examined by prospectively surveying resident work hours and activites. House staff completed a daily activity log for 30 days. The response rate was 93%.

*Findings.*—The average hours of work per week were 100 for interns, 97 for junior residents, and 95 for chief residents. The overall average of 98 hours a week significantly exceeded the current and proposed guidelines. Patient care and "scut," defined as work that could be done by other persons, accounted for 81% of time spent in the hospital (Fig 1–1). Removing scut work lowered the overall in-hospital time to 78 hours. Surgery residents were more satisfied than were house officers from other programs who rotated through surgery.

*Implications.*—Scut work is the logical place to reduce resident hours. It includes drawing blood, transporting patients, gaining intravenous access, ordering tests, and doing paperwork other than medical record-keeping. Resident hours could be reduced by integrating physician assistants into general surgery teams.

---

**Quantitative Increases in Surgical House Officer Clinical Activity as the Basis for Increased Work Loads in a University Hospital**
Zelenock GB, Holmes MM, Campbell DA Jr, Stanley JC, Greenfield LJ (Univ of Michigan, Ann Arbor)
*Surgery* 112:235–243, 1992                                                1–2

---

*Background.*—In the continuum of medical education, house officers (HO) are considered trainees in a very advanced educational program at the same time they are hospital employees. Surgical HOs participate in sophisticated learning experiences, including regular in-service testing. Medicine demands better, faster and more practice activity because of profound changes such as diagnosis-related group reimbursement patterns, greater patient acuity, more efficient use of clinical resources, and increasing reliance on clinical income to support salaries, research, and education. The hypothesis that clinical service demands on HOs have increased was examined. Objective and quantifiable measures influencing contemporary surgical HO practice were assessed.

*Method.*—The number of HO trainees, as well as the number of admissions, discharges, total inpatient and outpatient operations, clinic visits, and other clinical activities, were documented for a 10-year period. Significant differences during the 10 years were noted.

*Findings.*—Although the number of HOs during the 10-year study period was constant at about 122, total operations increased by 143% and inpatient procedures increased by 75%; annual hospital admissions, discharges, clinic visits, and operating room hours also increased significantly. The case mix index showed a twofold increase in the acuity of inpatient hospital care from 1.41 in 1985 to 1.71 in 1991. This was accompanied by a 125% increase in the number of surgical intensive care unit beds. Even though the number of HOs remained constant, there was a 49% staffing increase in the department of surgery faculty, a 118% increase in the clinical nursing staff, a 59% increase in the hospital administrative staff, and a 53% increase in hospital support staff. The number of medical students decreased by 16% during this period. The calculated workload increased from 91.2 hr/wk per HO in 1981 to 110.9 hr/wk per in 1991.

*Conclusion.*—During a 10-year study period, the baseline level of every clinical activity involving surgical patients at a university hospital increased, whereas the number of HOs remained constant. House officers may not necessarily be working more hours, but they are unequivocally doing more work than in past years. Greater numbers of HOs to share the burden is not a viable solution because the number of HOs at an institution is limited by residency review committees. Surgical educators must find solutions to excessive HO workloads before external regulatory intervention is imposed on the profession.

▶ The studies by Schwartz et al. (Abstract 1–1) and Zelenock et al. (Abstract 1–2) quantitate what those of us in medical education have known for some time. The problem in resident education is a fixed work force with ever-increasing administrative and patient care responsibilities. The safety of patient care will not be substantially improved by legislating a reduction in work hours of residents unless methods to concentrate the knowledge of these skilled individuals at the bedside are improved. In an era of shrinking medical budgets, an increased number of residents will not occur. Therefore, better utilization of paramedical personnel and better data retrieval are needed. Residents on call should have a team of individuals and computer-generated data at their disposal to increase the efficiency of patient care. Ideally, residents should be on call only for those patients for whom they provide care during the day. Many problems that require a physician visit at night can predictably be avoided if the same health care team provides 24-hour coverage and, with such a system, the in-house physician may actually get some sleep (assuming the hospital provides a comfortable, quiet location). Cross-covering or "floating coverage" requires the on-call physician to evaluate minor problems for unknown patients and fosters an attitude of "leave it for the guy on call" in the residents who have the night off.—E.M. Copeland, III, M.D.

---

**The Stresses of the Surgical Residency**
Bunch WH, Dvonch VM, Storr CL, Baldwin DC Jr, Hughes PH (Lakeshore Rehabilitation Hosp, Birmingham, Ala; Johns Hopkins Univ, Baltimore, Md; Univ of South Florida, Tampa; AMA, Chicago)
*J Surg Res* 53:268–271, 1992                                    1–3

---

*Introduction.*—Concern over surgical residents' work hours prompted a study of the stress experienced by these residents and whether such

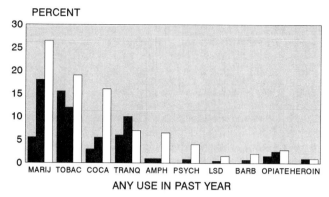

**Fig 1–2.**—Graph shows use of 10 substances by surgery residents, all residents, and college gradu-
ates. Surgery residents are less likely to have used these substances than are the other groups. *Filled
bars*, surgery residents; *middle bars*, all residents; and *open bars*, college graduates. *Abbreviations:
MARIJ,* marijuana; *TOBAC,* tobacco; *COCA,* cocaine; *TRANQ,* tranquilizers; *AMPH,* amphetamines;
*PSYCH,* psychedelics; *BARB,* barbiturates; (Courtesy of Bunch WH, Dvonch VM, Storr CL, et al: *J Surg
Res* 53:268–271, 1992.)

stress leads to excessive use of alcohol or drugs. Data were obtained
from a national survey of residents' workloads.

*Methods.*—The self-administered, 8-page, multiple-choice question-
nare contained 32 questions regarding stress and stress-related behav-
iors. It was sent to 3,000 residents selected from the American Medical
Association physician master file in the spring of 1987. The overall response rate of 60% provided answers from 1,754 physicians; 80 were
residents in general surgery and 179 were residents in various surgical
specialties.

*Results.*—Sixty-four percent of the responding residents were married
and 22% of the general surgical group and 12% of the specialty surgical
group were female. Sixty-three precent of the general surgery residents
rated their assigned hours as excessive much of the time, compared to
46% of the specialty residents, a significant difference in opinion. This
outcome was supported by an analysis of call schedules and assigned
hours. Sleep deprivation and exhaustion occurred significantly more often in general surgery residents than in the specialty group. Nearly half
of the former group stated that they dealt with much death and suffer-
ing, whereas the surgery specialty residents did not.

Surgery residents, both general and specialty, were more likely to have
used alcohol in the past month than other residents. The frequency of
use within the past month, however, was generally low and not different
from that of all residents. Significantly more residents in the surgical specialty group than general surgery residents had used marijuana, but the
use rate of all surgical residents was less than that of all residents or college graduates (Fig 1–2).

*Conclusions.*—These results can lead to an optimistic conclusion
about the stresses of surgical residencies. Severe stresses do exist, how-

ever, particularly for general surgical residents, and more research is required to fully understand how to avoid such stresses in the future training of new residents.

▶ General surgery residents have a heavier workload because the illness acuity of their patients is greater than that of specialty surgical residents who often take call at home. As a rule, surgical residents enjoy their work and realize that much of their quality surgical training takes place at night. Nevertheless, no one likes to be taken advantage of, as indicated by 63% of the respondents to this study's questionnaire. When the health care system realizes that tertiary care centers will require an increase in paramedical personnel to provide direct patient care, we would hope that this personnel will be assigned to the services with the sickest patients and not distributed evenly to all medical disciplines or to the service chief with the "silver" tongue.—E.M. Copeland, III, M.D.

---

**Experience as a Surgeon Determines Resident Knowledge**
Luchette F, Booth FMcL, Seibel R, Bernstein G, Ricotta J, Hoover E, Hassett JM (State Univ of New York, Buffalo)
*Surgery* 112:419–423, 1992                                                  1–4

---

*Background.*—Evaluations of residents' knowledge have shown that performance on a written examination is directly related to clinical experience. An increase in clinical experience improves the individual's cognitive knowledge base but not the basic science knowledge. The primacy of the operative experience in the graduate training environment was demonstrated by identifying the specific relationship between the operative experience of 42 residents at 1 institution and their performance on the American Board of Surgery Inservice Training Examination (ABSITE).

*Method.*—In a prospective study, the patient, operative procedure, and the residents involved in the operation were tracked by a computerized log. Report D of the ABSITE was used to assign each test item to specific operative procedures and to determine the frequency of the correct response for each item. The fraction of operative procedures (Fs) was determined for each category of surgical procedures (Fs = number of procedures as surgeon/total number of procedures). The frequency of the correct response was compared to the Fs by use of the Pearson correlation coefficient with significance at the 95% confidence level.

*Results.*—The 42 residents performed 8,357 surgical procedures in 12 months. Of the 209 test items on report D, 162 items could be assigned to 26 categories of surgical procedures. The frequency of the correct response, the total number of correct responses divided by the total number of responders for each item, correlated directly with the Fs. The resident performance on the ABSITE improved from 44% to 83% as operative experience increased from .11% to 8.36%. Knowledge appears directly related to experience.

*Conclusion.*—The data on the significant correlation of the residents' clinical experience and their performance on the ABSITE examination confirms the paradigm for the curriculum of a surgical residency. Procedural or clinical experience reinforces the knowledge base. ABSITE can be used to help to establish certification for a resident's clinical credentials. Inadequate ABSITE performance may be modified by changing the resident's clinical experience to increase the frequency of operative procedures.

▶ Retention of information comes from experience with it. To properly diagnose the disease, design the proper operation to cure it, and provide appropriate postoperative care requires a wealth of information. Then repetitively utilizing this information, particularly if it is a technical skill, further improves and expands one's knowledge of it. As a member of the American Board of Surgery, I am pleased that the ABSITE is constructed appropriately to help measure clinical credentials.—E.M. Copeland, III, M.D.

**Preliminary Assessment of a Scientific Curriculum in a Surgical Residency Program**
Safran DB, Crombie HD, Allen L, Ruby ST, Deckers PJ (Hartford Hosp, Hartford, Conn; Univ of Connecticut Health Ctr, Farmington)
*Arch Surg* 127:529–535, 1992                                          1–5

*Background.*—Recognizing the impact of recent scientific advances, the American Board of Surgery (ABS) has mandated that residency programs give greater attention to the teaching of basic science. A new basic science curriculum based on ABS guidelines and instituted for residents at the University of Connecticut (Farmington) during the 1990–1991 academic year was assessed.

*Methods.*—The central component of the curriculum was a weekly, 90-minute conference. Under the guidance of a faculty advisor with expertise in the area of discussion, a senior resident and a junior resident organized and presented the material. All residents were examined monthly by a written, multiple-choice test, followed by a review and discussion of the questions. Senior residents were also expected to participate in oral examinations. A 16-question survey was distributed to residents who completed the curriculum.

*Results.*—Thirty-five categorical residents and 15 preliminary residents were enrolled in the general surgical residency programs during the 1989-1990 academic year. Although performance on the monthly examinations improved, scores on the ABS In-Training Examination (ABSITE) declined in the group. The decline from previous scores, however, was not statistically significant. For the entire group of senior residents, performance on the oral examination was unchanged from 1 year to the next. Categorical residents showed greater improvement than preliminary residents. The curriculum was received positively with recommendations that assigned readings be shortened and attending physicians be more involved in the conferences.

*Conclusion.*—Academic growth needs to continue during the demanding years of a surgical residency. The disappointing results on the ABSITE may be attributed to the fact that this examination did not yet incorporate the scientific materials advocated by the ABS.

▶ The ABS has sought to emphasize basic science as applied to the practice of surgery. In this regard, many of the ABS questions might not appear to be "basic science" in the classic sense. Seminars prepared by the residents and well attended by faculty are quite popular, as identified by this study. Such active participation by everyone in the training program may not immediately improve ABSITE scores, but it will broaden and enhance the residency training program and lead to improved patient care.—E.M. Copeland, III, M.D.

---

**Relationships Between Surgical Ability Ratings and Spatial Abilities and Personality**
Deary IJ, Graham KS, Maran AGD (University of Edinburgh, Edinburgh, Scotland; Royal Infirmary of Edinburgh)
*J R Coll Surg Edin* 37:74–79, 1992                              1–6

---

*Background.*—Clinical skills in surgery cannot be accurately predicted by academic examination results or impressions made at an interview. Although measures of intelligence or cognitive knowledge are not significantly correlated with surgical skill, several studies suggest that a high level of spatial ability appears to be a prerequisite of success for surgeons. Twenty-two trainee surgeons were evaluated to determine which type of test correlated best with surgical performance.

*Methods.*—The study participants had a mean age of 31.6 years and a mean of 6.6 years of surgical training. Three aspects of spatial ability— spatial orientation, spatial scanning, and visualization—were evaluated with a standard test. The trainee surgeons were also given a computerized reaction time test involving response to pairs of 2-dimensional shapes; a stereoscopic vision test; a paper-and-pencil test that gives separate measures of verbal, numerical, and diagrammatic ability; and personality inventories. Consultant surgeons rated the trainees' operating ability and clinical decision-making.

*Results.*—The ability ratings of the surgical trainees were high. Intelligence test scores were not significantly correlated with surgical ability ratings. Only 1 subtest of spatial ability correlated with ability rating, and the correlation was in the opposite direction to that expected. There were trends suggesting that superior ratings were associated with the personality traits of introversion and conscientiousness and the spatial ability of stereoscopic depth perception.

*Conclusion.*—There were few significant results in this attempt to relate surgical skills to results of spatial ability and personality tests. Surgery is clearly more than a technical skill, and surgical skill may not be measurable directly.

▶ Accurately predicting clinical skills in surgery is a difficult task. Manual dexterity, for example, may improve through practice, but the rate and extent of this improvement are not predictable. Nevertheless, surgical residents should be closely monitored during the first 2 years of training to determine improvement in dexterity and the development of organizational skills. The field of general surgery is broad, and some residents may be more comfortable in a specialty with more narrow boundaries. Likewise, not everyone is technically proficient. The first 2 years of residency should be used to identify those individuals who are unsuited for general surgery and to channel them into a medical specialty where they will be more competitive with their peers, once in practice.

Although this study did not show a correlation between clinical skills in surgery and spatial ability, conscientiousness did have a positive correlation.—E.M. Copeland, III, M.D.

---

**Problem-Based Learning: An Effective Educational Method for a Surgery Clerkship**
Schwartz RW, Donnelly MB, Nash PP, Johnson SB, Young B, Griffen WO Jr
(Univ of Kentucky, Lexington; VA Med Ctr, Lexington)
*J Surg Res* 53:326–330, 1992                                      1–7

---

*Introduction.*—Medical educators have currently recommended changing the fundamental process of medical school education in the areas of basic science and clinical practice. Some have suggested the inclusion of problem-based learning (PBL) as a format to aid the development of clinical knowledge. Student performance on modified essay examinations (MEE) and the National Board of Medical Examiners Part II (NBME II) examination was evaluated after completion of a PBL curriculum.

*Methods.*—Seventy-eight students were exposed to 4 successive 12-week junior surgery clinical clerkships, with 42 students completing a traditional training method and 36 students assigned to the PBL method. All students had about 4 hours of directed study daily, with the remainder of time available for self-directed activities. The PBL sessions were in a tutorial format conducted by a faculty member. The students reviewed 28–30 cases during the 12 weeks. Students in the traditional program attended 6 45-minute lectures each week, conducted in a Socratic format (SI) and containing twice as many topics as in the PBL program.

*Results.*—In the essay examination, the SI students made more errors in 3 areas than did the PBL students, with significantly more mistakes in differential diagnosis and interpretation of clinical data. The PBL students also performed better than SI students in ordering appropriate laboratory and diagnostic studies. No significant differences were observed between the groups in the NBME-II examination, although the PBL students tended to score higher on the surgery subtest.

*Conclusions.*—Medical students in the PBL program performed significantly better than did the students in the SI curriculum format with regard to clinical problem solving and retaining clinical information.

▶ Problem-based learning designed to simulate clinical situations should be more valuable than didactic lectures or teaching using an oral examination style. Unfortunately, the latter 2 methods are much easier to accomplish and are therefore used frequently. Similar to retention of information by residents, students will learn more by active participation in a clinical problem than by simply being told about it in a lecture.—E.M. Copeland, III, M.D.

---

**Measuring and Managing Quality of Surgery: Statistical vs Incidental Approaches**
McGuire HH Jr, Horsley JS III, Salter DR, Sobel M (Virginia Commonwealth Univ, Richmond)
*Arch Surg* 127:733–738, 1992                                             1–8

---

*Introduction.*—For generations, surgeons have voluntarily scrutinized their performance and have assumed that the evaluation scores of their outcome were the same as those reported by other surgeons using the same techniques. A statistical approach to quality management involves comparing rates of desired or unwanted side effects in samples of procedures to predetermined standards. The incidental approach involves reviewing patients who have complications and asking how the problems might have been avoided.

*Methods.*—Weekly reports and monthly conferences dealing with surgical complications were reviewed for the period 1977–1990 at a VA medical center. Apart from statistical analysis, representatives of all surgical specialities reviewed each complication and attributed it to 1 of 6 causes if possible.

*Statistical Approach.*—Data on a total of 44,603 major operations indicated that 5.4% of patients had complications after 6.3% of procedures. Mortality in the same hospital admission was 1.7%. Forty-eight operations were common enough, or complicated enough, to serve as indices of surgical safety.

*Incidental Approach.*—Most common errors, including nosocomial infections and surgical wound problems, were discussed critically in staff conference. When the need was apparent, memorandums dealing with such measures as hand washing, changing dressings safely, removing catheters at an early stage, and limiting the use of antibiotics were sent to staff members. Unique events led on occasion to global improvements in patient care.

*Conclusions.*—Statistical methods produce data too slowly to protect patients currently under treatment. Statistical data measured quality during periods of several years and compared the findings to national norms. Statistical analysis was, therefore, only of value to avoid claims of unsafe practice. The incidental approach, however, when comprehensive, appeared to improve surgical knowledge and patient safety by allowing an in-depth review of patients with complicated and heterogenous diseases.

▶ The incidental approach used by McGuire and associates is the classic morbidity and mortality (M&M) conference held in most medical schools. For such a conference to achieve the excellent results reported in this study, attendance by faculty and residents must be near 100% and all complications must be listed for review. Quality assurance monitors and trending of complications should be blended into the complications' conference for the incidental approach to be maximally effective and to produce data immediately valuable for patient safety and future planning.—E.M. Copeland, III, M.D.

---

**Quality Assurance and Morbidity and Mortality Conference**
Thompson JS, Prior MA (Univ of Nebraska, Omaha; Creighton Univ, Omaha)
*J Surg Res* 52:97–100, 1992                                                   1–9

---

*Introduction.*—Some surgeons contend that an institution's regularly scheduled morbidity and mortality (M&M) conference assures quality control of surgical programs, thus rendering other forms of assessment and monitoring unnecessary. The effectiveness of the M&M conference in assuring quality care in the areas of infection control and surgical case review was assessed.

*Methods.*—All adverse patient care reports in the survival service records between 1989 and 1990 were reviewed. These data were then presented and assessed at the M&M conference and compared to information resulting from the quality assurance measures used in the institution, e.g., infection reporting, care review, and continuous reassessment of complications and deaths.

*Results.*—Of the 602 adverse outcomes, peer review practices identified only 95 cases. Of these 95 reports, only 70 (74%) were discussed at the M&M conference. Of the 69 cases of wound infections, the nursing staff initially reported 37. During the surgical case review process, 99 procedures did not pass the primary screening, and 49 of the 99 procedures failed the justification process. Of the total adverse events, 14 were found by subsequent peer review and 5 at the M&M conference.

Ninety-five problems and 63 deaths were reported only at the M&M conference. Significantly more physicians attended the general surgery section of the M&M meeting than the surgical specialty areas, with 74% of all residents and 33% of surgical staff attending the conference. The M&M conference and the peer review of charts correlated well for the assignment of level of care.

*Conclusions.*—The M&M conference, routinely held at health care institutions, benefits patient care through the quality assurance program. Many adverse events were first reported at the meeting and had not been identified by other monitoring programs.

▶ Attendance at M&M conference was poor; only 33% of surgical staff attended. Likewise, several adverse events identified by peer review of the medical record were not reported at the M&M conference. Nevertheless, there was excellent agreement about level of care when M&M conference data were compared to quality assurance data. Information from this study underscores the need for blending the multiple methods of insuring high quality of patient care within any institution.—E.M. Copeland, III, M.D.

---

**Autopsy in General Surgery Practice**
Stothert JC Jr, Gbaanador G (Univ of Texas, Galveston)
*Am J Surg* 162:585–589, 1991                                        1–10

---

*Introduction.*—The autopsy rate in most hospitals has declined in the past 50 years, from approximately 50% to the present 10% to 15%. The procedure is expensive, thought to yield little additional information, and may raise issues for litigation. At the University of Texas Medical Branch, however, autopsies continue to be performed frequently. The procedure's educational value to students and residents in the general surgical program was evaluated.

*Methods*—The charts of all patients who died on the surgical services from 1984 through 1988 were evaluated and compared with autopsy findings. Discrepancies between clinical impressions and the anatomical diagnosis were categorized as class I to class IV. Class I discrepancies were errors that would have changed therapy and possibly improved survival; class II errors were missed major diagnoses having an equivocal impact on survival; class III discrepancies consisted of information that could not be diagnosed clinically; and class IV included totally unsuspected diagnoses unrelated to the cause of death.

*Results.*—Autopsies were performed in 73% of the 628 deaths that occurred on the surgical services during the 5-year study period. Class I diagnostic discrepancies were found in 5% to 10% of patients studied and class II errors in 10% to 30%. Classes III and IV diagnostic discrepancies, of intellectual interest only, were discovered in virtually all autopsies. Most class I discrepancies were infectious (30% to 40%), pulmonary (10% to 20%), or cardiovascular (10% to 20%).

*Conclusion.*—The autopsy, once the "gold standard" by which clinical impressions were confirmed, has fallen out of use. But, as the results of this study demonstrate, diagnostic errors are commonplace. Considerations of cost and fear of litigation should not allow this important educational tool to become a rare event. A formal presentation of autopsy findings, followed by discussion of possible errors in diagnosis and management, is an invaluable part of surgical training.

▶ Sophisticated noninvasive diagnostic tests are thought to have made autopsy obsolete, yet a minimum of 15% of patients in this study had autopsy findings that were unsuspected and might possibly have changed therapy and/or outcome. It would seem that correlating the results of autopsy with sophisticated noninvasive studies would produce valuable information about the reasons for false positive or false negative tests, not to mention the value of the information learned as a teaching tool and as a quality assurance monitor. Autopsy should be reinstituted!—E.M. Copeland, III, M.D.

---

**Efficacy of Preadmission Testing in Ambulatory Surgical Patients**
Golub R, Cantu R, Sorrento JJ, Stein HD (Flushing Hosp Med Ctr, Flushing, NY; Albert Einstein College of Medicine, Bronx, NY)
*Am J Surg* 163:565–571, 1992                                                    1–11

---

*Background.*—The proportion of operations done on an ambulatory basis at the study center increased from 24% in 1985 to 40% in early 1990. The usefulness of preoperative testing in ambulatory patients was assessed.

*Methods.*—The records were reviewed for 325 patients who had preadmission testing before ambulatory surgery during a 10-week period in 1988.

*Findings.*—At least 1 laboratory abnormality was found in 84% of patients. Serial multiple analysis results were abnormal nearly two thirds of the time, and 38% of urinalysis results were abnormal. One fourth of the patients had an abnormal ECG, and 19% had abnormal chest radiographs. Only 3 patients appeared to benefit from preadmission testing. Fully 96% of abnormalities were ignored by attending physicians. Most abnormal values were only a few points outside the normal range or were predictable from the patient's history. All patients with potentially serious abnormalities were older than age 50 or had a history of heart disease.

*Discussion.*—Preadmission screening of patients scheduled for ambulatory surgery had a negligible effect on surgicial morbidity. A workup to

Recommendations for Preadmission Testing for Ambulatory Surgery in the Literature

| | [18] | [5] | [6] | [16] | [4] | [32] | [17] | Present Series |
|---|---|---|---|---|---|---|---|---|
| Hematocrit | H&P All women Men > 60 yr | Spun | Yes | > 40 yr | Yes | Yes | All women | Major blood loss |
| PT, PTT, platelets | H&P | | H&P | | H&P | H&P | H&P, vasc | H&P |
| Urinalysis | | Dip | H&P | | Yes | | Dip | |
| Electrolytes | H&P | | K+ | > 60 yr & major | H&P | H&P | H&P | H&P |
| Glucose | H&P | | Yes | > 60 yr & major | H&P | H&P | Yes | H&P |
| BUN, creatinine | H&P | | H&P | > 60 yr & major | H&P | H&P | | H&P |
| Liver profile | H&P | | H&P | | H&P | | | H&P |
| Chest roentgenogram | > 60 yr, H&P | | H&P | > 60 yr & major | H&P | H&P | > 40 yr, H&P, chest case | H&P |
| Electrocardiogram | > 60 yr, ± > 40 yr, H&P | H&P | H&P | > 50 yr | H&P | H&P | Men > 40 yr, Women > 55 yr | H&P, > 50 yr |

*Abbreviations: H&P,* as indicated by history and physical examination; *PT,* prothrombin time; *PTT,* partial thromboplastin time; *BUN,* blood urea nitrogen; *major,* major surgery planned; K+, potassium; *Vasc,* vascular or cardiac procedure; *Dip,* dipstick.

(Courtesy of Golub R, Cantu R, Sorrento JJ, et al: *Am J Surg* 163:565–571, 1992.)

assess screening abnormalities may lead to unnecessary delay and expense. Previously recommended policies are shown in the table. It was recommended instead that patients older than 50 years have ECG, and that the hematocrit be measured if major blood loss is expected. Other tests should be ordered selectively on the basis of the history, examination, and proposed procedure.

▶ I agree with the conclusions of this study that screening of healthy asymptomatic patients for disease before an ambulatory surgicial procedure is inefficient and may result in unnecessary expense and delay in therapy for the primary problem. The majority of disease processes will be discovered during the history and physical examination, which emphasizes the continued importance of these evaluations.—E.M. Copeland, III, M.D.

## Admission Stool Guaiac Test: Use and Impact on Patient Management

Gomez JA, Diehl AK (Univ of Texas, San Antonio)
*Am J Med* 92:603–606, 1992
1–12

*Introduction.*—The practice of obtaining a stool guaiac test during the admission physical exmination is widespread, but it has never been evaluated in terms of its yield of unexpected diagnoses. The use admission stool guaiac (ASG) testing was documented to determine the diagnostic yield of this test and to evaluate its potential benefits.

*Methods.*—The study included 264 patients admitted to general medicine wards, telemetry, and intensive care units in a 1-month period.

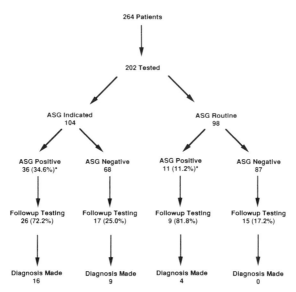

**Fig 1–3.**—Results, follow-up testing, and number of gastrointestinal diagnoses in patients receiving ASG tests. * P < .001. (Courtesy of Gomez JA, Diehl AK: *Am J Med* 92:603–606, 1992.)

There were 144 men and 120 women (mean age, 50 years). Members of the house staff performed ASG tests using a single Hemoccult card and stool obtained during admission rectal examination. Each test was categorized as being indicated or routine according to established criteria.

*Findings.*—An ASG test was performed in 20 patients, or 77%. The ASGs were more likely to be done in men than in women and in patients admitted to ward as opposed to intensive care services. They were done in 84% of patients with clinical indications and in 70% of those with no indications. The test was positive in 35% of patients with clinical indications and in 11% of those without. Of the 104 patients with indications, 25 were eventually found to have gastrointestinal lesions, most of which were important. In contrast, only 4 of 98 patients tested routinely had diagnoses established, and all but 1 of these were benign (Fig 1–3). Clinical indications were present in 4 of 5 patients with cancer; in the other patient the diagnosis was made only after experiencing copious rectal bleeding occurred after aspirin and heparin treatment.

*Conclusions.*—It is suggested that ASG testing is best reserved for patients with clinical indications for such a test. Otherwise, the test is of questionable value and only infrequently leads to important diagnoses in patients without such indications. Further study is needed to clarify the value of the routine ASG test.

▶ A single Hemoccult test on admission is a valuable teaching tool because it focuses the trainee on a potentially important diagnostic sign—blood in the stool. This study shows it to be of little diagnostic value in asymptomatic patients, a result that would probably be predictable if thought were given to it. However, this study should not detract from the importance of detection of fecal occult blood when the test is done properly, or from the value of the rectal and pelvic examination as an important component of a complete physical examination.—E.M. Copeland, III, M.D.

---

**A Randomized Comparison of Patient-Controlled Versus Standard Analgesic Requirements in Patients Undergoing Cholecystectomy**
Kenady DE, Wilson JF, Schwartz RW, Bannon CL, Wermeling D (Univ of Kentucky, Lexington; VA Med Ctr, Lexington)
*Surg Gynecol Obstet* 174:216–220, 1992                                                        1–13

---

*Introduction.*—Patient-controlled analgesia (PCA) reportedly is superior to standard regimens in providing pain relief. The use of PCA was compared with the use of standard intramuscular administration of narcotics in patients undergoing cholecystectomy.

*Methods.*—To obtain a homogeneous study group, only patients with chronic disease were selected. Participants were randomly assigned to either PCA (morphine intravenously) or morphine intramuscularly. Twice as many patients had PCA as had morphine intramuscularly. The final sample included 35 patients in the PCA group and 18 in the group treated intramuscularly. Nurses recorded morphine requirements and assessed the patients' degree of pain; participants were interviewed about their pain experience.

*Results.*—The 2 groups did not differ significantly in average period of hospitalization, daily dosage of morphine, or total morphine used. Patients who received PCA, however, reported less distress from pain during the first 2 postoperative days and were less groggy on the first postoperative day. Also, patients who received PCA reported less interference with both postoperative breathing and pulmonary recovery.

*Conclusion.*—Standard postoperative delivery of analgesics resulted in a long delay between the patient's request for medication and delivery by the nursing staff. The use of PCA allows a larger dose of narcotic when needed so that patients who receive PCA spend significantly less time in pain than patients who receive standard intramuscular therapy.

▶ The technique of PCA is becoming widely used. The results of this study do not show a dramatic difference between morphine administered by standard intramuscular injection versus the PCA pump. The majority of the differences were subjective. Possibly, a crossover study (using patients as their own controls) might better elucidate the differences between delivery techniques. This study demonstrates that intramuscular morphine is still a worthy tool to reduce postoperative pain.—E.M. Copeland, III, M.D.

## Ondansetron Is Effective in Decreasing Postoperative Nausea and Vomiting

Dershwitz M, Rosow CE, Di Biase PM, Joslyn AF, Sanderson PE (Massachusetts Gen Hosp, Boston; Glaxo, Inc, Research Triangle Park, NC)
*Clin Pharmacol Ther* 52:96–101, 1992                    1–14

*Objective.*—Ondansetron is a selective 5-$HT_3$ receptor antagonist with antiemetic properties. Its efficacy has been demonstrated in animal models as well as in humans, particularly in patients receiving cancer chemotherapy. The safety and efficacy of ondansetron were assessed when used prophylactically against postoperative nausea and vomiting in patients undergoing abdominal operations.

*Patients.*—Of 50 women having intra-abdominal and extra-abdominal gynecologic procedures, 26 were randomized to 2 doses of ondansetron, 8 mg intravenously and 24 were given placebo. The first dose was given immediately before induction of general anesthesia, and the second dose was given 8 hours later. The number of emetic episodes was recorded for 24 hours after the operation, and the patients were asked to rate their nausea on a scale from 0 to 10. Rescue therapy with droperidol or prochlorperazine was administered to patients with intractable nausea or intractable vomiting.

*Results.*—Fifteen of the 26 ondansetron-treated patients (58%) and 1 of the 24 placebo-treated patients (4%) did not have any emetic episodes and did not require rescue therapy. In the placebo-treated group, the median number of emetic episodes was greater in patients who underwent extra-abdominal procedures than in those who had intra-abdominal procedures, but the difference did not reach statistical significance. In the ondansetron-treated group, the drug was more effective in those who had extra-abdominal procedures. Ondansetron also improved the patients' subjective nausea rating. Both groups had similar rates of minor adverse effects.

*Conclusions.*—Ondansetron is a highly effective antiemetic when used prophylactically before general anesthesia in patients undergoing intra-abdominal or extra-abdominal gynecologic operations.

▶ Having an effective antiemetic is a powerful tool. However, its routine use should be avoided. Nausea and vomiting are important symptoms of surgical illness and should not be eliminated from the diagnostic armamentarium of the physician lest mechanical small bowel obstruction, acute gastric dilatation, acalculus cholecystitis, pancreatitis, and the like go undetected for a dangerously long period of time postoperatively.—E.M. Copeland, III, M.D.

## Geographic Variation in the Use of Breast-Conserving Treatment for Breast Cancer

Nattinger AB, Gottlieb MS, Veum J, Yahnke D, Goodwin JS (Med College of

Wisconsin, Milwaukee; Univ of Wisconsin, Milwaukee)
*N Engl J Med* 326:1102–1107, 1992                                    1–15

*Introduction.*—Breast-conserving treatment for breast cancer has increased in the past decade; however, it remains unknown how extensively this treatment has been adopted in various regions of the United States and whether its use can be predicted by hospital and patient characteristics. Medicare data were used to assess regional and hospital differences in the use of breast-conserving surgery.

*Methods.*—Medicare claims for inpatient care provided to 36,982 women aged 65–79 years in 1986 were reviewed. In this age range, the percentage of women undergoing breast-conserving surgery was constant. In all of the women, local or regional breast cancer was treated by mastectomy or breast-conserving surgery (local excision, quadrantectomy, or subtotal mastectomy). Hospital characteristics were derived from an American Hospital Association survey.

*Results.*—Breast-conserving surgery was performed in approximately 12% of patients and mastectomy was performed in 88%. Breast-conserving treatment was used in 20% of patients in the Middle Atlantic states and in 17% in New England, compared with 6% in the East South Central states and 7% in the West South Central states (Fig 1–4). Patients in urban areas were more likely to undergo breast-conserving treatment than those in rural areas. This type of treatment was also more common in teaching hospitals, large hospitals, and hospitals with on-site radiation therapy or geriatric services (table). Most of the regional differences re-

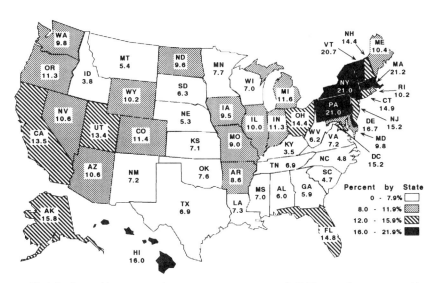

**Fig 1–4.**—Rates of breast-conserving surgery among women aged 65–79 years who were covered by Medicare and who underwent surgery for local or regional breast cancer in 1986, according to state. (Courtesy of Nattinger AB, Gottlieb MS, Veum J, et al: *N Engl J Med* 326:1102–1107, 1992.)

Use of Breast-Conserving Surgery According to
Hospital Characteristics

| CHARACTERISTIC | PERCENT OF PATIENTS† | ODDS RATIO (95% CI) |
|---|---|---|
| Medical school affiliation (any vs. none) | 38.5 | 1.4 (1.3–1.5) |
| Member of Council of Teaching Hospitals (vs. not a member) | 19.1 | 1.7 (1.6–1.9) |
| Full-time house staff (any vs. none) | 34.1 | 1.8 (1.7–1.9) |
| No. of hospital beds (≥500 vs. <50) | 20.6 | 2.5 (1.9–3.3) |
| No. of Medicare discharges (≥6000 vs. <1500) | 21.3 | 1.8 (1.6–2.0) |
| Radiation therapy (available vs. not available) | 46.1 | 1.4 (1.3–1.4) |
| Geriatric services (available vs. not available) | 25.8 | 1.4 (1.3–1.5) |
| Cancer center (available vs. not available) | 45.0 | 1.3 (1.2–1.4) |
| Women's center (available vs. not available) | 19.1 | 1.0 (0.9–1.1) |
| Investor-owned (vs. not-for-profit) | 9.6 | 1.0 (0.9–1.1) |

Note: This table includes data on women aged 65-79 years who were covered by Medicare; only patients for whom data were available on each hospital characteristic have been included in the separate analyses. Odds ratios are for the use of breast-conserving surgery. CI denotes confidence interval.

† The percentage of patients who were treated in hospitals with that particular characteristic. The comparisons used in calculating the odds are shown in parentheses for each characteristic.

(Courtesy of Nattinger AB, Gottlieb MS, Veum J, et al: N *Engl J Med* 326:1102-1107, 1992.)

mained, however, after adjustment for hospital and patient characteristics.

*Conclusion.*—There is considerable regional variation in the use of breast-conserving treatment among older women, independent of differences in hospital characteristics. Black women are less likely to undergo breast-conserving treatment.

▶ The data indicating that survival after breast conservation surgery in properly selected patients is equal to mastectomy have been available now for some time. The operation's limited use is an indicator that education occurs primarily in medical centers during medical school and residency training. Also, the procedure requires easy access to radiation therapy, which may not be available in smaller communities. Change in established surgical technique in the community comes slowly (and, in most cases, appropriately slowly) unless forced on the practicing surgeon by the economic pressures of new technology, e.g., laparoscopic surgery. The demographics of this study underscore the importance of sound, basic medical education in medical school and during residency training as the cornerstone of quality medical practice in the country, because patterns of care learned in training are difficult to change in practice. Postresidency continuing medical education cannot be depended on to make up for incomplete basic education.—E.M. Copeland, III, M.D.

## A Quantitative, Qualitative, and Critical Assessment of Surgical Waste: Surgeons Venture Through the Trash Can

Tieszen ME, Gruenberg JC (Saginaw Cooperative Hosps, Inc, Saginaw, Mich)
*JAMA* 267:2765–2768, 1992                                                        1–16

*Introduction.*—In November 1988, Congress enacted the Medical Waste Tracking Act to assess medical waste in 10 states. With the increasing amount of medical waste, including infectious waste, and the

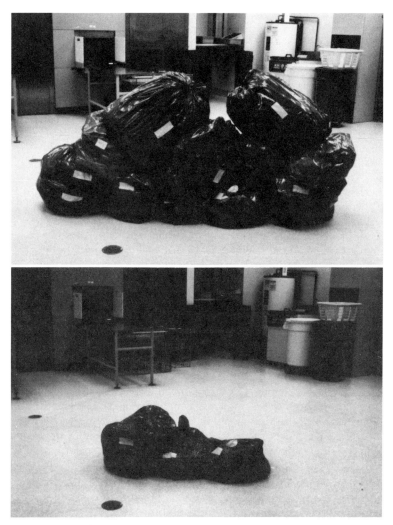

**Fig 1–5.**—Volume of waste from 4 operations was reduced by 93% after removal of disposable linen, paper, and recyclable plastic. (Courtesy of Tieszen ME, Gruenberg JC: *JAMA* 267:2765–2768, 1992.)

costs of disposing of these materials, new or alternative methods of disposal or reduction must be implemented. The surgical waste generated by several common surgical procedures was evaluated quantitatively and qualitatively, the categories of waste that might be readily separated for alternative disposal practices or substitution were defined, and changes in surgical waste output that elimination or alternative handling methods might bring about were examined.

*Setting.*—Surgical waste from 5 types of surgical procedures—operations on the back, heart, abdomen, joints, and herniorrhaphies—were identified prospectively at a single tertiary community teaching hospital. Measurements were made of the weight, volume, and percentage of disposable linen, paper, and miscellaneous waste.

*Results.*—Surgical waste from 27 cases (all 5 types of operations) weighed 610.5 lb and occupied 171.6 cu ft. The total waste varied widely for different types of procedures, from 8.5 lb per hernia case to 43.01 lb per cardiac surgery procedure. By weight, disposable linens accounted for 39% of total waste; paper, 7%; plastic, 26%; and miscellaneous waste, 27%. By volume, disposable linen and paper accounted for 69%; plastic, 23%; and miscellaneous waste, 7%. In a subset of 4 operations, removal of disposable linen, paper, and plastic dramatically reduced weight by 73% and volume by 93% (Fig 1–5).

*Discussion.*—Nationwide, the total hospital waste is estimated to be 8 $\times$ $10^8$ lb per year. The surgical waste from the 5 types of operation included in this study contributes only .012%. Surgical waste is a collection of readily identifiable and recyclable materials that can be reduced through recycling and converting from disposable to reusable linens.

---

**Cost Containment in the Operating Room: Use of Reusable Versus Disposable Clothing**
DiGiacomo JC, Odom JW, Ritota PC, Swan KG (Saint Francis Med Ctr, Trenton, NJ; UMDNJ-New Jersey Med School, Newark)
*Am Surg* 58:654–656, 1992                                         1–17

---

*Introduction.*—The benefits and convenience of disposable vs. reusable operating room attire must be weighed against the environmental problems of waste disposal and pollution as well as cost effectiveness for the hospital. The costs incurred by the use of disposable or reuseable attire in the operating suites of 2 teaching hospitals were compared.

*Methods.*—The annual operating room budgets for a fiscal year at 2 New Jersey hospitals were reviewed. The annual cost of disposable attire was determined by adding the amount spent on disposable clothing and the estimated cost of disposal. For reusable operating room attire, the annual cost was determined by adding annual purchases with laundry and/or sterilization costs for the operating room gowns and scrub suits. A review of operating room records determined that the 2 hospitals per-

Comparison of Hospital A and Hospital B

|  | Hospital A | Hospital B |
|---|---|---|
| Number of beds | 496 | 443 |
| Operative procedures/year* | 5,927 | 9,657 |
| Type of operating room | Disposable | Reusable |
| Annual cost | $155,664 | $35,680 |

* Total operative procedures in Hospital B included 4,390 major and 5,267 minor operations.

(Courtesy of DiGiacomo JC, Odom JW, Ritota PC, et al: *Am Surg* 58:654-656, 1992.)

formed similar types of operative procedures. Rates of nosocomial infection in the 2 institutions were comparable.

*Findings.*—In 1980, Schwartz documented that disposable gowns cost 5 times more than reusable gowns. The findings in this study were similar. The cost per gown per case for disposable gowns was $2.45 compared with $.68 for reusable gowns. On an annual basis, costs were $155,664 for disposable attire and $35,680 for reusable attire (table). The savings with the reusable gowns are even greater when the cost of medical waste is considered.

*Conclusion.*—The use of reusable scrub suits and gowns resulted in a savings of $119,984 compared with the use of disposable attire, even though the institution using disposables performed 3,730 fewer operative procedures. Hospitals should reevaluate the use of disposables to reduce operating costs and the amount of medical waste generated.

**In-Use Evaluation of Surgical Gowns**
Quebbeman EJ, Telford GL, Hubbard S, Wadsworth K, Hardman B, Goodman H, Gottlieb MS (Med College of Wisconsin, Milwaukee)
*Surg Gynecol Obstet* 174:369–375, 1992                                    1–18

*Introduction.*—There is an increased demand for protective measures in the operating room. Surgical gowns must provide a barrier for the patient from the bacteria of operating room personnel and protect personnel from deadly viruses in the blood and body fluids of patients. Various gowns were evaluated for the occurrence of blood strikethrough, defined as visible blood of any amount found on the inside surface of the garment.

*Methods.*—Three experienced operating room nurses were present at 234 operations for the sole purpose of documenting blood exposure on surgical gowns. All gowns, the scrub suit, foot and ankle wear, and exposed areas of skin were inspected for blood contamination. All person-

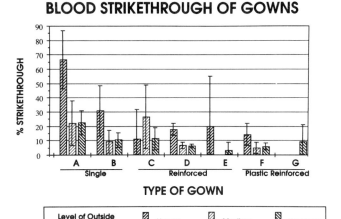

**Fig 1–6.**—The percentage of gown areas that had strikethrough for the areas with heavy or medium blood contamination on the outside of the gown. The bar labeled *All* is the total of all strikethrough divided by the total areas with small, medium, or heavy contamination. The *vertical bars* represent 95% confidence intervals. (Courtesy of Quebbeman EJ, Telford GL, Hubbard S, et al: *Surg Gynecol Obstet* 174:369–375, 1992.)

nel were observed, but only the surgeon and first assistant had sufficient amounts of blood contamination to be included in the analysis.

*Results.*—The surgeons and first assistants wore 535 gowns during the observed operations. Nine areas were examined on each gown, for a total of 4,815 individual areas. Most areas (54%) showed no contaimination and only 10% had heavy contamination. The amount of blood contamination was similar between the 7 different types of gowns (6 disposable and 1 reusable). An additional gown made of a spun bond polyethylene allowed free penetration of blood and was removed from use during the study. The risk of strikethrough increased with greater amounts of blood on the outside of the gown (Fig 1-6) and the length of time the gown was worn. Gowns reinforced with a second layer of material or coated with plastic offered significantly more protection than those composed of only a single layer of material. The forearm was the most frequently contaiminated area.

*Conclusion.*—Further improvements in gown design are needed to prevent nonsterile contact between surgeon and patient. One of the gowns was unacceptable for any operating room use. Plastic coating did not prevent fluid penetration in all gown areas.

▶ Surgical waste made up only a small portion of total hospital waste. Nevertheless, surgical waste was a collection of easily identifiable and potentially recyclable materials. Medical waste disposal is possibly more costly than quality control of reusable linens. Several studies have now shown the cost effectiveness of reusable versus disposable operating attire. Although plastic-reinforced gowns are not yet totally impervious to body fluids, such high-quality recyclable linens are significantly less permeable than are single-layer, lightweight, disposable gowns, are more cost effective, and may decrease the risk to the surgeon of exposure to infectious diseases.—E.M. Copeland, III, M.D.

---

**Percutaneous Injuries During Surgical Procedures**
Tokars JI, Bell DM, Culver DH, Marcus R, Mendelson MH, Sloan EP, Farber BF, Fligner D, Chamberland ME, McKibben PS, Martone WJ (Ctrs for Disease Control, Atlanta, Ga; Mount Sinai School of Medicine, New York City; Cook County Hosp, Chicago; Cornell Univ, Manhasset, NY; Christ Hosp and Med Ctr, Oak Lawn, Ill)
*JAMA* 267:2899–2904, 1992                                                    1–19

---

*Purpose.*—Surgical personnel are at risk of infection by bloodborne pathogens when percutaneous injuries occur via needles or sharp instruments contaminated with a patient's blood. Conversely, patients may be at risk of such infection during surgical and dental procedures performed by infected health care workers. The precise events leading to transmission of infection are usually not clear. The numbers and circumstances of percutaneous injuries that occur during surgical procedures were examined.

*Methods.*—During a 9-month period in 1990, nurses or operating room technicians with no other duties in the operating room observed 1,382 surgical procedures performed at 4 teaching hospitals. Each observer documented the number and circumstances of percutaneous injuries among surgical personnel, and the number of times surgical instruments that had injured a worker recontacted the patient's surgical wound. Procedures eligible for observation were performed on adults in 5 surgical services.

*Results.*—Of 8,153 procedures eligible for observation, 1,382 (17%) were observed. During the observed procedures, 99 percutaneous injuries were witnessed and recorded. Seventy-six of the 99 injuries were caused by suture needles. In 24 cases, the sharp object that caused the injury was held by a co-worker. The nondominant hand was injured in 62 instances, and the palmar surface of the distal forefinger was the most commonly injured area. Among the 13 procedure groups observed, the risk of injury ranged from 1.6% during certain orthopedic procedures to 21.3% during vaginal hysterectomy. Of the 99 injuries, 88 were sustained by resident or attending surgeons. There were 29 recontacts. In 28 of these recontacts, a sharp object that had percutaneously injured a worker later recontacted the patient.

*Conclusions.*—Percutaneous injuries occur regularly during surgery. The incidence varies with the procedure performed. Many of these injuries may be preventable by changes in surgical technique and equipment.

▶ The majority of injuries during an operation were to the surgeon or first assistant and were secondary to a suture needle. This probably means that hand retraction was being used rather than instrument retraction. Injuries from sharp knife blades have been greatly reduced by more liberal use of cautery dissection. The surgeon and assistants should keep their hands out of the wound when suturing is underway. Also, when practical, the needle should be removed from the suture before a knot is tied. Obviously, any instrument that has been contaminated should be discarded immediately.—E.M. Copeland, III, M.D.

---

**Response to Plasma Exchange and Splenectomy in Thrombotic Thrombocytopenic Purpura: A 10-Year Experience at a Single Institution**
Onundarson PT, Rowe JM, Heal JM, Francis CW (Univ of Rochester, Rochester, NY; American Red Cross, Rochester, NY)
*Arch Intern Med* 152:791–796, 1992                                                1–20

---

*Background.*—Thrombotic thrombocytopenic purpura (TTP) is a progressive and fatal disease in the absence of treatment, but plasma exchange provides effective therapy. Patients who fail to respond to plasma exchange, however, or who have relapses after an initial response have poor outcomes. A study of 27 patients treated with plasma exchange for TTP was conducted to determine which patients fail to respond to plasma exchange and the outcomes of those who had relapses after an initial response.

*Methods.*—Patients with TTP diagnosed between 1980 and 1990 at a single center were studied retrospectively. All underwent exchange of a single plasma volume for fresh frozen plasma daily until the platelet count had risen to at least $100 \times 10^9$/L. A response was defined as such a rise associated with improvement in the patient's clinical condition.

*Results.*—More than three quarters of the patients (78%) responded to plasma exchange; all of the nonresponders died within 10 days of diagnosis, after a mean of 7 exchanges. In 20 of 21 responders, a rise in the platelet count of $30 \times 10^9$/L occurred within 5 days of treatment initiation. In 13 of 27 patients, sustained remission without additional therapy occurred; 8 (30%) had at least 1 relapse. All patients who had relapses eventually attained lasting remission after additional plasma exchange therapy. Four patients had splenectomy during their first to third relapses; all had a complete and sustained response without additional therapy. The only favorable prognostic indicator identified was the initial response to plasma exchange, which was invariably associated with long-term survival. A literature review, including 224 patients with TTP who underwent plasma exchange, showed that 81% responded initially, 19% were refractory, and 27% of responders eventually relapsed.

*Conclusions.*—Plasma exchange can provide excellent initial therapy for TTP. Refractoriness to plasma exchange is apparent early, is associated with a grave prognosis, and should prompt immediate additional therapy to include the possibility of splenectomy.

▶ The value of splenectomy for TTP has been debated for years. It would appear that patients with TTP are segregated into those who respond to plasma exchange and those who do not (and die). Those who relapse after initially responding to plasma exchange often require many exchanges to obtain an adequate platelet count. Splenectomy appears valuable in this group, often resulting in prompt and sustained remissions.—E.M. Copeland, III, M.D.

---

## Phase I-II Trial of Erythropoietin in the Treatment of Cisplatin-Associated Anemia

Miller CB, Platanias LC, Mills SR, Zahurak ML, Ratain MJ, Ettinger DS, Jones RJ (Johns Hopkins Oncology Ctr, Baltimore, Md; Univ of Chicago)
*J Natl Cancer Inst* 84:98–103, 1992                                          1–21

*Background.*—Anemia may result from many causes in patients receiving cisplatin-containing chemotherapy, but erythropoietin deficiency seems to play an important role. Animal studies suggest that recombinant human erythropoietin (epoetin) can reverse cisplatin-associated

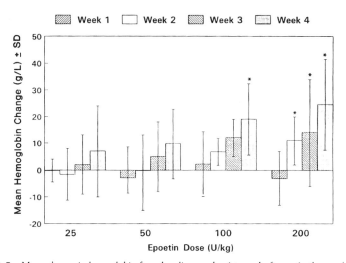

**Fig 1–7.**—Mean change in hemoglobin from baseline on day 1 to end of epoetin therapy (week 4). *Asterisk* indicates statistical significance. (Courtesy of Miller CB, Platanias LC, Mills SR, et al: *J Natl Cancer Inst* 84:98–103, 1992.)

anemia. A phase I-II clinical trial was conducted to evaluate the safety and effectiveness of epoetin treatment.

*Methods.*—The sample comprised 21 patients in whom anemia developed in association with cisplatin chemotherapy. There were 14 men and 7 women (mean age, 51 years) with cancer in a wide variety of sites. All had a hemoglobin level of less than 110 g/L. Patients were given epoetin at escalating doses of 25, 50, 100, or 200 units per kg intravenously 5 times a week for 4 weeks.

*Results.*—In the patients receiving the 2 highest doses, hemoglobin levels increased significantly after 4 weeks of treatment; there was an increase of 19 g/L in the group given 100 units per kg and an increase of 24 g/L in those given 200 units per kg (Fig 1–7). Twelve patients achieved a clinical response, defined as an increase of more than 10 g/L. Their mean increase was 25 g/L over the level at the same point in their chemotherapy cycle preceding treatment. The response to epoetin could not be predicted by either the serum erythropoietin level or the hemoglobin level. Treatment was well tolerated with no severe dose-dependent side effects. Two patients had hypertension, which responded to standard antihypertensive therapy.

*Conclusions.*—Epoetin has promise as a safe and effective treatment for cisplatin-associated anemia. The best responses were achieved at doses of 100 and 200 units per kg.

▶ Although this study is a small phase I-II study of only 21 patients, it demonstrates significant improvement in hemoglobin levels in cancer patients receiving cisplatin chemotherapy as long as the dose of erythropoietin is more than 100 units per kg. There are 2 significant points brought up by this study. The minimum effective dose of erythropoietin appears to be around 100 units per kg for several weeks. (1). The second point is that pretreatment erythropoietin levels do not predict individual patient response, as has been the case in some other disease states, e.g., infection with HIV (2).

Further, erythropoietin, along with granulocyte-colony-stimulating factor and other growth factors will be used more frequently to minimize the side effects of chemotherapy-based regimens. These growth factors will take on even greater significance as medical oncologists increase the doses of multidrug regimens in an effort to eradicate metastatic disease.—T.J. Eberlein, M.D.

*References*

1. Platnias LC, et al: *J Clin Oncol* 9:2021, 1991.
2. Fischl M, et al: *N Engl J Med* 322: 1488, 1990.

# 2  Critical Care

## Introduction

The role of oxygen debt and suboptimal oxygen delivery in the development of organ failure continues to be investigated. The importance of maintaining physiologically adequate levels of oxygen delivery to meet the increased metabolic needs of both high-risk surgical and trauma patients was clearly illustrated in several reports. Specifically, the magnitude of the oxygen debt occurring during surgery was found to correlate with the development of organ failure and predict mortality. Furthermore, in prospective studies, the incidence of organ failure and mortality was reduced in patients resuscitated to supranormal levels of oxygen delivery compared to patients resuscitated to normal levels. Taken together, these results indicate that basing hemodynamic goals of resuscitation on values established for healthy individuals frequently results in under resuscitation in the critically ill or injured. That is, what is normal for healthy man is neither normal nor appropriate for injured man. These and previous studies strongly mandate the early (prophylactic when possible) use of pulmonary artery catheters to optimize both oxygen delivery and consumption in patients at risk of experiencing multiple organ failure.

Although the pulmonary artery wedge pressure (PAWP) is a good indicator of volume status in most patients, in some who are critically ill or septic, PAWP may not adequately reflect preload. Recent advances in pulmonary artery catheter technology now allow the right ventricular end-diastolic volume (RVEDI) to be measured. Based on a clinical series comparing the accuracy of PAWP versus RVEDI in assessing preload, it appears that the RVEDI is a more accurate index of fluid requirements in certain patients. Other cardiovascular topics reviewed include the use of continuous arteriovenous hemofiltration as adjuvant therapy in patients with established adult respiratory distress syndrome, the incidence and prognostic significance of perioperative ventricular arrhythmias in patients undergoing noncardiac surgery, and the need for scheduled replacement of central venous catheters.

The concept that the 1990s will be characterized by the transition of molecular biology from the laboratory to the clinic is clearly evident in the fields of inflammation and infection. Studies investigating the potential clinical benefits of natural cytokine antagonists, such as interleukin-1 receptor antagonist and anticytokine antibodies are appearing with increasing regularity. At the same time, increasing progress is being made in the basic physiology of inflammation, injury, and the biology and therapy of septic shock.

The role of gut injury as an inducer or potentiator of distant organ injury, systemic infection, and multiple organ failure is an area of increasing interest and study. Although it is now clear that gut injury can potentiate injury to other distant organs, especially the liver and lung, and that loss of intestinal barrier function to luminal bacteria is associated with systemic infection, the mechanisms responsible for these phenomena remain to be fully determined. Nonetheless, there is evidence incriminating cytokines, inflammatory factors, activated neutrophils, and endotoxin as the messengers that are responsible for distant organ injury.

Historically, the decision of when to transfuse blood was guided largely by the patient's hemoglobin concentration and, as a rule of thumb, if the hemoglobin or hematocrit dropped below 10 or 30, respectively, prophylactic transfusions were administered almost routinely. This arbitrary, nonphysiologic approach to blood transfusion no longer appears valid, because blood transfusions are not without danger and in some patients the risks of transfusion clearly outweigh the benefits. The potential benefits of raising the hemoglobin level in the critically ill or injured at the risk of organ failure developing has been assessed, and in fully volume-resuscitated patients receiving cardiac inotropic support, the administration of blood to increase the hemoglobin to values of 10 g/dL or greater have not been associated with improved oxygen consumption, even though oxygen delivery is distress increased. Consequently, the decision to transfuse in anemic patients with adult respiratory distress syndrome, multiple organ failure, or septic shock must be judged on a patient-to-patient basis and should be predicated on signs of supply-dependent oxygen consumption.

Lastly, a study is included documenting the major adverse impact on the clinical outcome of potentially preventable iatrogenic complications occurring after admission to the intensive care unit.

Edwin A. Deitch, M.D.

---

### Role of Oxygen Debt in the Development of Organ Failure Sepsis, and Death in High-Risk Surgical Patients

Shoemaker WC, Appel PL, Kram HB (Univ of California, Los Angeles)
Chest 102:208–215, 1992                                                    2–1

---

*Introduction.*—Trauma and postoperative patients reportedly have initial reductions of cardiac output and oxygen consumption $\dot{V}O_2$, with subsequent increases in the postoperative period after the hemodynamic crisis. Increasing the $\dot{V}O_2$ with administration of fluids and inotropic therapy improves survival. Tissue oxygen deficits were investigated in the

Data on Tissue Oxygen Deficit

| Data | Nonsurvivors (n = 64) | Survivors with Organ Failure (n = 31) | Survivors with no Organ Failure (n = 158) |
|---|---|---|---|
| $\dot{V}O_2$ deficit, L/m$^2$ | | | |
| Intraoperative | 12.0 $\pm$ 1.3 | 11.8 $\pm$ 1.6 | 5.7 $\pm$ 0.9 |
| Maximum | 33.2 $\pm$ 4.0 | 21.6 $\pm$ 3.7 | 9.2 $\pm$ 1.3 |
| Time to maximum | | | |
| $\dot{V}O_2$ deficit, h | 17.8 $\pm$ 2.2 | 10.1 $\pm$ 2.7 | 4.1 $\pm$ 0.6 |
| Time to net cumulative positive $\dot{V}O_2$, h | 48.6 $\pm$ 3.5 | 29.2 $\pm$ 4.7 | 17.9 $\pm$ 1.6 |

Note: Table values are means $\pm$ SEM.
(Courtesy of Shoemaker WC, Appel PL, Kram HB: *Chest* 102:208-215, 1992.)

postoperative period in a series of high-risk surgical patients and related to the development of organ failure and systemic disorders.

*Methods.*—The study subjects were 253 unselected high-risk surgical patients whose average age was 59 years. Oxygen consumption was measured at frequent intervals in all patients before, during, and immediately after surgery. The rate of $\dot{V}O_2$ deficit was calculated by subtracting $\dot{V}O_2$ need, estimated from the patient's resting preoperative control values and corrected for temperature and anesthesia, from the measured $\dot{V}O_2$. The calculated oxygen deficit was correlated with multiple organ failure, complications, and outcome. A prospective series included a control group maintained at normal circulatory values and a protocol group maintained at the supranormal $\dot{V}O_2$ values based on results in survivors from the retrospective series.

*Results.*—There were 64 deaths, all in patients with organ failure. At its maximum, 18 hours after surgery, the cumulative $\dot{V}O_2$ deficit in this group was 33 L/m$^2$. Thirty-one patients with organ failure survived—their average maximum $\dot{V}O_2$ deficit was 22 L/m$^2$, occurring 10 hours postoperatively. For the 158 survivors with no organ failure or other complications, the maximum cumulative $\dot{V}O_2$ deficit was 9 L/m$^2$, and it occurred 4 hours after surgery (table). In the prospective study, the protocol group had a significant reduction in oxygen debt—8 L/m$^2$ versus 17 L/m$^2$ in the control group—and lower mortality—4% versus 33%.

*Conclusions.*—These findings show a strong relationship between the magnitude and duration of $\dot{V}O_2$ deficit in high-risk patients in the intraoperative and early postoperative periods and subsequent organ failure and death. Mortality may be decreased by preventing or minimizing the oxygen debt through augmentation of naturally occurring compensations that increase oxygen delivery. This may be done at the bedside by increasing oxygen delivery to supranormal values. More study is needed to determine the specific criteria for evaluating and titrating the adequacy of therapy in a wide range of clinical circumstances.

▶ Intermediary metabolism and energy production have an absolute dependence on oxygen, and oxygen cannot be stored intracellularly. Thus, regardless of cause, inadequate oxygen availability rapidly leads to cellular dysfunction and ultimately to cell death, with the net result being organ dysfunction. Because the role of inadequate oxygen availability in the pathogenesis of tissue and cellular injury is well established, it is not difficult to conceptualize how prolonged periods of oxygen debt can lead to organ injury.

The value of this study is twofold. First, it clearly shows that there is a definite correlation between the maximal oxygen debt that develops in the perioperative period and organ failure as well as death. Secondly, in a prospective fashion, the authors show that it is possible to decrease the incidence of organ failure and improve survival by maintaining oxygen delivery at supranormal levels. The physiologic goals used in the hyperdynamic group were a cardiac index greater than 4.5 L/min $\cdot$ m$^2$, oxygen delivery greater than 600 mL/min $\cdot$ m$^2$, and oxygen consumption greater than 170 mL/min $\cdot$ m$^2$.

Based on this and an increasing number of other studies, it seems prudent to maintain supranormal levels of oxygen delivery in high-risk patients during the operative and perioperative periods. In this situation, an ounce of prevention may be worth much more than a pound of cure.—E.A. Deitch, M.D.

---

## Incommensurate Oxygen Consumption in Response to Maximal Oxygen Availability Predicts Postinjury Multiple Organ Failure
Moore FA, Haenel JB, Moore EE, Whitehill TA (Denver Gen Hosp, Denver, Colo)
*J Trauma* 33:58–67, 1992                                                 2–2

Incidence of Multiple Organ Failure

|  | Number of Patients with MOF (%) | |
|---|---|---|
|  | Baseline V$o_2$ <150 mL/min$\cdot$m$^2$ | Baseline V$o_2$ >150 mL/min$\cdot$m$^2$ |
| 12-Hour V$o_2$ <150 mL/min$\cdot$m$^2$ | 9/11 (82%) | 3/4 (75%) |
| 12-Hour V$o_2$ >150 mL/min$\cdot$m$^2$ | 3/10 (30%) | 1/14 (7%) |

Note: The incidence of MOF was stratified by the patients' baseline V̇o$_2$ (less than 150 vs. greater than 150) and 12-hour V̇o$_2$ (less than 150 vs. greater than 150).
(Courtesy of Moore FA, Haenel JB, Moore EE, et al: *J Trauma* 33:58–67, 1992.)

*Background.*—Although multiple organ failure (MOF) is the main cause of late postinjury death, its exact pathogenesis has eluded intensive study. It was suggested that untreated flow-dependent oxygen consumption ($\dot{V}O_2$) might be a risk factor. The response of high-risk trauma patients to a protocol aimed at eradicating flow dependency was evaluated to determine whether inadequate $\dot{V}O_2$ is a factor in postinjury MOF.

*Methods.*—The analysis included 39 patients with known risk factors for MOF. Most (83%) were men, and the mean age was 36 years. Risk factors were massive transfusion in 20 patients, multiple fractures in 15, and combined flail chest/pulmonary contusion in 4. Patients were enrolled in an established resuscitation protocol with the aim of maximizing oxygen delivery to more than 600 mL/min·m², with a $\dot{V}O_2$ goal of more than 150 mL/min·m². Low-dose inotropic support was given if the oxygen delivery goal was not achieved.

*Results.*—In 38% of patients the $\dot{V}O_2$ goal was not reached by 12 hours. In 9 of 11 patients with baseline and 12-hour $\dot{V}O_2$ values less than the target, MOF developed, compared with only 1 of those in whom the target $\dot{V}O_2$ was maintained (table). Lactate levels were significantly elevated in patients who failed to respond, suggesting that their aerobic metabolism was defective. Despite maximal efforts to enhance peripheral oxygen availability, the blunted $\dot{V}O_2$ response predicted MOF. In patients with a 12-hour $\dot{V}O_2$ less than the target value and a lactate level more than 2.5 mmol/L, odds ratio of MOF was 25.6

*Conclusions.*—Trauma patients with a blunted $\dot{V}O_2$ response appear to be at risk for MOF. This early inability to consume oxygen may be explained by inadequate flow, maldistribution of flow, or defective cellular $O_2$ utilization. The initial shock insult is significant in causing late MOF or priming the host for its development.

▶ This study reiterates the important point that there is an association between oxygen delivery, oxygen consumption, and organ failure. However, it also illustrates the frustrating fact that it is not always possible to achieve the desired levels of oxygen delivery or consumption, try as we may. The fact that the patients in this study in whom MOF developed failed to respond to attempts to increase oxygen delivery and consumption highlights the complexity of this syndrome. These results also indicate that, although oxygen delivery and consumption are important prognostic factors, the development of MOF is caused by more than just the level of oxygen delivery. For a review of the MOF syndrome, see my 1992 study (1).—E.A. Deitch, M.D.

*Reference*

1. Deitch EA: *Ann Surg* 216:117, 1992.

## Prospective Trial of Supranormal Values as Goals of Resuscitation in Severe Trauma

Fleming A, Bishop M, Shoemaker W, Appel P, Sufficool W, Kuvhenguwha A, Kennedy F, Wo C-J (Charles R Drew Univ of Medicine & Science, Los Angeles, Calif)

*Arch Surg* 127:1175–1181, 1992                                        2–3

*Objective.*—In a previously reported series of trauma patients, the mean oxygen delivery ($DO_2$), oxygen consumption ($\dot{V}O_2$), and cardiac index (CI) values were higher in patients who survived and in patients with

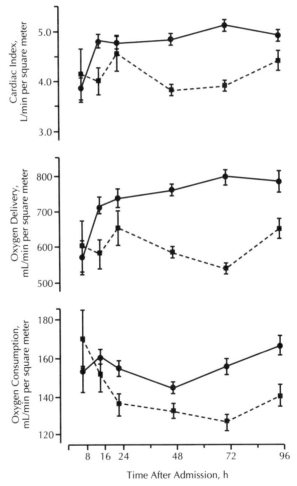

**Fig 2–1.**—Hemodynamic and oxygen transport patterns in resuscitation of trauma patients. *Bars* indicate mean ± SEM; *solid lines*, protocol patients; and *dashed lines*, control patients. (Courtesy of Fleming A, Bishop M, Shoemaker WC, et al: *Arch Surg* 127:1175–1181, 1992.)

fewer organ failures than in those who died. These values were kept supranormally high as a goal of resuscitation in patients with severe trauma to determine whether this approach would increase survival and decrease the incidence of shock-related organ failure.

*Methods.*—Sixty-seven patients were studied during a 6-month period; the 59 males and 8 females (mean age, 30 years) had a mean Trauma Score 12 and a mean Injury Severity Score of 27. All had lost at least 2,000 mL of blood. Patients were randomized to control and protocol groups, the controls receiving resuscitation according to conventional criteria, with the goal of attaining normal values in all hemodynamic measurements. In the protocol group, the goal was to maintain supranormal values determined empirically from the patterns of a previous series. These values were at least 4.52 L/min/m² for CI, at least 670 mL/min/m² for $DO_2$ and at least 166 mL/min/m² for $\dot{V}O_2$.

*Results.*—Forty-four percent of the control group died, compared with 24% of the protocol group. The control group had a mean of 1.59 organ failures, compared to .76 in protocol patients. Intensive care unit stay was also shorter in the protocol group (5 versus 12 days), as was the mean number of days requiring ventilation (4 versus 11).

*Conclusions.*—Increased survival and decreased morbidity were demonstrated in severely injured patients with attainment of supranormal CI, $DO_2$, and $\dot{V}O_2$ values. These measures appear to compensate for the patients' increased metabolic requirements and previous oxygen debt (Fig 2–1). The improvement in survival is even better in patients who lose greater amounts of blood and those in whom supranormal values are achieved within 24 hours.

▶ This prospective study clearly shows that normal hemodynamic values as determined in healthy individuals are inadequate in the severely stressed, injured patient. In this circumstance, resuscitation to "normal" hemodynamic values results in underresuscitation. Thus, in these hypermetabolic patients, supranormal levels of oxygen delivery and consumption, plus maintenance of a hyperdynamic circulation, is the goal. Based on what we now know, the answer to the question, should high-risk patients be managed without a pulmonary artery catheter and close attention to cardiac output and oxygen, is a resounding "no". Therapy based on traditional hemodynamic markers, such as blood pressure, pulse, and urine output, in these patient populations is neither accurate nor acceptable.—E.A. Deitch, M.D.

---

**End-Diastolic Volume: A Better Indicator of Preload in the Critically Ill**
Diebel LN, Wilson RF, Tagett MG, Kline RA (Wayne State Univ, Detroit, Mich; Detroit Receiving Hosp)
*Arch Surg* 127:817–822, 1992                                        2–4

*Introduction.*—Clinicians usually optimize the preload status of the cardiac output (CO) and oxygen delivery in patients critically ill or seriously injured, using the pulmonary artery wedge pressure (PAWP) as a monitoring test. New developments in flow-directed pulmonary artery catheter technology have allowed direct measurement of right ventricular end-systolic volume and right ventricular end-diastolic volume (RVEDV).

*Study Design.*—The RVEDV index (RVEDVI) and the PAWP, with additional hemodynamic variables, were compared in 29 critically ill patients (mean age, 52 years) undergoing surgery. Eighteen had laboratory-confirmed sepsis. The 29 patients had 146 sets of complete hemodynamic data available for analysis.

*Results.*—Based on mean hemodynamic values from 131 analyses from the first 21 patients, circulation appeared hyperdynamic with relatively normal mean filling pressures (PAWP and CVP), whereas the mean pulmonary vascular resistance (PVR) approached the upper limit of the reference range. Significant correlations were observed when comparing the RVEDVI, PCWP, and the CVP versus cardiac index. The RVEDVI and the CVP, and the RVEDVI and the PAWP, weakly correlated with each other. Of the 146 hemodynamic studies carried out, 24 assessments among 8 patients suggested possible fluid overload with the PAWP higher than 18 mm Hg. Only 1 of these 8 patients had a high RVEDVI, whereas the remaining 7 individuals had sepsis and required ventilation. In 75 of the other analyses among 19 patients, the PAWP produced relatively low values, reflecting a preload status in direct contrast to the RVEDVI at some point in the clinical course of the illness in 15 of these patients. Fifteen patients underwent fluid challenge study (22 assessments), which found that those with a high PAWP responded to the challenge with an increase in cardiac index more often than did those with a low PAWP.

*Conclusions.*—The RVEDVI provides the more accurate assessment and serves as a better predictor of the volume status and the preload recruitable increases in cardiac output than the PAWP.

▶ The importance of this clinical study is that it focuses our attention on the limitations of *pressure* measurements in evaluating the *volume* status of the heart. Although Starling clearly states that the preload status of the heart is a function of volume, because of limitations in technology, we have based fluid therapy on pressure measurements (CVP or PAWP). Filling pressures do correlate with volume status, but in the critically ill this relationship can be lost to the extent that PAWP no longer is an accurate predictor of preload status. As shown in this study, in some patients, measurements of right ventricular volume may reflect preload status more accurately than PAWP. As more studies are performed comparing the accuracy of RVEDVI vs. PAWP measurements in septic and critically ill patients, the clinical utility of the new modified Swan-Ganz catheter described in this publication will be determined. Until then, it is important to remember that, although PAWP is reasonably accurate in most patients, this measurement has limitations. Thus my advice is, in case of doubt, give fluids and base further therapy on the patient's cardiac response.—E.A. Deitch, M.D.

## Continuous Arteriovenous Hemofiltration Countercurrent Dialysis (CAVH-D) in Acute Respiratory Failure (ARDS)

Garzia F, Todor R, Scalea T (State Univ of New York, Brooklyn)
*J Trauma* 31:1277–1284, 1991                                             2–5

*Background.*—In patients with adult respiratory distress syndrome (ARDS), the balance between intravascular volume, oxygen transport, and arterial oxygenation is delicate and controversial. The use of continuous arteriovenous hemofiltration (CAVH) can remove serum and low-molecular-weight toxins from the intravascular space. The application of countercurrent dialysis (CAVH-D) clears additional circulating toxins

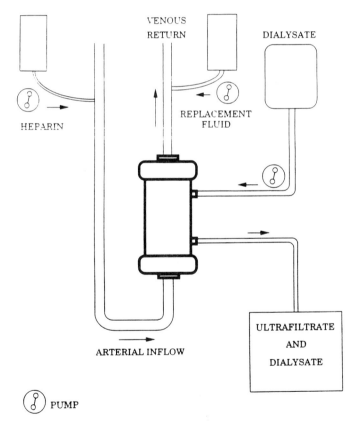

**Fig 2–2.**—The circuit used for CAVH-D. (Courtesy of Garzia F, Todor R, Scalea T: *J Trauma* 31:1277–1284, 1991.)

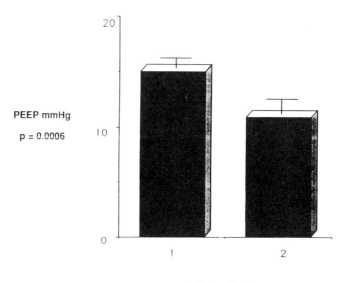

1. Before CAVH/D

2. After CAVH/D

**Fig 2–3.**—Positive end-expiratory pressure before and after CAVH-D. (Courtesy of Garzia F, Todor R, Scalea T: *J Trauma* 31:1277–1284, 1991.)

that may be responsible for ARDS (Fig 2–2). The results of CAVH-D in 14 nonoliguric patients with severe refractory ARDS were reviewed.

*Patients.*—The 14 nonoliguric patients were edematous and in marked positive fluid balance but not intravascularly overloaded before CAVH-D. Patients underwent transfemoral CAVH-D for a mean of 65.2 hours and cleared a mean of 480 mL of filtrate per hour.

*Results.*—Three patients were grossly unstable when CAVH-D was begun, their mean cardiac index being 2.3 L/min/m$^2$; all had a low mean oxygen consumption. Although their CAVH-D filters cleared a mean of 600 mL/hr, they required constant fluid resuscitation to maintain adequate filling pressures. These 3 patients died of cardiogenic shock and ARDS within 3 days. The remaining 11 patients had a significant response to CAVH-D. Their mean $FIO_2$ was weaned from 0.73 to 0.45 and positive end-expiratory pressure from 14.3 cm to 8.9 cm (Fig 2–3). The peak airway pressure fell from a mean of 60 mm Hg to 45 mm Hg. There was no significant change in the cardiac index or wedge pressure, but oxygen consumption rose from a mean of 279 mL/m to 409 mL/m (Fig 2–4). The only complication was bleeding in 1 patient when the tubing became disconnected from the vascular catheter.

*Conclusion.*—Continuous arteriovenous hemofiltration countercurrent dialysis can be an effective alternative in the treatment of patients with ARDS, especially those who have been at least partially stabilized. It is safe, can be managed by the surgical staff, and is associated with signif-

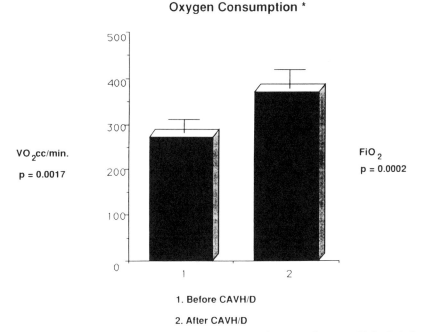

## Oxygen Consumption *

VO$_2$cc/min.

p = 0.0017

FiO$_2$

p = 0.0002

1. Before CAVH/D

2. After CAVH/D

**Fig 2–4.**—Oxygen consumption before and after CAVH-D. (Courtesy of Garzia F, Todor R, Scalea T: *J Trauma* 31:1277–1284, 1991.)

icant improvement in respiratory variables without requiring a drop in preload, which may potentially compromise oxygen transport.

▶ When our cars are not running right, we may decide it is time for an oil change. This same approach is reported in this article, and it has been tried sporadically in severely injured burn patients, patients with poisonings or drug overdoses, and, most recently, in patients with multiple organ failure. The basic concept behind the use of CAVH-D in these patient populations is twofold: first, that circulating substances or factors present in the plasma are contributing to the disease process, and, second, that removal of these tissue-injurious factors will improve organ function.

The results of this uncontrolled clinical trial indicate that CAVH-D can improve cardiac output and pulmonary function in a high percentage of patients with established ARDS. On the other hand, 55% of the patients whose ARDS initially responded to CAVH-D relapsed and, ultimately, refractory ARDS developed. The overall survival rate in this series was just 36%. Thus I bring this technique to your attention neither to completely condone it or support it, but as a tool that may be helpful in the occasional patient with early but refractory ARDS.—E.A. Deitch, M.D.

## Ventricular Arrhythmias in Patients Undergoing Noncardiac Surgery

O'Kelly B, Browner WS, Massie B, Tubau J, Ngo L, Mangano DT, for the Study of Perioperative Ischemia Research Group (VA Med Ctr, San Francisco, Calif)

*JAMA* 268:217–221, 1992                                                    2–6

*Background.*—Among patients undergoing noncardiac surgery, the management of ventricular arrhythmias during and after surgery depends partly on knowledge of the incidence and prognostic importance of these disturbances. Because such information is largely lacking, however, operative management of perioperative arrhythmias is unclear for the 7 million patients with cardiac disease who undergo noncardiac surgery each year. A prospective study was undertaken to assess the incidence, clinical predictors, and prognostic importance of perioperative ventricular arrhythmias.

*Methods.*—Of 230 consecutive men scheduled for major noncardiac operations, 54% were at high risk of coronary artery disease and the rest were known to have it. Continuous ambulatory ECG monitoring was used to record cardiac rhythm for a mean of 21 hours in the preoperative period, 6 hours in the intraoperative period, and 38 hours in the postoperative period. Adverse cardiac outcomes were evaluated without knowledge of arrhythmias.

*Results.*—In 44% of the patients, frequent or major ventricular arrhythmias, defined as more than 30 ventricular ectopic beats per hour or ventricular tachycardia, occurred, 21% preoperatively, 16% intraoperatively, and 36% postoperatively. Arrhythmias increased in severity in only 2% of the patients intraoperatively but in 10% postoperatively. Smokers and patients with a history of congestive heart failure were more likely to have preoperative ventricular arrhythmias, as were those with ECG evidence of myocardial ischemia. Patients with preoperative arrhythmias had an increased incidence of intraoperative and postoperative arrhythmias. Nonfatal myocardial infarction or cardiac death occurred in 9 patients. Those events were not significantly more common in patients with perioperative arrhythmias.

*Conclusions.*—This study reports a 44% incidence of frequent ventricular ectopic beats or nonsustained ventricular tachycardia among high-risk patients undergoing noncardiac surgery. When occurring with no other signs of myocardial infarction, however, these arrhythmias may not call for aggressive perioperative monitoring or treatment.

▶ The importance of this study is severalfold. First, it documents that almost half of high-risk patients undergoing noncardiac surgery will have frequent ventricular ectopic beats or nonsustained episodes of ventricular tachycardia. Second, it provides information that antiarrhythmic therapy is not needed in the absence of signs or symptoms of myocardial infarction. Because adverse outcomes were not associated with arrhythmias occurring during any of the monitoring periods, the results of this study, taken together with increasing clinical information that prophylactic antiarrhythmic therapy in patients with premature ventricular contractions (PVCs) is dangerous, must make us rethink the risk:benefit ratio of treating asymptomatic ventricular arrhythmias. Thus, in my mind, this article helps to settle the issue of which postoperative patients with symptomatic PVCs require antiarrhythmic therapy. The answer is, very few.—E.A. Deitch, M.D.

**A Controlled Trial of Scheduled Replacement of Central Venous and Pulmonary-Artery Catheters**
Cobb DK, High KP, Sawyer RG, Sable CA, Adams RB, Lindley DA, Pruett TL, Schwenzer KJ, Farr BM (Univ of Virginia, Charlottesville)
*N Engl J Med* 327:1062–1068, 1992          2–7

*Introduction.*—Prolonged central venous catheterization increases the incidence of infection in critically ill patients. Changing catheters every 3 days to reduce the rate of infection has been advocated, but it has not been demonstrated conclusively whether this is effective. It is also not known whether it is safer to change the catheter over a guidewire or insert it at a new site. The efficacy of replacing the central venous catheter every 3 days, using either a new puncture site or inserting it at a new site, was assessed.

*Methods.*—The study included 160 adult intensive care unit (ICU) patients who required a central venous or pulmonary artery catheter for more than 3 days. After stratification by medical or surgical ICU confine-

Incidence Rates of Infectious and Mechanical
Complications, According to the Method of
Catheter Replacement

| TYPE OF REPLACEMENT AND COMPLICATION | NEW PUNC-TURE SITE (N = 882 DAYS) | GUIDE-WIRE ASSISTANCE (N = 1340 DAYS) |
|---|---|---|
| *no./1000 days of catheter use* | | |
| Scheduled replacement | | |
| Bloodstream infection | 3 | 6 |
| Colonization | 17 | 16 |
| Mechanical | 14 | 4 |
| Replacement when clinically indicated | | |
| Bloodstream infection | 2 | 3 |
| Colonization | 10 | 8 |
| Mechanical | 8 | 3 |

*Note:* There were no statistically significant differences; data include complications that occurred during the first 3 days of catheterization.
(Courtesy of Cobb DK, High KP, Sawyer RG, et al: N Engl J Med 327:1062–1068, 1992.)

ment, patients were randomized into 4 groups. Group 1 had catheter replacement every 3 days by insertion at a new site, group 2 had replacement every 3 days by exchange over a guidewire, group 3 had replacement when indicated by insertion at a new site, and group 4 had replacement when indicated by exchange over a guidewire. Semiquantitative cultures were performed on 523 catheters.

*Results.*—There was a 5% rate of catheter-related bloodstream infections, a 16% rate of catheter colonization, and a 9% rate of major mechanical complications. Rates of bloodstream infection were 3/1,000 days in group 1, 6/1,000 days in group 2, 2/1,000 days in group 3, and 3/1,000 days in group 4. After the first 3 days, patients assigned to guidewire exchange had a 6% rate of bloodstream infections compared with none in the other groups. The rate of mechanical complications in patients assigned to insertion at new sites was 5%, versus 1% in the other groups.

*Conclusions.*—Replacing central venous catheters every 3 days does not prevent infection. Although using a guidewire increases risk of bloodstream infection, insertion at new sites increases the risk of mechanical complications (table).

Pending further research, the recommendation is to place central venous catheters with optimal aseptic procedures and leave them in place until a change is indicated. Such indications include fever of unknown source and catheter malfunction.

▶ How often should central lines be changed? Can they be changed safely over guidewires or should new sites be used? This and another recent study provide the answer to these questions (1) which is that routine catheter changes are not indicated, and that changing the catheter over a guidewire is an acceptable alternative to placing the catheter in a new site in most patients.—E.A. Deitch, M.D.

*Reference*

1. Hagley, et al: *Crit Care Med* 20:1426, 1992.

---

**Recombinant Interleukin-1 Receptor Antagonist (IL-1ra): Effective Therapy Against Gram-Negative Sepsis in Rats**
Alexander HR, Doherty GM, Venzon DJ, Merino MJ, Fraker DL, Norton JA (Natl Cancer Inst, Bethesda, Md)
*Surgery* 112:188–194, 1992                                   2–8

---

*Background.*—Despite advances in diagnosis and treatment, the mortality rate associated with bacterial sepsis remains high. Recent studies have implicated interleukin-1 (IL-1) as a mediator of the lethal effects of endotoxin shock or bacterial sepsis. The therapeutic value of a human

IL-l receptor antagonist (IL-lra) against gram-negative sepsis was assessed in rats.

*Methods.*—Gram-negative sepsis was induced in the animals by cecal ligation and puncture (CLP) following placement of indwelling carotid arterial and superior vena cava catheters. Three hours later, the rats were assigned to receive either IL-lra (10 mg/kg intravenous bolus followed by 5 mg/kg/hr) or an equal volume of vehicle intravenously for 24 hours. The animals were monitored for 30 hours, at which time the survivors were killed.

*Results.*—All animals appeared ill 3 hours after CLP. The survival rate at 30 hours was greater in treated rats (71%) than in controls (20%). There was significantly less hypothermia, bradycardia, and hypotension in IL-lra–treated animals than in controls 24 hours after CLP. Histologic studies of liver tissue showed necrosis and bacteria in animals treated with vehicle but not in those receiving IL-lra.

*Conclusion.*—Treatment with a recombinant human Il-lra ameliorated the acute hemodynamic and fatal effects of gram-negative septicemia produced by CLP in rats, a clinically relevant model of intra-abdominal sepsis. The findings strongly support the use of Il-lra in the treatment of human life-threatening septic shock.

▶ This study supports the use of IL-lra in the treatment of patients with life-threatening infections, and phases II and III clinical studies testing IL-lra are now in various stages of progress.

The transition from antibiotics to cytokine antagonists is based on the recognition that the host is being injured by the production of an excessive inflammatory response to the invading bacteria rather than by the bacteria themselves. This realization that the host is destroying itself, rather than being destroyed by bacteria, has led to a research shift from attempts limited to finding more effective ways to kill bacteria to attempts to limit that host's uncontrolled or excessive inflammatory response. The identification, production, and experimental and clinical testing of substances such as IL-lra, which dampen the host's inflammatory response, are the fruits of this labor. Undoubtedly, IL-lra or conceptually similar substances that block the deleterious effects of endogenously produced cytokines will ultimately become part of our everyday therapeutic armamentarium.—E.A. Deitch, M.D.

---

**Tumor Necrosis Factor-α Induces Vascular Hyporesponsiveness in Sprague-Dawley Rats**
Takahashi K, Ando K, Ono A, Shimosawa T, Ogata E, Fujita T (Univ of Tokyo, Japan)
*Life Sci* 50:1437–1444, 1992                                                    2–9

---

*Background.*—The cytokine tumor necrosis factor-α (TNF-α) appears to be an important mediator of local and systemic inflammatory re-

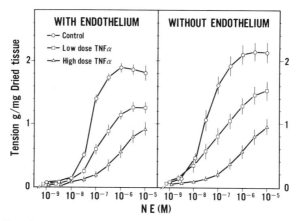

**Fig 2–5.**—Effect of TNF-α on contractions to norepinephrine in rat aortic rings. Contractions are expressed as tension (g) per milligram dried tissue. Contractions were studied in aortic rings from rats treated with saline (*circles*), low-dose TNF-α (*squares*), and high-dose TNF-α (*triangles*). Treatment with TNF-α significantly depressed contractions in rings both with (**left,** $n = 7$) and without (**right,** $n = 6$) endothelium. (Courtesy of Takahashi K, Ando K, Ono A, et al: *Life Sci* 50:1437–1444, 1992.)

sponses, including septic shock. Reduced systemic vascular resistance and decreased responsiveness to vasoconstrictors both may contribute to progressive cardiovascular insufficiency in septic patients.

*Methods.*—In an attempt to delineate the mechanisms of TNF-α-induced hypotension, the effects of recombinant human TNF-α on cardiovascular function were examined in rats given either TNF-α, 0.006 or 0.06 mg/kg/h, or a saline placebo. In addition, aortic tissues were exposed to vasoconstrictors in vitro.

*Findings.*—The high dose of TNF-α significantly reduced mean arterial pressure, and both doses increased the heart rate. Contractile responses of aortic rings to norepinephrine were depressed by TNF-α in vitro in a dose-dependent manner, whether or not the endothelium was present (Fig 2–5).

*Conclusions.*—Administration of TNF-α to rats induced nonspecific vascular hyporesponsiveness, which may help to explain the hypotensive effect of this cytokine.

▶ Studies investigating the potential mediators and basic pathophysiology of septic shock are of unquestioned importance, because the annual incidence of septic shock exceeds 200,000 patients a year and is responsible for up to 100,000 deaths annually. One particularly frustrating factor contributing to the refractory nature of septic shock is the inability to pharmacologically reverse the profound vasodilatory state of these patients. In fact, the combination of decreased systemic vascular resistance and depressed vascular responsiveness to vasoconstrictive agents is characteristic of septic shock. Why does this phenomenon occur? Why are these patients refractory to vasoconstrictive agents? Could this refractory vasodilated state be mediated via cytokines such as TNF? The answers to these questions are important if we expect to develop new and effective therapeutic agents.

In this light, the results of the current study provide firm evidence that TNF-induced decreased mean arterial blood pressure is associated with depressed vascular contractility to adrenergic as well as nonadrenergic agents. Because anti-TNF antibodies are available and are beginning to be tested clinically, it is now possible to test the hypothesis that TNF plays a role in the vascular hyporesponsiveness of septic shock.—E.A. Deitch, M.D.

---

**Administration of Anti-TNF Antibody Improves Left Ventricular Function in Septic Shock Patients: Results of a Pilot Study**
Vincent J-L, Bakker J, Marécaux G, Schandene L, Kahn RJ, Dupont E (Erasme Univ Hosp, Brussels, Belgium)
*Chest* 101:810–815, 1992                                                2–10

---

*Background.*—Three recent observations have led to the identification of tumor necrosis factor-α (TNF, or cachectin), a macrophage-derived cytokine, as a potentially important mediator of septic shock. First, TNF blood levels in severely septic patients have been related to the severity of acute disease and the likelihood of death; second, in animal studies, the administration of TNF reproduced the hemodynamic, metabolic, and pathologic findings associated with endotoxic shock; and third, administering anti-TNF to animals counteracted the deleterious effects of endotoxin and improved survival from gram-negative sepsis. A pilot study was undertaken to test the responses of 10 patients to a murine monoclonal antibody against TNF.

*Method.*—Murine monoclonal anti-TNF antibody was administered to 10 patients after initial resuscitation during the first 24 hours of septic shock.

*Results.*—Treatment with murine monoclonal anti-TNF antibody resulted in a reduction in heart rate and an increase in the left ventricular stroke work index (LVSWI), indicating improvement in ventricular function in the absence of change in cardiac filling pressures. There was concurrent improvement in arterial oxygenation in 6 of the 10 patients, but these changes appeared to be transient.

*Conclusion.*—Tumor necrosis factor is released early in septic shock, and anti-TNF antibody may need to be administered early to have any effect. The use of murine monoclonal anti-TNF antibody produced no adverse effects and resulted in transient improvement in ventricular function and arterial oxygenation.

▶ The improvement in cardiac function after administration of anti-TNF antibody in this pilot clinical study validates recent experimental work indicating that TNF plays a significant role in the myocardial depression observed in septic shock. Of equal importance was the lack of side effects observed after anti-TNF antibody administration. Thus the results of this phase I study further support the initiation of multi-institutional studies directed at assessing the clinical efficacy of anti-TNF antibodies in patients with life-threatening infections or septic shock.

One of the things I liked about this study in particular was that the authors chose to study physiologic end points rather than just survival, because mortality may be too crude a marker of therapeutic efficacy in these complex patients.—E.A. Deitch, M.D.

---

**Effect of Amrinone on Tumor Necrosis Factor Production in Endotoxic Shock**
Giroir BP, Beutler B (Howard Hughes Med Inst, UT Southwestern Med Ctr, Dallas, Tex)
*Circ Shock* 36:200–207, 1992                                                    2–11

---

*Background.*—Because many pathophysiologic mechanisms of endotoxic shock are caused by the macrophage-derived mediator tumor necrosis factor (TNF), methods of inhibiting the production or activity of TNF are under study. Whether the noncatechol inotrope amrinone can diminish TNF production occurring in response to endotoxin challenge was investigated.

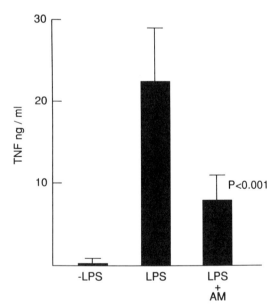

Fig 2–6.—Effect of amrinone (AM) on TNF production in endotoxin-challenged mice. Serum was obtained for assay 90 minutes after endotoxin administration. Tumor necrosis factor values are plotted as the mean; *error bars* represent the standard deviation. The *P* value was calculated by a 2-tailed Student's *t* test. (Courtesy of Giroir BP, Beutler B: *Circ Shock* 36:200–207, 1992.)

Effect of Amrinone on 24-Hour Survival in
Endotoxin-Challenged Mice

| Group | 24 Hours Alive | Dead |
|---|---|---|
| Amrinone + LPS | 13 | 11 |
| Saline + LPS | 4 | 24 |

Note: P value calculated by a 2-tailed Fisher's exact test. $P = .0046$.
(Courtesy of Giroir BP, Beutler B: *Circ Shock* 36:200–207, 1992.)

*Observations.*—In vivo and in vitro experiments showed that amrinone strongly inhibited lipopolysaccharide-induced production of TNF. Evidence of this inhibition was noted in murine macrophages, in macrophage cell lines, in vivo, and in cells containing a reporter gene construct that substitutes the chloramphenicol acetyl transferase coding sequence for the TNF coding sequence and introns. In endotoxin-challenged mice, amrinone reduced TNF production by more than 65% (Fig 2–6); amrinone pretreatment also significantly improved survival (table). The inhibitory effects of amrinone were apparent at the level of mRNA accumulation. The production of TNF was increased considerably by the abrupt removal of amrinone or pentoxifylline from the culture medium before lipopolysaccharide stimulation.

*Conclusions.*—Amrinone is a strong inhibitor of lipopolysaccharide-induced TNF production at concentrations that are easily attained in vivo. It appears to have anti-inflammatory as well as inotropic properties, which may make it suitable for use in septic shock and other serious bacterial infections. After discontinuation of therapy, amrinone and other phosphodiesterase inhibitors may increase sensitivity to lipopolysaccharide.

▶ The importance of this study is that it shows us that certain nonadrenergic inotropic agents may exert beneficial effects independent of their direct effect on the heart.

Amrinone is currently used in the management of cardiogenic shock but not septic shock. Yet, based on the results of this study and previous work indicating that amrinone improves myocardial performance and oxygen delivery in dogs challenged with endotoxin, it appears possible that this drug may be beneficial in selected patients refractory to adrenergic inotropes. However, because of the rebound increase in endotoxin-induced TNF production observed after amrinone is stopped, caution must be exercised in clinical studies investigating the utility of this or similar drugs to augment cardiac function during septic shock. Caveats aside, this experimental study may be providing us with a peak into a new future therapy for patients in septic shock.—E.A. Deitch, M.D.

### Plasma Endothelin Levels Are Increased During Septic Shock

Voerman HJ, Stehouwer CA, van Kamp GJ, Strack van Schijndel RJM, Groeneveld ABJ, Thijs LG (Free Univ Hosp, Amsterdam)
*Crit Care Med* 20:1097–1101, 1992                                        2–12

*Background.*—During septic shock, the increased cardiac output cannot compensate for decreased peripheral vascular tone. This causes hypotension and may even result in death. Overall vasodilation may be caused by the increased production or release of endothelium-derived relaxing factors. In the midst of the overall vasodilation, however, regional vasoconstriction can occur in, for example, the renal vascular bed. An endothelium-derived vasoconstricting peptide, endothelin, has been identified. If endothelin also is released during septic shock, the regional balance between vasoconstricting and vasodilating compounds might determine the vascular response of various tissues, e.g., the kidney. To determine whether endothelin is involved in the pathophysiology of septic shock, a prospective study of endothelin levels was carried out in 6 patients with severe sepsis.

*Methods.*—Serial measurements of plasma endothelin levels were made for 8 days in 6 patients with severe sepsis admitted to an intensive care unit. The results were correlated with hemodynamic, renal, and therapeutic variables.

*Results.*—Initial plasma endothelin concentrations were significantly elevated in the patients compared with normal controls. The endothelin levels were significantly correlated with the Acute Physiology and Chronic Health Evaluation II score. Multiple regression analysis indicated that plasma endothelin concentrations were predicted by dopamine doses but not by mean arterial pressure (MAP). Plasma endothelin concentrations predicted the decrease in creatinine clearance, independently of MAP. The pooled value for correlations between endothelin levels and creatinine clearance, during the course of disease, was significant.

*Conclusions.*—During septic shock, endothelial injury by activated leukocytes and the infusion of catecholamines may increase endothelin release or production. This process may be involved in the renal vasoconstriction seen in septic shock and may increase the severity of this condition.

▶ Why is it that the blood flow to certain organs such as the kidney and gut is inordinately decreased at a time when systemic vascular resistance is decreased? One possible explanation is endothelin.

Endothelin is a recently discovered, endothelium-derived peptide with vasoconstricting properties. Endothelin is produced by endothelium and macrophages in response to a variety of stimuli and appears to play a major role in the normal regulation of tissue blood flow. Thus, although preliminary, the results of the above study indicating that the production of endothelin is increased during septic shock even at a time when the systemic vascular resistance was low, plus their findings of a weak, but statistically significant, inverse correlation between endothelin levels and creatinine clearance, support the authors' hypothesis that, during septic shock, renal dysfunction is related to endothelin-induced vasoconstriction of the renal circulation. Although speculative, there is some merit to this hypothesis, because endothelial-derived vasodilatory and vasoconstrictive products (e.g., nitric oxide and endothelin, respectively) are involved in the regulation of regional blood flow. Consequently, disruption of the normal balance between these vasoactive substances could lead to regional alterations in blood flow.—E.A. Deitch, M.D.

---

**Heat-Shock Gene Expression Excludes Hepatic Acute-Phase Gene Expression After Resuscitation From Hemorrhagic Shock**
Schoeniger LO, Reilly PM, Bulkley GB, Buchman TG (Johns Hopkins Univ, Baltimore, Md)
*Surgery* 112:355–363, 1992                                    2–13

---

*Introduction.*—Critically ill patients often experience multiple organ dysfunction syndrome (MODS) as the cause of death. At the cellular level, gene expression and heat-shock proteins as part of the heat-shock response may create a path toward cell injury and organ malfunctioning. A study of the gene transcription rates was undertaken using a nuclear runoff assay in porcine liver specimens from animals that underwent hemorrhagic shock and resuscitation, leading to the heat-shock expression.

*Methods.*—Sedated female piglets underwent ventilation, femoral cutdown, and shock induction via a 40% blood volume hemorrhagic shock procedure over 1–2 hours. The animals were then resuscitated. Liver biopsy specimens were obtained for a nuclear runoff assay to measure heat-shock protein (hsp) and acute-phase reactant gene expression after the hemorrhage shock and after resuscitation. The nuclear runoff assay measures the gross total incorporation of $^{32}P$-uridine triphosphate in the sample.

*Results.*—The 6 animals experienced a 50% decrease in cardiac output and splanchnic blood flow after induction of hemorrhage. These values returned to near baseline after resuscitation. The livers of individually hemorrhaged pigs synthesized RNA that encoded either the acute-phase reactants (APR) or hsp-72, the major heat-shock protein. No animals transcribed both classes of genes simultaneously. Transcription of hsp-72 mRNA was not observed in the sham-operated animals. In the hsp-72 transcriptional responder group the hsp-72 increased by 11-fold compared with findings in the sham-operated animals.

*Conclusions.*—Different classes of stress protein genes are not transcribed simultaneously. Induction of hsp transcription appears to eliminate the increased expression of acute-phase reactant genes and thereby influences survival after stress.

▶ The major goal of this study was to determine in shocked animals whether the gene expression of both acute-phase reactants and the major hsp can be induced simultaneously. The answer to this important question appears to be, no.

This question is important because the primary function of the acute-phase proteins and hsp-72 appears to be somewhat different. The acute-phase proteins serve to protect the *host* from the effects of inflammation, whereas the function of the hsps is to protect the *cell*. Thus, simplistically stated, if the liver cells shut off acute-phase protein synthesis to produce more hsps, they are acting to save themselves at the expense of the host; from the host's point of view, this is a somewhat selfish thing to do.—E.A. Deitch, M.D.

---

**A Study of the Relationships Among Survival, Gut-Origin Sepsis, and Bacterial Translocation in a Model of Systemic Inflammation**
Deitch EA, Kemper AC, Specian RD, Berg RD (Louisiana State Univ, Shreveport)
*J Trauma* 32:141–147, 1992                                                    2–14

---

*Background.*—Multiple organ failure (MOF), with or without sepsis, can exist in a patient with no identifiable focus of infection. A number of factors may have a role in the development of MOF, including uncontrolled inflammation, gut barrier failure, and sepsis. The inflammatory

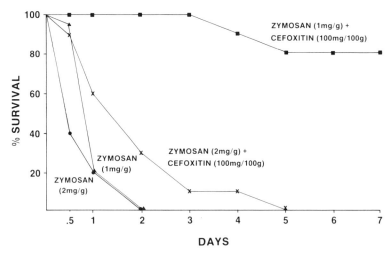

**Fig 2–7.**—Cefoxitin (100 mg/ 100 g) significantly prolonged and increased survival (*P* < .01) of mice challenged with zymosan at a dose of 1 mg/g. In contrast, cefoxitin did not prolong or increase survival when the dose of zymosan administered was 2 mg/g. Ten animals tested per group. (Courtesy of Deitch EA, Kemper AC, Specian RD, et al: *J Trauma* 32:141–147, 1992.)

agent, zymosan, was used to induce a systemic inflammatory state in mice, and the importance and interrelationships among factors involved in the development of MOF were assessed.

*Methods.*—Specific pathogen-free mice were given either saline solution or 1 of 3 doses of zymosan: .1, .5, or 1.0 mg/g. The spread of bacteria from the gut to the mesenteric lymph nodes, liver, spleen, and blood was measured, as was survival, after zymosan challenge. The ability of inhibition (allopurinol or tungsten) of xanthine oxidase to prevent bacterial translocation was measured, as was the ability of cefoxitin to improve survival.

*Results.*—At the 2 lower, nonlethal doses, zymosan resulted in injury to the intestinal mucosa, increased intestinal xanthine oxidase activity, and promoted bacterial translocation to the systemic organs in a dose-dependent fashion. Animals given allopurinol and those given a tungsten diet had reduced mucosal injury and bacterial translocation at a zymosan dose of .1, but not .5, mg/g. Cefoxitin, 1 mg/g, decreased the 7-day mortality of high-dose zymosan from 100% to 20%, suggesting that its lethal effects were related to sepsis of gut origin (Fig 2–7). Survival was not improved by antibiotics at a zymosan dose of 2 mg/g.

*Conclusions.*—In mice, the inflammatory agent zymosan appears to induce gut barrier failure and systemic infection in a dose-dependent fashion. The magnitude of the inflammatory insult—in this case, the dose of zymosan—appears to affect the mechanism of bacterial translocation and the relationship of gut-origin sepsis to survival.

▶ The importance of this article is several-fold. First, it documents that an inflammatory agent can lead to gut barrier failure and systemic infection. As an aside, this process of gut barrier failure leading to the escape of bacteria from the gut to systemic organs and tissues has been termed bacterial translocation. Second, this study illustrates that there is a dose-dependent relationship between the magnitude of the inflammatory insult and the extent of bacterial translocation and death. Third, gut-derived bacterial sepsis appears to play a causal role in the lethal effects of zymosan, because antibiotic treatment improves survival. However, the protective effect of antibiotics was lost when the dose of zymosan was increased from 1 mg/g to 2 mg/g, thus mortality no longer appeared to be directly related to the presence of translocating bacteria. This latter experimental observation is consistent with the clinical observation that in the severely critically ill or injured who contract secondary infections, antibiotic therapy is frequently ineffective.

Based on experimental studies such as this one, there has been a surge of interest in the causal role of gut barrier failure in the development of systemic infections and MOF. One clinically attractive aspect of the gut hypothesis is that bacterial translocation would explain the apparent paradox of why no septic focus can be identified clinically or at autopsy in more than 30% of bacteremic patients with MOF dying with clinical sepsis. Furthermore, the presence of gut-derived portal or systemic endotoxemia may contribute to the development of a septic state in patients without infection.

Thus the gut hypothesis of MOF clarifies how patients can have enteric bacteremias in the absence of an identifiable focus of infection or become septic in the absence of microbiological evidence of infection.—E.A. Deitch, M.D.

### Liver Injury Is a Reversible Neutrophil-Mediated Event Following Gut Ischemia

Poggetti RS, Moore FA, Moore EE, Bensard DD, Anderson BO, Banerjee A (Denver Gen Hosp, Denver, Colo; Univ of Colorado, Denver)
*Arch Surg* 127:175–179, 1992                                                      2–15

*Objective.*—Gut ischemia/reperfusion (I/R) may play an important role in the pathogenesis of multiple organ failure. Simultaneous liver and lung dysfunction may occur as a primary systemic event after gut I/R, rather than as a sequential cascade of organ failure. The temporal relationship between distant organ dysfunction and mesenteric I/R was examined and the role of the neutrophil in this process assessed.

*Methods.*—Rats, both normal and neutrophil depleted by means of vinblastine sulfate injection, were subjected to 45 minutes of superior mesenteric artery occlusion. Blood samples, livers, and lungs from the animals were analyzed after 0, 6, and 18 hours of reperfusion. Pulmonary and liver injury was assessed by iodine-125 ($^{125}I$) albumin leak; the hepatic mitochondrial redox state was assessed by serum acetoacetate/3-hydroxybutyrate (AcAc/3-OHB).

*Findings.*—There was no change in the $^{125}I$-albumin lung/blood ratio after 45 minutes of occlusion (Fig 2–8). At 6 hours of reperfusion, the normal rats showed significant increases in $^{125}I$-albumin/lung blood ratio

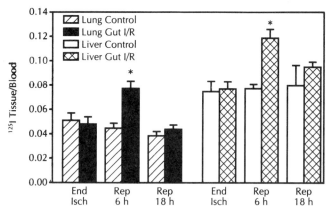

**Fig 2–8.**—Iodine-125 albumin tissue/blood ratios (lung and liver): end of 45 minutes of intestinal ischemia (*Isch*); after 6 hours of intestinal reperfusion (*Rep*); and after 18 hours of intestinal reperfusion. *Asterisk* indicates $P < .05$; I/R = ischemia/reperfusion. (Courtesy of Poggetti RS, Moore FA, Moore EE, et al: *Arch Surg* 127:175–179, 1992.)

and [125]I-albumin liver/blood ratio and a significant decrease in AcAc/3-OHB. These changes were not noted at 6 hours in the neutrophil-depleted animals.

*Conclusions.*—In this study, intestinal I/R caused simultaneous liver and lung injury. This injury was present at 6 hours but was reversed by 18 hours and was mediated by neutrophils. Further studies of this mechanism are needed to develop early therapy to prevent the "multiple organ failure cascade."

▶ The importance of this study is that it documents that an isolated episode of gut ischemia can result in the capillary leak syndrome plus promote lung and liver dysfunction. As such, these results add further support to the hypothesis that injury to the gut can promote injury to other organs, and imply that by preventing or reducing the magnitude of gut injury it may be possible to prevent or reduce injury to other organs.—E.A. Deitch, M.D.

---

**Early Gut Ischemia in Experimental Fecal Peritonitis**
Rasmussen I, Haglund U (Univ Hosp, Uppsala, Sweden)
*Circ Shock* 38:22–28, 1992                                                2–16

---

*Purpose.*—The intestinal mucosa is highly susceptible to hypoxic injury. The splanchnic area is of extreme importance in sepsis because organ injury may lead to serious systemic effects and further aggravate the shock state. Assessment of tissue oxygenation in the gastrointestinal tract would therefore be extremely useful. The usefulness of the tonometric technique in monitoring the intestinal mucosal pH was investigated in a porcine model of septic shock induced by fecal peritonitis.

*Methods.*—Peritonitis was induced by instillation of a standardized amount of autologous feces into the abdominal cavities of 6 pigs. Saline solution was instilled into the abdominal cavities of another 6 pigs who served as sham controls. Splanchnic oxygen delivery was estimated by measuring the portal venous blood flow and the calculated arterial oxygen saturation. Oxygen consumption of the viscera, including the gut, pancreas, and spleen, was estimated by measuring the portal venous blood flow and the difference between the calculated arterial oxygen saturation and the measured portal venous oxygen saturation. Oxygenation of the intestinal mucosa was also monitored by the tonometric technique. Lactate levels in arterial and portal blood were measured. The animals were followed for 5 hours and then killed with potassium chloride.

*Results.*—All animals survived the 5-hour experimental period. Septic shock induced by peritonitis caused a significant increase in systemic and gastrointestinal oxygen consumption (Fig 2–9). Oxygen consumption was maintained at a high level despite a falling oxygen delivery during the second half of the 5-hour experimental period. Despite an elevated oxygen consumption and even though normal oxygen delivery was main-

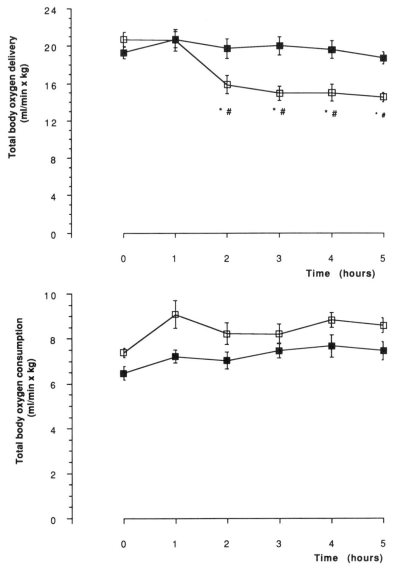

**Fig 2–9.**—Total body oxygen delivery and consumption in animals subjected to peritonitis (*open boxes*) and sham controls (*filled boxes*). Mean values ± SEM. # Values are significantly (P < .05) different from the baseline values for the same group. * Values are significantly (P < .05) different between the groups. (Courtesy of Rasmussen I, Haglund U: *Circ Shock* 38:22–28, 1992.)

tained in the early part of the septic period, the intestinal intramucosal pH was already reduced after 1 hour of peritonitis and very significantly so after 2 hours (Fig 2–10). Furthermore, an early increase in splanchnic oxygen consumption was evident simultaneously with the fall in the in-

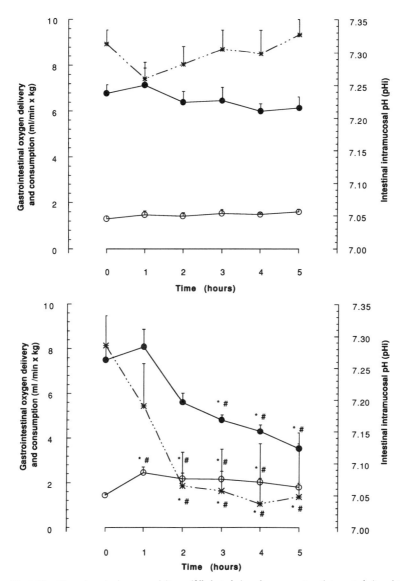

**Fig 2–10.**—Gastrointestinal oxygen delivery (*filled circles*) and consumption (*open circles*) and intramucosal pH (*) in controls (**top**) and in animals subjected to peritonitis (**below**). Mean values ± SEM. # Values are significantly different (*P* < .05) from the baseline value for the same group. * Values are significantly (*P* < .05) different between the experimental and the control group. (Courtesy of Rasmussen I, Haglund U: *Circ Shock* 38:22–28, 1992.)

testinal intramucosal pH. Arterial pH and lactate levels did not detect the inadequate regional tissue oxygenation.

*Conclusions.*—Measurement of the intestinal intramucosal pH via the tonometric technique is an indirect, minimally invasive, and sensitive method for detecting changes in splanchnic oxygenation during early sepsis.

---

### Reevaluation of Current Transfusion Practices in Patients in Surgical Intensive Care Units

Babineau TJ, Dzik WH, Borlase BC, Baxter JK, Bistrian BR, Benotti PN (New England Deaconess Hosp, Boston, Mass; Harvard Med School, Boston)
*Am J Surg* 164:22–25, 1992                                                    2–17

---

*Background.*—Wide concern about complications from packed red blood cell transfusion has prompted reassessment of conventional transfusion practices. Despite recent attempts to more clearly define indications for transfusion, especially in critically ill patients, transfusions still are ordered when a patient's hemoglobin level is below 10 g/dL.

*Objective.*—The impact of red blood cell transfusion on oxygen consumption was studied in 30 critically ill postoperative patients who received 33 transfusions to correct hemoglobin levels of less than 10 g/dL.

*Results.*—In the group as a whole, red blood cell transfusion did not appreciably alter oxygen consumption (table). Only one fourth of the transfusions increased oxygen consumption by more than 20%. The

Red Cell Transfusion and Oxygen Metabolism

|  | Pretransfusion * (n = 33) | Posttransfusion * (n = 33) | p Value (*t*-test) |
|---|---|---|---|
| Hgb (g/dL) | 9.4 ± 0.2 | 10.4 ± 0.3 | <0.001 |
| DO$_2$ (mL/min/m$^2$) | 401 ± 20 | 433 ± 21 | 0.01 |
| VO$_2$ (mL/min/m$^2$) | 117 ± 4 | 115 ± 5 | NS |
| SaO$_2$ (%) | 96 ± 1 | 95 ± 1 | 0.005 |
| SvO$_2$ (%) | 67 ± 1 | 70 ± 1 | 0.005 |
| Extract (%) | 31 ± 1 | 28 ± 1 | 0.003 |
| CI (L/min/m$^2$) | 3.2 ± 0.2 | 3.2 ± 0.2 | NS |
| MAP (torr) | 78 ± 3 | 81 ± 3 | NS |
| SVR (dynes · s) | 956 ± 49 | 1026 ± 63 | NS |
| Heart rate (beats/min) | 94 ± 3 | 92 ± 3 | NS |

*Abbreviations: Hgb,* hemoglobin; *CI,* cardiac index; *MAP,* mean arterial pressure; *SVR,* systemic vascular resistance; *SaO$_2$,* arterial oxygen saturation; *SvO$_2$,* venous oxygen saturation; *DO$_2$,* oxygen delivery; *VO$_2$,* oxygen consumption; *Extract,* oxygen extraction ratio.
* All transfusion values are mean ± standard error.
(Courtesy of Babineau TJ, Dzik WH, Borlase BC, et al: *Am J Surg* 164:22–25, 1992.)

mean oxygen consumption rose by 7% in septicemic patients but declined by 9% in those who were not septic.

*Conclusions.*—The policy of administering transfusions to patients solely on the basis of a hemoglobin level of less than 10 g/dL is questionable. With such a policy, many patients, especially nonseptic patients, will have no substantial rise in oxygen consumption.

▶ Blood transfusions cost money, take time, and are associated with an increasing number of recognized adverse consequences, including, most recently, immune suppression. Thus today we can no longer accept the concepts that, when in doubt, it is better to transfuse or that a little blood never hurt anyone. Instead, the decision to transfuse blood must be based on objective evidence of physiologic benefit. The results of this study and several other clinical studies appearing in the past 5 years do not support the concept of arbitrarily maintaining a hemoglobin of 10 g/dL or greater in patients in the intensive care unit. At the current time, my practice is not to prophylactically transfuse hemodynamically stable patients with hemoglobin levels greater than 7 g/dL, with the exception of those with coronary artery disease, especially if the anemia is inducing signs or symptoms of cardiovascular dysfunction. The role of transfusion therapy in anemic patients with adult respiratory distress syndrome, multiple organ failure, or septic shock is judged on a patient-to-patient basis and is predicated on signs of supply-dependent oxygen consumption.—E.A. Deitch, M.D.

---

**Blood Transfusion Impairs the Healing of Experimental Intestinal Anastomoses**

Tadros T, Wobbes T, Hendriks T (Univ Hosp, Nijmegen, The Netherlands)
*Ann Surg* 215:276–281, 1992                2–18

---

*Background.*—The cell-mediated immune response appears to be impaired by blood transfusion. Because patients undergoing gastrointestinal surgery commonly need transfusions as a result of anemia or blood loss, it is important to establish the effect of transfusions on intestinal repair.

*Methods.*—The ileum and colon of adult male Lewis rats were resected and then either an everted or end-to-end anastomosis was constructed. The animals were given either saline or heparinized blood from Lewis or Brown Norway rat donors, 3 ML administered intravenously immediately after operation. Three days or 1 week after surgery, the rats were killed and the strength of their anastomoses tested by measuring the bursting pressure.

*Results.*—None of the control animals had anastomotic abscesses or generalized peritonitis, but the incidence of these complications was increased in the animals that received transfusions, especially allogeneic transfusions. Anastomotic strength was significantly reduced at 3 days in rats that received transfusion from either Lewis or Brown Norway rats. For inverted ileal anastomoses, average bursting pressures were 79 mm Hg in controls, 46 mm Hg in rats receiving Lewis rat blood transfusion, and 21 mm Hg in those receiving Brown Norway rat blood transfusion. At 1 week the site of rupture was significantly more common within the anastomotic line in transfused animals.

*Conclusions.*—Blood transfusion impairs the healing of experimental intestinal anastomoses in rats and increases their vulnerability to intra-abdominal sepsis. This may result from some alteration in the local or systemic immune response to the intestinal trauma of surgery. These findings could have important clinical effects that warrant further study.

▶ This study speaks for itself. This is one more reason to avoid prophylactic transfusions in hemodynamically stable, asymptomatic patients.—E.A. Deitch, M.D.

---

**Outcome in Critical Care Patients: A Multivariate Study**
Ferraris VA, Propp ME (Albany Med Ctr, Albany, NY)
*Crit Care Med* 20:967–976, 1992                                    2–19

---

*Introduction.*—Several severity indices have been used to assess and predict death in the intensive care unit (ICU), among them the Acute Physiology and Chronic Health Evaluation (APACHE II) classification score. Patient chart data were evaluated to further determine the variables responsible for an unfavorable outcome for ICU patients.

*Methods.*—The charts of patients who had stayed in the ICU for more than 72 hours or who died within the first 72 hours in the unit were reviewed retrospectively for 26 variables representing chronic health status, physiologic condition, and iatrogenic complications associated with drug therapy, ventilatory treatment, invasive procedures, or general interventions.

*Results.*—Of the 26 variables assessed, 9 were significantly related to adverse patient outcome, including age, physiologic status, APACHE II score, number of repeat ICU admissions, respiratory complications, sepsis, renal failure, disseminated intravascular coagulation, and any iatrogenic complication. These data resulted from assessment of the charts of 46 patients who improved and 64 who did not improve (52 deaths and 12 unimproved patients). The final logistic regression analysis revealed 5 variables that significantly related to negative patient outcome: the APACHE II score; deteriorating respiratory failure, sepsis, and/or renal failure in the ICU; and iatrogenic complications during the patient's ICU stay. A relatively frequent iatrogenic complication appeared to be related to drug complications, e.g., aminoglycoside toxicity. Twenty-one iatrogenic drug complications occurred in 64 patients who did not improve, whereas only 3 such complications occurred in the 46 patients who improved.

*Conclusion.*—Patients remaining in the ICU for longer than 72 hours often experience complications associated with inappropriate drug treatment. They may have significantly more adverse outcomes, many of which could be prevented.

▶ Most indexes used to predict outcome in the ICU are based on patient variables obtained at or shortly after arrival in the unit. In general, such indexes ignore events that occur after the patient has arrived in the ICU, yet post-ICU admission events influence survival.

The strength and novel aspect of this study are that the authors evaluated the potential impact of iatrogenic events on outcome. One of the most interesting findings was that for patients who remained in the ICU for more than 72 hours, events occurring after ICU admission reflected an adverse outcome better than ICU admission status, as determined by APACHE II scores. In spite of the limitations of the retrospective nature of this study, the basic message is important. That is, because potentially preventable iatrogenic complications significantly influence survival, by identifying and subsequently reducing their incidence it should be possible to improve the outcome of patients admitted to the ICU.—E.A. Deitch, M.D.

---

### Attitudes of Medical Students, Housestaff, and Faculty Physicians Toward Euthanasia and Termination of Life-Sustaining Treatment

Caralis PV, Hammond JS (VA Med Ctr, Miami, Fla; Univ of Medicine and Dentistry of New Jersey, New Brunswick)
*Crit Care Med* 20:683–690, 1992
2–20

---

*Introduction.*—Recent legislative actions and court decisions have extended the acceptance of death and may have weakened prohibitions against euthanasia, but little is known about physicians' attitudes toward changes in their traditional role of prolonging life. A study via questionnaire was undertaken to define the views of 360 faculty physicians, housestaff, and medical students toward living wills, do-not-resuscitate orders, and termination of life support.

*Responses.*—Three-fourths of the respondents considered withholding life-support measures to be consistent with passive euthanasia, and most found this to be preferable to active euthanasia. Half of the respondents would accede to a patient's wish not to receive lifesaving treatment, but very few would accede if a patient asked for help in dying. Only 6% of respondents would be willing to end a patient's life by giving medication to arrest respiration. Responses to the case vignettes provided in the questionnaire indicated that faculty valued disease-based information most highly when considering decisions, whereas housestaff and students focused more on quality-of-life factors. Respondents were most willing to take "active" action when a patient was terminally ill.

*Overview.*—It is not easy to balance personal liberty and patient autonomy with professional integrity and the state's interest in preserving life. At a minimum, physicians can no longer be indifferent about issues of euthanasia.

▶ I refer this article and its accompanying editorial to you, not because I want to preach what is ethically correct, but because of the increasing importance of ethics-based decision making in all aspects of medical care.—E.A. Deitch, M.D.

# 3 Burns

## Introduction

In the United States, it is estimated conservatively that more than 2.5 million persons seek medical care for burn injuries each year. More than 100,000 of these patients are hospitalized, and about 12,000 burn victims die of their injuries each year. Despite continuing progress in this field, burn injuries remain a common cause of death, and only motor vehicle accidents produce more accidental deaths. In addition, the prevention and treatment of the cosmetic, functional, and emotional sequelae in these patients continue to pose major challenges (1).

In many ways, the first line of battle is fought at the level of the burn wound. One of the major factors limiting survival in patients with extensive and deep burns is the lack of available donor sites for grafting. Futilely watching patients die of the ravages of their burn injuries while waiting for previously harvested donor sites to heal and be ready for reuse is a relatively common occurrence. Consequently, the development of alternative methods to permanently close the excised burn wound has been an area of active research. Although this problem has not been solved, several options are in various stages of development. The options covered in this section include the use of in vitro cell culture methods to grow cultured epithelial autografts from a 1 cm-skin biopsy specimen, intermingled skin grafts, and microskin autografts placed under pigskin xenografts. The use of a living dermal substitute to potentially reduce hypertrophic scar formation and contracture in patients receiving widely meshed skin grafts is also described (Abstract 3–5), as are options in surgical technique for facial and electrical burns (Abstracts 3–6 and 3–7). The latter 2 articles were chosen, because most burn victims have non–life-threatening burns in which the goal of care is the production of a healed wound with optimal function and cosmesis. Another article (Abstract 3–8) deals directly with the burn wound in an experimental study using liposomes to more effectively deliver antimicrobial agents to the injured site.

Studies investigating the pathophysiology, mediators, and mechanisms of pulmonary and other organ injury, as well as infection, continue to shed light on the underlying biology of burn-induced morbidity and mortality. Because of experimental studies indicating that an exaggerated cytokine-mediated inflammatory response may lead to organ injury and mediate (potentiate) the hypermetabolic response, clinical studies investigating the cytokine response of thermally injured patients have been carried out. Although, to some extent, the results of these studies are confusing and in some cases contradictory, as a whole they indicate that certain cytokine patterns are of prognostic importance. For example, persistent elevations in interleukin-6 levels were associated with increased mortality in one study (Abstract 3–9), whereas the inability to maintain elevated interleukin-1$\beta$ levels were a poor prognostic sign in a second study (Abstract 3–10). Interestingly, the administration of interleukin-1$\beta$ improved survival in burned mice subjected to an infectious challenge.

Studies investigating the potential relationships between oxygen delivery, oxidant-mediated organ injury, and inflammatory-induced leukocyte-mediated endothelial injury are helping to clarify the pathophysiology of burn-induced distant organ injury and the development of multiple organ failure, as well as provide clues for the creation of more optimal resuscitative regimens. Additionally, evidence supporting the role of the gut as a reservoir for systemic infections, and the clinical benefits of orally administered antibiotics to prevent gut-origin sepsis, was documented in two clinical studies (Abstracts 3–16 and 3–17). Lastly, attention continues to focus on optimal methods of ventilation in patients with smoke inhalation injury, the risk of HIV infections, and the long-term psychosocial consequences of thermal injury.

**Edwin A. Deitch, M.D.**

*Reference*

1. Deitch EA: N *Engl J Med* 323:1249, 1990.

---

**Addendum: Multicenter Experience With Cultured Epidermal Autograft for Treatment of Burns**
Odessey R (BioSurface Technology, Inc, Cambridge, Mass)
*J Burn Care Rehabil* 13:174–180, 1992                                    3–1

---

*Background.*—Since 1989, BioSurface Technology, Inc, has provided more than 37,000 cultured epidermal autografts (CEAs) for more than 240 patients in 79 different burn centers. This multicenter experience has a follow-up period of up to 2.5 years.

*Clinical Data.*—The CEAs were used primarily to treat extensive burns, with an average size of 70% of total body surface area; half were full-thickness burns. In the 104 patients with complete data, the average final "take" of CEA was approximately 60%. Half of the patients had a final take of 70% or greater, and 22% had a final take of at least 90%. Sixteen per cent of patients had a final take of less than 30%, and many of these cases were associated with wound infection. The final take was associated with early excision (less then 10 days after burn injury) (78%) and temporary coverage with cadaveric homograft that was allowed to engraft (71%). When an engrafted homograft was only partially excised, leaving a layer of "allodermis" as the graft bed for the CEA, the final take averaged 90% in 14 patients. Final graft take was not affected by the burn size, extent of full-thickness injury, or patient's age.

*Discussion.* —These CEAs are more sensitive to the effects of infection in the wound bed than are split-thickness skin grafts. This may result from the high vulnerability of the cultured cell sheet to bacterial proteases and cytotoxins during the first weeks of treatment and maturation. Early excision of the wound bed or temporary coverage with a cadaveric homograft can significantly improve graft take.

▶ Since the first successful use of CEAs in 1981 (1), the concept of using tissue-culture methods to produce sheets of cultured epithelial skin grafts have caught the imagination of the surgical community. With this technique it is possible to expand a 1-cm skin biopsy specimen up to 10,000-fold over a 30-day period and thereby solve the problem of lack of donor sites. The current study presents the uncontrolled results reported by the company that sells CEAs. If this technique sounds almost too good to be true, it may be.

These results are generally somewhat better than those of most other reports (see Abstract 3–2). In my experience, when CEAs take and survive, they can be lifesaving; however, we have not yet reached the stage when CEA survival can be achieved consistently. Further work is necessary to define the optimal technical approach to achieving consistent CEA graft take. The modification originally described by Cuono (2) in which the CEA is placed on to the dermis portion of previously applied cadaver skin rather than a fully excised burn wound may improve graft take.

Currently, my approach, and the general consensus of most major burn centers, is that CEA technology should be used only in patients with extensive and deep burns involving more than 60% to 70% of their body surface area and should not be used in patients with smaller burns whose wounds can be covered using more standard techniques.—E.A. Deitch, M.D.

*References*

1. O'Connor NE, et al: *Lancet* 1:75, 1981.
2. Cuono CB, et al: *Plast Reconstr Surg* 80:626, 1987.

---

**Cultured Epithelial Autografts: Three Years of Clinical Experience With Eighteen Patients**
Clugston PA, Snelling CFT, Macdonald IB, Maledy HL, Boyle JC, Germann E, Courtemanche AD, Wirtz P, Fitzpatrick DJ, Kester DA, Foley B, Warren RJ, Carr NJ (Vancouver Gen Hosp, Vancouver, BC, Canada)
*J Burn Care Rehabil* 12:533–539, 1991                                                    3–2

---

*Introduction.* —Patients with major burns often have an increased catabolism that can lead to a higher risk of death and complications. Cultured epithelial autografts (CEAs) have promoted wound healing in many burn patients. The results of CEAs used to treat 18 patients with burns were reveiwed.

*Methods.*—The 18 patients had a mean age of 37 years and a mean total body surface area (TBSA) burn of 49%. The split-thickness skin graft was harvested when it reached about 4 cm². After formation of a single-cell suspension of keratinocytes, the CEA was attached to fine-meshed vaseline gauze for application. Follow-up continued for 13 days to 18 months after the CEA application using random biopsy sampling.

*Results.*—In 6 patients there was a successful "take" of more than 65%, and in 12 the "take" was less than 40%; 7 patients had no CEA remaining. Perioperative wound cultures demonstrated that all injury sites hosted microorganisms; *Staphylococcus epidermidis* and *Pseudomonas aeruginosa* were present in those with poor CEA outcomes. The use of CEAs did not reduce the length of hospital stay or the number of autograft harvests.

*Conclusion.*—Cultured epithelial autographs should be used in body areas where proper wound care and the treatment of blister formation can easily take place. Physicians should carefully record the data for each patient using this adjunctive procedure to optimize the method's success.

▶ This report, in which only about a third of patients derived clinical benefit from the use of CEAs, is consistent with most reports in the literature (1). It is included to serve as a counterweight to the report by Odessey (Abstract 3–1).—E.A. Deitch, M.D.

*Reference*

1. Munster A, et al: *Ann Surg* 211:676, 1990.

---

**Increased Survival Rate in Patients With Massive Burns**
Xiao J, Chai B-R, Kong F-Y, Peng S-G, Xu H, Wang C-G, Suo H-B, Huang D-Q (Burn Ctr of 205 Hosp, Jin Zhou, Liao Ning, China)
*Burns* 18:401–404, 1992                                           3–3

---

*Objective.*—Survival is now possible in more severely burned patients, with reports of successful treatment even in those with more than 90% full-skin-thickness burns. The treatment techniques responsible for such improvement were reviewed.

*Methods.*—During a 20-year period, 113 patients with massive burns—defined as a burn of at least 50% of the total body surface area (TBSA)—were treated. Patients seen in the latter decade of this experience were aggressively treated in the early resuscitation period by fluid resuscitation, pulmonary support, and early wound management, and in the post-resuscitation period by careful use of fluids, nutrition, and continued

Comparison of Rates of Mortality With Different Burn Sizes

| | 1970s | | | 1980s | | |
|---|---|---|---|---|---|---|
| TBSA (%) | No. | Deaths | % | No. | Deaths | % |
| 50–59 | 17 | 2 | 17.6 | 12 | 0 | 0* |
| 60–69 | 11 | 5 | 45.45 | 16 | 1 | 6.25 |
| 70–79 | 11 | 8 | 72.73 | 11 | 2 | 18.18 |
| 80–89 | 11 | 4 | 36.36 | 8 | 1 | 12.5 |
| 90–99 | 6 | 6 | 100.00 | 10 | 4 | 40.00 |
| Totals | 56 | 25 | 44.6 | 57 | 8 | 14.00* |

* $P < .01$ compared with 1970s.
(Courtesy of Xiao J, Chai B-R, Kong F-Y, et al: *Burns* 18:401–404, 1992.)

wound management. The patients underwent a series of eschar excisions between 3–14 days after injury; tourniquets were used for all excisions. Each operation excised 15% to 20% of TBSA. Wounds were then grafted with a large sheet of allograft. The next day, slits in the allograft were transformed into rectangular "windows" made to fit the autografts, which were then inlaid.

*Results.*—Survival improved significantly with the more recent protocol, from 55% to 86%. The 2 groups were not different in any characteristic except for survival and tracheotomy rate—tracheotomy was avoided in the early part of the experience because it was believed to cause lung infection. The greatest improvements in survival were in patients with full-thickness burns covering more than 59% TBSA (table).

*Conclusions.*—Patients with massive burns treated by a new, aggressive protocol favoring early excision and grafting using the technique of intermingled skin grafts experienced improvements in survival. These improvements are attributed to the early treatment of inhalation injury, sepsis, and multiorgan failure.

▶ This article was chosen because it illustrates the technique of intermingled skin grafts, a technique first described by Yang et al. (1) This method has been widely accepted in China where burn centers can obtain large sheets of fresh cadaver skin on demand. However, because of sociologic and political differences between China and the United States, the accessibility of large sheets of fresh cadaver skin in the United States is limited. Nonetheless, this approach has stimulated interest in developing alternative methods of using expanded autografts in patients with massive burn injuries.—E.A. Deitch, M.D.

*Reference*

1. Yang CC, et al: *Burns* 6:141, 1980.

### Microskin Autograft With Pigskin Xenograft Overlay: A Preliminary Report of Studies on Patients

Lin S-D, Lai C-S, Chou C-K, Tsai C-W, Wu K-F, Chang C-W (Kaohsiung Med College, Taiwan, Republic of China)
Burns 18:321–325, 1992                                                      3–4

*Background.*—The technique of microskin grafting, which requires a specially prepared allograft, is limited by the scarcity of allograft skin and the associated expense and storage facilities. Pigskin xenografts were used successfully in rabbits to replace the allograft in microskin grafting. This technique was investigated in humans.

*Methods.*—The study sample comprised 16 patients aged 2–88 years, with full-thickness skin defects that needed resurfacing by skin grafting. There were 9 burn patients, 5 who had traumatic avulsion wounds, and 2 with diabetic ulcers. The range of ratios of recipient to donor site expansion was from 8:1 to 12:1. A carefully prepared split-thickness pigskin graft (STPSG) was laid over autogenous microskin graft (MSG) pieces, sutured into position, covered by conventional dressings, and immobilized (Fig 3–1). The autogenous donor skin was obtained from the inguinal region, and the donor site was closed primarily.

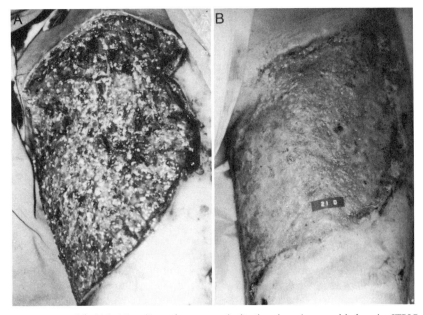

**Fig 3–1.—A,** left thigh. Microskin grafts were evenly distributed on the wound before the STPSG was overlaid. The autogenous donor skin came from the right inguinal area. **B,** the grafted wound on day 21 was completely resurfaced with well-differentiated stable neoepithelium. (Courtesy of Lin S-D, Lai C-S, Chou C-K, et al: *Burns* 18:321-325, 1992.)

*Results.*—By the first dressing change at 6 or 7 days, firm adherence of the STPSG to its wound was observed in all 16 patients. On histologic examination, the MSG was found to have proliferated actively beneath its STPSG overlay. Time until full resurfacing ranged from 13 to 21 days, depending on the expansion ratio used for the individual patient. There were 2 pseudmonas infections, and no patient required further grafting.

*Conclusions.*—An STPSG preparation was found to be safe for clinical application. Even though it undergoes scattered lytic and desquamatory changes, the STPSG overlay used in this technique provides a suitable environment for epithelialization of autogenous MSG. It offers a good alternative to allografts when they are not available. The STPSG is easier to obtain and harvest and less expensive to prepare than an allograft.

▶ One novel surgical approach to limited donor sites is use of the microskin autograft technique described in this report. In this approach, after the donor skin has been cut into small pieces and spread evenly over the wound, it is covered by pigskin, under which the micrografts are allowed to heal and co-alesce. The results achieved with this technique are very encouraging and represent a modification of the sandwich grafting technique popularized by Alexander et al. (1) in which widely meshed autograft (6–9:1) is covered by meshed cadaver skin. The major limitation of the current study is the relatively small size of the burn wounds (mean area grafted, 14% of the body surface). However, as more widespread experience with this technique is obtained, it may become a valuable adjunct to the surgical care of the burn patient.—E.A. Deitch, M.D.

*Reference*

1.   Alexander JW, et al: *J Trauma* 21:433, 1981.

---

**Clinical Trials of a Living Dermal Tissue Replacement Placed Beneath Meshed, Split-Thickness Skin Grafts on Excised Burn Wounds**
Hansbrough JF, Doré C, Hansbrough WB (Univ of California, San Diego)
*J Burn Care Rehabil* 13:519–529, 1992                                    3–5

---

*Background.*—Full-thickness burn wounds associated with extensive thermal injury are often closed with meshed and expanded split-thickness skin grafts (MESTSGs) when sufficient unburned skin for autografting is not available. The MESTSG closes full-thickness wounds by epithelialization without dermis, and the absence of dermal tissue may contribute to hypertrophic scarring, wound contraction, and instability of the skin. Initial experience with a new living dermal substitute placed on excised burn wounds beneath MESTSGs was reviewed.

*Methods.*—Dermagraft is a living tissue composed of neonatal human fibroblasts that are cultured on polyglactin acid mesh. Surgical excision of burn wounds was performed in 17 patients aged 6 to 69 years by a mean of 4.29 days after thermal injury. The mean burn size was 23.8% of the total body surface area. The wounds were excised to subcutaneous fat in 9 patients, to fascia in 3, and to a combination of deep dermis and fat in 5. Experimental and control wound sites were randomly selected; control sites received MESTSGs only. One patient received MESTSGs on both sites. Study sites measured approximately 10 × 20 cm. Each wound was examined and photographed at 9 days and 14 days after grafting, and again at 1, 3, 6, and 12 months thereafter. Wound biopsy specimens were obtained at 14 days and at 3, 6, and 12 months after grafting.

*Results.*—By day 28 after grafting, both control and test sites had undergone "take" to the wounds. Three months after grafting, both sites showed a mesh pattern, but the "take" was somewhat less pronounced at the Dermagraft-treated sites. Wound biopsy specimens obtained 14 days after Dermagraft and MESTSG placement showed no sign of rejection of the cultured allogeneic fibroblasts. The inflammatory reaction to the mesh fibers was minimal. Fourteen days after grafting, immunohistochemical staining revealed continuous basement membrane formation beneath healed epithelium in skin graft interstices at the epithelial-Dermagraft junction. Mesh fibers in the wound were biodegraded by hydrolysis, and absorption was complete within 60 to 90 days.

*Conclusions.*—Dermagraft appears to be a safe and effective dermal replacement when placed on full-thickness burn wounds beneath MESTSGs. Further studies of its safety and efficacy are ongoing.

▶ A common and major problem after split-thickness skin grafting, especially with the use of widely meshed skin grafts placed on fat or fascia, is the development of hypertrophic scars or contracture formation. The frequent development of these complications has generally been considered to be related to the fact that the skin graft lacks an adequate amount of dermis. Consequently, the development of a living or artificial dermal replacement is of major importance. The results of this phase I human clinical trial of Dermagraft documents the potential clinical feasibility of using meshed split-thickness skin grafts in combination with a dermal substitute, such as Dermagraft.

Although encouraging, in the absence of long-term results attesting to the cosmetic or functional superiority of the Dermagraft-treated burns, the jury is still out on the clinical value of this material. Nonetheless, the importance of this article is that it illustrates a potential avenue for reducing the cosmetic and functional sequelae observed in patients requiring widely meshed skin grafts.—E.A. Deitch, M.D.

---

**Primary Pressure Grafts in Early Reconstruction of Deep Facial Burns**
Rougé D, Chavoin JP, Nicoulet B, Gavroy JP, Costagliola M (CHU Rangueil, Toulouse, France; Centre de Rééducation du Docteur Ster, Lamalou les

Bains, France)
*Burns* 18:336–339, 1992                                            3–6

*Purpose.*—In patients with deep facial burns, reconstruction is especially difficult because both appearance and function must be considered. The surgeon must minimize damage to the donor area and perform the reconstruction as early as possible. Full-skin-thickness pressure grafts were used as primary treatment for deep facial and hand burns in 8 women. Less than 20% of body area was affected.

*Methods.*—Primary reconstruction was done in 3 steps: total excision of necrotic tissue around day 3, followed by development of good granulation tissue by days 10–12; raising of a made-to-measure full-thickness skin graft in an area not generally exposed; and continuous compression of the graft for 10 days. The surgeons made sure that the graft was totally revascularized before removing the compression mask.

*Results.*—All grafts took successfully, and all patients were pleased with the esthetic results. The quality of the full-thickness graft prevented contraction and retraction and the resultant deformation and asymmetry.

*Conclusions.*—With this full-thickness pressure graft technique, burned tissue is replaced early after the injury with skin of normal thickness and quality. Esthetic reconstruction after severe facial burns is no longer an unrealistic aim, and research in this area must continue.

▶ A picture is worth a thousand words. This aphorism is clearly supported by the photographs in the original full-length article that illustrate the clinical results obtained using a full-thickness skin graft in combination with immediate pressure therapy in the patient with severe facial burns.—E.A. Deitch, M.D.

## Early Free-Flap Coverage of Electrical and Thermal Burns

Chick LR, Lister GD, Sowder L (Univ of Utah, Salt Lake City)
*Plast Reconstr Surg* 89:1013–1021, 1992                              3–7

*Background.*—Surgeons are often reluctant to perform early coverage of high-voltage electrical injuries and severe thermal burns because of the clinical concept of progressive tissue necrosis. Recent studies suggest, however, that progressive gross tissue necrosis does not occur. The results of early flap coverage were reviewed in 5 patients with severe electrical and thermal injuries of the extremities.

*Patients.*—There were 3 high-voltage electrical injuries, 1 injury caused by a laminating heat press, and 1 combination electrical and avulsion injury. Two patients had flaps placed on both hands, for a total of 7 free flaps. Burn sites were radically débrided, with removal of all nonviable or questionably viable burn tissue except for intact nerves, tendons, and bone. This removal was followed immediately by free-flap reconstruction.

*Outcomes.*—All 7 flaps survived with no wound healing difficulties. One patient required removal of silicone spacers from the metacarpophalangeal joints at 10 months because of a draining infection. Three of the 5 patients returned to gainful employment. Of 8 dysfunctional digital nerves, 5 recovered 2-point discrimination of less than 10 mm. Of 3 first web spaces covered with free flaps, none had any contracture after 1 year, and all had more than 90 degrees of abduction and full opposition.

*Conclusions.*—In patients with electrical and severe thermal burns, early extensive débridement and flap coverage improve results and reduce morbidity compared with serial débridements. The concept of progressive gross tissue necrosis is an outdated one that should not affect surgical principles. Radical débridement of all questionably nonviable tissues is essential, except for intact tendons, nerves, and bone, in which anatomical continuity is more important than apparent viability.

▶ The concept that early excision and skin grafting is the optimal treatment of deep second- and third-degree burns is widely accepted. However, this approach to electrical and very deep thermal burns that involve bony and/or tendinous structures has not been as widely applied. These case reports argue for an equally early and aggressive approach to wound closure in patients with complicated burn injuries. I have come to agree strongly with this approach in the past several years.—E.A. Deitch, M.D.

## Liposome Delivery of Aminoglycosides in Burn Wounds

Price CI, Horton JW, Baxter CR (Univ of Texas, Southwestern Med Ctr, Dallas)
*Surg Gynecol Obstet* 174:414–418, 1992                                                3–8

*Introduction.*—Creams and ointments containing antimicrobial agents are an established part of burn wound management. Disadvantages of this therapy include a short duration of activity, adverse effects from systemic absorption, and the need for frequent cleaning of the burn area to remove carrier residue. The potential advantages of liposomal delivery of antimicrobial agents were evaluated.

*Methods.*—Liposomes, which are artificially constructed lipid membrane-bound spheres, have been used as drug delivery vehicles for many years. Because liposomes are biodegradable, the need to remove drug carrier is reduced. Radiolabeled [125]I-phenyldecanoic acid was used in the formulation of small unilamellar liposomes. Rats subjected to a 10% total body surface area full-thickness burn were treated with topical application of .3 mL of tobramycin entrapped in [125]I-liposomes. The animals were sacrificed at 24, 48, and 72 hours after burn injury and examined for serum and tissue tobramycin levels and tissue concentration of [125]I-liposomes.

*Results.*—Although serum tobramycin concentrations were low at each sampling period, significant levels of the agent were present in the burn tissues. More than 90% of recovered liposomes remained at the site of initial application. The animals' splanchnic organs had no more than 2% of the recovered [125]I-liposomes at any time period.

*Conclusion.*—Tobramycin tissue concentrations at the burn sites and the lack of systemic absorption of the agent confirm the value of liposomes in delivering antimicrobials to burn wound areas. Liposome delivery might allow the use of agents with potential systemic toxicity.

▶ One of the great challenges in burn care has been to control bacterial growth in the burn wound. Since the introduction of silvadene and sulfamylon to control burn wound bacterial growth 20 years ago, little new has emerged in this field. This is not because of a lack of new antimicrobial agents, or because burn wound sepsis no longer occurs, but, instead, to some extent, because of inefficient or ineffectual delivery systems. For example, either the drugs do not penetrate the burn eschar well, or they penetrate too well and reach possibly toxic systemic levels. One potential solution to this problem is the use of liposomes as a delivery system—thus the importance of this experimental study.—E.A. Deitch, M.D.

---

**Interleukin 6—A Potential Mediator of Lethal Sepsis After Major Thermal Trauma: Evidence for Increased IL-6 Production by Peripheral Blood Mononuclear Cells**
Schlüter B, König B, Bergmann U, Müller FE, König W (Ruhr-Universität Bochum, Germany; Universitätsklinik "Bergmannsheil"Bochum)
*J Trauma* 31:1663–1670, 1991                                          3–9

---

*Introduction.*—Sepsis is the main cause of late posttraumatic mortality in severely burned patients. In addition to tumor necrosis factor-$\alpha$(TNF-$\alpha$) and interleukin-1, recent evidence suggests that interleukin-6 (IL-6) may act as a mediator of the acute host response to trauma and infection. Plasma levels of IL-6 were determined in 21 patients with severe burn injuries.

*Observations.*—The patients' injuries involved 24% to 75% of total body surface area. Fourteen patients survived, and 7 died. Survivors, both with and without suspected sepsis, had peak IL-6 levels of 251 pg/mL in the first 3 days after injury. These values returned to the normal range, 26 pg/mL, from day 30 to day 50. In contrast, those who did not survive had permanent elevations, up to 1,921 pg/mL, until they died of sepsis and consecutive multiple organ failure on days 10 to 19 (Fig 3–2). Interleukin-6–specific messenger RNA expressed in the peripheral blood

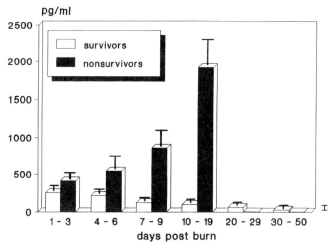

**Fig 3–2.**—Post-traumatic course of IL-6 plasma levels after major thermal trauma. There were 14 survivors and 7 nonsurvivors. The data represent the mean ± SEM of different determinations within the indicated time intervals. (Courtesy of Schlüter B, König B, Bergmann U, et al: *J Trauma* 31:1663–1670, 1991.)

mononuclear cells of patients in vivo and in vitro was high compared with that of healthy donors.

*Conclusions.*—Interleukin-6 may be a mediator of lethal sepsis in patients with severe burn injuries. The kinetics of IL-6 plasma levels in these patients are closely related to their clinical outcome. It remains to be determined whether IL-6, like TNF-α, acts through secondary release of final effector molecules.

▶ The famous Pogo cartoon, saying that "We have met the enemy and he is us" is nowhere more relevant than in a discussion of the biology of injury and inflammation.

Recognition that the clinical manifestations of sepsis, such as fever, leukocytosis, hypermetabolism, and a hyperdynamic circulatory response, are mediated by factors released from our own cells and not by invading microorganisms has been one of the major conceptual advances in the past decade. In this light, the role of cytokines, such as tumor necrosis factor, IL-1, and IL-6, as well as other factors in the pathogenesis of organ injury and burn-induced morbidity and mortality, has become of increasing interest. Because it is potentially possible to therapeutically modulate the cytokine response, studies such as this one, which are directed at elucidating the cytokine response to injury, are of importance. In fact, Zhu et al. (1) have recently implicated elevated levels of IL-6 in the development of impaired cell-mediated immunity and have hypothesized that the increased susceptibility to infection in burn patients may be related to greatly elevated levels of IL-6.—E.A. Deitch, M.D.

*Reference*

1. Zhu D, et al: *Arch Surg* 127:65, 1992.

---

**Circulating Interleukin-1$\beta$ and Tumor Necrosis Factor-$\alpha$ Concentrations After Burn Injury in Humans**
Cannon JG, Friedberg JS, Gelfand JA, Tompkins RG, Burke JF, Dinarello CA
(Tufts Univ, Boston, Mass; Harvard Med School, Boston)
*Crit Care Med* 20:1414–1419, 1992                                    3–10

---

*Objective.*—Burn wounds are an important source of cytokines, including interleukin-1$\beta$ (IL-1$\beta$) and tumor necrosis factor-$\alpha$ (TNF-$\alpha$). Plasma cytokine levels are related to overall illness severity, mortality, and certain clinical parameters, but their prognostic significance is unclear. A prospective study was undertaken to determine whether plasma cytokine levels after burn trauma are related to clinical outcome.

*Methods.*—Thirty-one patients aged 18–94 years had second- or third-degree burns covering 10% to 95% of their body surface area. Plasma IL-1$\beta$ and TNF-$\alpha$ levels were measured at 2 days and 10 days after admission to the burn unit, and the findings were correlated with age, burn size, severity of illness as measured by the Acute Physiology and Chronic Health Evaluation (APACHE II) score, body temperature, white blood cell count, and survival.

*Results.*—The initial APACHE II scores ranged from 1 to 25; the median score was 10. The initial mean plasma IL-1$\beta$ and TNF-$\alpha$ values were increased, and IL-1$\beta$ and TNF-$\alpha$ levels both significantly correlated with body temperature at the time of blood sampling. Also, the mean initial plasma TNF-$\alpha$ concentration was inversely related to the white blood cell count. On day 10, the APACHE II scores ranged from 3 to 24, and the median score was 9. Although plasma cytokine levels fluctuated considerably throughout the course of hospitalization, the transient increases in these levels did not correlate with any clinical signs or with overall illness severity as determined by the APACHE II scores. Seven patients died, but their plasma cytokine levels did not differ significantly from those in survivors matched for age and burn size. Patients who died, however, had significantly lower final IL-1$\beta$ levels than did survivors measured at the same time after admission to the burn unit.

*Conclusions.*—Plasma cytokine values in burn patients correspond with certain host responses early in the course of disease, but the correlations disappear as the illness progresses. Circulating IL-1$\beta$ and TNF-$\alpha$ levels are poor prognostic indicators of clinical outcome. The low plasma IL-1$\beta$ values found in patients who died, however, suggest that IL-1$\beta$ is an essential mediator of host defenses.

▶ The results of this study highlight how confusing the interpretation of plasma cytokine levels can be. Yet, the authors' observation that the later development of low rather than elevated circulating IL-1$\beta$ levels correlated with increased mortality is of more than academic interest. First of all, this observation is consistent with increasing evidence that cytokines at modestly to moderately elevated levels exert beneficial effects on wound healing, intermediary metabolism, and the response to infection, and it is only when the cytokine response becomes excessive that deleterious effects predominate. Additionally, the concept that elevated IL-1$\beta$ levels may be necessary for normal antibacterial host defenses is consistent with experimental studies described in Abstract 3–11.—E.A. Deitch, M.D.

---

## Modulation of Macrophage Hyperactivity Improves Survival in a Burn-Sepsis Model

O'Riordain MG, Collins KH, Pilz M, Saporoschetz IB, Mannick JA, Rodrick ML (Brigham and Women's Hosp–Harvard Med School, Boston, Mass)
*Arch Surg* 127:152–158, 1992                    3–11

*Background.*—Thermal injury increases macrophage activity, which leads to increased serum cytokine levels. Cytokine overproduction has been implicated as a major cause of morbidity and mortality in previously healthy persons with acute sepsis. The effects of sustained cytokine overproduction in disease, however, have not been well studied, and interventions to normalize cytokine levels after major injury have not been attempted previously. The effects of normalizing cytokine overproduction on survival in a murine-sepsis burn model were studied.

*Methods.*—Burned mice were randomly allocated to receive intraperitoneal injection with recombinant human interleukin-1$\beta$ (rhIL-1$\beta$) alone, indomethacin sodium alone, or rhIL-1$\beta$ plus indomethacin sodium, given for 6 days after injury. On day 10, burned mice underwent cecal ligation and puncture and were monitored for the development of sepsis and survival. Interleukin-1 (IL-1), interleukin-6 (IL-6), and tumor necrosis factor-$\alpha$ (TNF-$\alpha$) production were measured at baseline and 10 days after the burn injury.

*Results.*—Ten days after the burn injury, the untreated controls had significantly increased IL-1, IL-6, and TNF-$\alpha$ serum levels compared with baseline values, whereas burned mice treated with a combination of rhIL-1$\beta$ and indomethacin had normal cytokine values. Survival after cecal ligation and puncture was 22% in untreated controls, 52% in mice treated with rhIL-1$\beta$ plus indomethacin, 31% in mice treated with rhIL-1$\beta$ alone, and 27% in mice treated with indomethacin alone.

*Conclusions.*—Controlling macrophage hyperactivity with a combination of rhIL-1β plus indomethacin improves survival from subsequent sepsis in burned mice. This therapeutic approach may have clinical application in burn patients.

▶ The results of this experimental study, taken together with those reported in Abstract 3-10, illustrate that the cytokine response can be beneficial. Studies of this type serve to highlight the complexity of the host's response to injury and infection. They also serve to warn against therapeutic strategies directed at globally shutting off the cytokine response. It is wise to remember that Mother Nature may be a pain, but she is not a fool.—E.A. Deitch, M.D.

---

**Oxygen Consumption Early Postburn Becomes Oxygen Delivery Dependent With the Addition of Smoke Inhalation Injury**
Demling RH, Knox J, Youn Y-K, LaLonde C (Longwood Area Trauma Ctr, Boston, Mass)
*J Trauma* 32:593–599, 1992                    3–12

*Introduction.*—When inhalational injury is combined with burn injury, oxygen consumption becomes dependent on oxygen delivery. This might help to explain the greater deficit in systemic oxygenation and more marked instability that characterize combined injury, as well as the increased risk of lung and other organ failure.

*Objective and Methods.*—Relationships among oxygen delivery and oxygen consumption were examined in yearling sheep subjected to moderate smoke inhalation injury and a third-degree, 15% body surface, burn injury. The study began 3 hours after injury, when carboxyhemoglobin levels had returned to baseline. In control animals, oxygen delivery was reduced by 25% by removing blood and in burned animals by decreasing the rate of fluid infusion. Lung oxidant production was assessed by estimating tissue levels of malondialdehyde.

*Observations.*—In controls and animals with a burn alone, a 25% decrease in oxygen delivery was compensated for by an increase in oxygen extraction, maintaining oxygen consumption constant. Thus oxygen consumption was independent of oxygen delivery. After combined surface burn and inhalation injury, however, oxygen consumption decreased in proportion to oxygen delivery with a correlation coefficient of .9, indicating delivery-dependent oxygen consumption. Lung lipid peroxidation was markedly increased in this setting.

*Conclusion.*—Oxygen consumption becomes pathologically dependent on oxygen delivery with the combination of burn and inhalation injury. This process increases the potential for tissue hypoxemia and organ injury and is associated with evidence of increased lung tissue oxidant production.

▶ The rationale for this study is the clinical observation that the combination of a surface burn and a lung injury from smoke inhalation produces a marked increase in morbidity and mortality compared to either injury alone. The results of this study documenting that oxygen consumption post burn becomes oxygen-delivery dependent with the addition of smoke inhalation injury helps to explain why these individuals require volumes of fluid resuscitation that are 30% to 50% greater than those required for a similarly sized burn in the absence of inhalation injury. The clinical importance of this study is that it upholds the concept of providing as much fluid and inotropic therapy as it takes to maintain an adequately high level of oxygen delivery to fully support oxygen consumption.—E.A. Deitch, M.D.

---

**Relationship Between Hepatic Blood Flow and Tissue Lipid Peroxidation in the Early Postburn Period**
LaLonde C, Knox J, Youn Y-K, Demling R (Longwood Area Trauma Ctr, Boston, Mass)
*Crit Care Med* 20:789–796, 1992                                      3–13

---

*Objective.*—Burn injury is followed by increased inflammation in distant organs and increased oxidant-induced lipid peroxidation, particularly in the liver—even if shock is absent. The effects of burn injury on hepatic blood flow were examined in anesthetized sheep with a 40% body surface third-degree burn.

*Methods.*—After burn injury, the animals were resuscitated with fluid to restore ventricular filling pressure and cardiac output to baseline levels. The animals were resuscitated for 6 hours with Ringer's lactate alone, Ringer's solution plus 5% hydroxyethyl starch, or Ringer's solution and starch to which was complexed deferoxamine to prevent oxidant release. Hepatic blood flow was estimated by the galactose infusion method and lipid peroxidation in the liver determined by its malondialdehyde content.

*Results.*—Hepatic blood flow was reduced by half within 4–5 hours after burn injury despite resuscitation with Ringer's lactate. Tissue malondialdehyde content increased in these animals. Resuscitation with hydroxyethyl starch restored effective hepatic blood flow to control levels, but the malondialdehyde content remained increased. Lipid peroxidation did not occur when deferoxamine was given, and liver blood flow was 80% above control values.

*Discussion.*—Apparently, optimal resuscitation does not prevent a marked fall in effective hepatic blood flow shortly after burn injury. Increased lipid peroxidation also is evident. Use of an iron chelator increases liver blood flow and prevents lipid peroxidation in the liver.

▶ The goal of fluid resuscitation is to restore blood flow to the peripheral tissues as well as to maintain central hemodynamic stability. Recent studies, such as this one, indicate that our current fluid resuscitation regimens fail to adequately restore organ microvascular blood flow, even though they prevent hypotension, and therefore may not be optimally effective in preventing burn-induced organ injury.

The use of agents such as deferoxamine to prevent oxidant-mediated tissue injury and maintain microvascular blood flow during the resuscitative phase of burn injury is conceptually attractive. However, the benefits of this approach must await clinical trials.—E.A. Deitch, M.D.

---

**Inhibition of Leukocyte-Endothelial Adherence Following Thermal Injury**

Mileski W, Borgstrom D, Lightfoot E, Rothlein R, Faanes R, Lipsky P, Baxter C (Univ of Texas, Southwestern Med School, Dallas; Boehringer Ingelheim Pharmaceuticals Inc, Ridgefield, Conn)
*J Surg Res* 52:334–339, 1992                                                     3–14

*Background.*—Progressive microvascular injury in the marginal zone of stasis surrounding cutaneous burns can result in extension of tissue loss. Leukocytes, particularly polymorphonuclear neutrophils (PMNs), are central mediators of microvascular injury that depend, in part, on PMN adherence to the vascular endothelial cell surface. It is hypothesized that inhibition of PMN-endothelial adherence by using monoclonal antibodies directed to the leukocyte CD18 adhesion complex or its endothelial ligand, intercellular adhesion molecule-1 (ICAM-1, CD54), may reduce

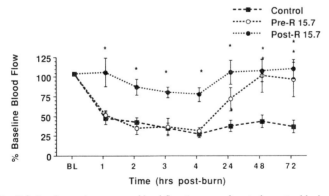

**Fig 3–3.**—Relative changes in cutaneous blood flow in zones of stasis determined by laser Doppler blood flow meter are presented as percentage of baseline values (mean ±standard error of mean) for controls (number = 12), animals given monoclonal antibody R 15.7 prior to burn injury (pre-R, number = 5) and animals given R 15.7 at 30 minutes after burn injury (post-R 15.7, number = 6. *P <.05. (Courtesy of Mileski W, Borgstrom D, Lightfoot E, et al: *J Surg Res* 52:334–339, 1992.)

the microvascular injury in the marginal zone of stasis after thermal injury.

*Methods.*—A model of thermal injury was developed with the use of New Zealand White rabbits. Two sets of 3 full-thickness burns separated by 2 zones 5 × 30 mm in size were produced on the backs of the animals. Cutaneous blood flow was measured at the burned skin sites, marginal zones, and shaved unburned skin for 72 hours in control animals, in animals given monoclonal antibody to the PMN CD18 complex R 15.7 before or after burn injury, and in animals given the anti-ICAM-1 antibody R 6.5 before or after burn injury.

*Findings.*—Cutaneous blood flow in the marginal zone of stasis between burn contact sites was significantly increased in the antibody-treated animals during the 72-hour observation period. In contrast, reductions in blood flow in the initial postburn injury persisted throughout the observation period in control animals. At 72 hours after burn all antibody-treated animals had blood flow in the zone of stasis at or above baseline levels, whereas control animals had levels equal to 34.7% of baseline (Fig 3–3). Post burn administration of antibodies was as effective as, if not better than, preburn administration in preserving blood flow. Visual evidence of burn extension in the marginal zones of stasis was evident in 41% of zones in control animals, compared with 5% to 20% of zones in the antibody-treated animals.

*Conclusion.*—Inhibition of PMN adherence improves microvascular perfusion in the marginal zone of stasis after thermal injury and also prevents extension/-progression of the size of the burn. It appears that PMNs may play a role in the pathogenesis of microvascular injury after thermal injury.

▶ This important study illustrates the major potential clinical benefit of studies directed at the basic biology of inflammation. Knowledge derived from these basic science studies documenting the role of neutrophil-endothelial interactions in the evolution of microvascular and tissue injury are now being translated to the clinical arena. Studies, such as this one, illustrating the potential of molecular and cellular biology-based therapy to modify the natural history of burn wound injury are exciting and document the feasibility of pharmacologically modulating burn depth. Progress is our most important product.—E.A. Deitch, M.D.

---

**Peripheral Lymphocyte Membrane Fluidity After Thermal Injury**
Tolentino MV, Sarasua MM, Hill OA, Wentworth DB, Franceschi D, Fratianne RB (MetroHealth Med Ctr, Cleveland, Ohio; Case Western Reserve Univ, Cleveland)
*J Burn Care Rehabil* 12:498–504, 1991                                      3–15

*Objective.*—Thermal injury induces a host of immunologic and hormonal alterations, including an increase in serum cortisol levels. Previous studies have demonstrated altered lymphocyte function in burn patients that renders them more susceptible to infection. An examination was made of the in vitro changes in lymphocyte membrane fluidity that result from cortisol exposure and these changes correlated with those observed in patients with thermal injury.

*Methods.*—Blood samples were obtained within 6 hours of thermal injury from 36 patients with burn injuries aged 16–81 years and from 9 healthy controls aged 24–53 years. Peripheral blood lymphocytes (PBLs) were extracted by standard techniques and lymphocyte membrane fluidity was measured by spectofluorometry. In additional studies, the effects of acute and long-term cortisol exposure on lymphocyte membrane fluidity of normal human PBLs were measured and correlated with the result observed in the thermally injured patients.

*Results.*—Peripheral blood lymphocyte membrane fluidity in patients with burns covering less than 30% of total body surface area (TBSA) did not differ significantly from that in normal controls, whereas PBL membrane fluidity in patients with more extensive burns was significantly increased when compared with that in normal controls. The changes in membrane fluidity observed in these burn patients were similar to those observed in control PBLs incubated in cortisol.

*Conclusions.*—Major thermal injury covering more than 30% of the TBSA causes alterations in PBL membrane fluidity that may result from exposure to increased cortisol concentrations.

▶ This article was chosen because I was intrigued by the concept that burn-induced alterations in cell membrane fluidity could provide a unifying hypothesis to explain the etiology of altered lymphocyte function observed in patients with major thermal injuries. Although undoubtedly there are signals other than cortisol (e.g., cytokines, oxidants, complement products) that can lead to altered membrane fluidity, once fluidity becomes abnormal, problems are likely to occur, because many, if not all, physiologic cellular activities are initiated at the level of the membrane. This article also illustrates the increasingly recognized fact that the immune and endocrine systems talk to and modulate each other. Thus it is to be expected as we begin to modulate the metabolic response that we will see changes (not all beneficial) in the immune as well as in other systems.—E.A. Deitch, M.D.

---

**Selective Intestinal Decontamination for Prevention of Wound Colonization in Severely Burned Patients: A Retrospective Analysis**
Manson WL, Klasen HJ, Sauer EW, Olieman A (Lab for Public Health, Groningen, The Netherlands; Roman Catholic Hosp, Groningen)
*Burns* 18:98–102, 1992                                3–16

*Background.*—Infection is a common complication of thermal injury. Despite protective measures, burns become colonized with both gram-positive and aerobic gram-negative organisms, including enteric bacteria. Despite the presence of enteric microorganisms at the burn site, little attention has been directed to the gastrointestinal tract as a resevoir of colonizing bacteria in the burn patient. Selective intestinal decontamination (SDD) is a well-established method of removing potentially pathogenic microorganisms from the digestive tract in immunocompromised patients. The effect of SDD on wound colonization in burn patients was investigated in a 10-year study.

*Methods.*—The series included 91 patients with at least 25% of their total body surface covered by burns. They received polymyxin orally; 63 patients also received cotrimoxazole and amphotericin B.

*Results.*—Cotrimoxazole decreased the incidence of Enterobacteriaceae wound colonization from 71% to 11% and eliminated colonization with *Proteus*. Amphotericin B decreased the incidence of yeast wound colonization from 39% to 10%. There was a close relationship between burn wound colonization and gastrointestinal tract colonization. No resistant bacterial strains were detected.

*Conclusions.*—Selective intestinal decontamination appears to be an effective method for preventing wound colonization by gastrointestinal microorganisms.

---

**Prevention of Infection in Burns: Preliminary Experience With Selective Decontamination of the Digestive Tract in Patients With Extensive Injuries**

Mackie DP, van Hertum WAJ, Schumburg T, Kuijper EC, Knape P (Red Cross Hosp, Beverwijk, The Netherlands)
*J Trauma* 32:570–575, 1992                    3–17

---

*Background.*—Selective decontamination of the digestive tract (SDD) may be helpful in preventing infection in burn-injured patients. It has been used routinely at the study institution since 1988 in patients with burns over more than 30% of the body surface and in those with inhalation injury.

*Protocol.*—Adult patients received 80 mg of tobramycin, 100 mg of polymyxin E, and 500 mg of amphotericin B orally 4 times daily, either in capsule form or as a suspension flushed into the nasogastric tube. Ventilated patients receive the antibiotics in the form of a 2% paste applied to the buccal cavity 4 times daily. Patients also receive 1 g of cefotaxime 4 times daily parenterally for 4 days.

*Results.*—Results in 31 patients with more than 30% body surface burns treated with SDD were compared to those in 33 patients treated earlier who were managed conventionally. Fewer of the SDD-treated patients had their wounds colonized by *Pseudomonas* or Enterobacteria-

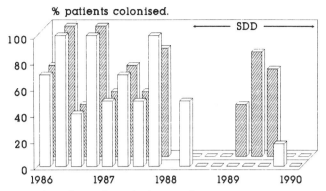

**Fig 3–4.**—Quarterly incidences of wound colonization by gram-negative microorganisms. The *open bars* represent enteric bacteria; the *filled bars* represent *Pseudomonas aeruginosa*. (Courtesy of Mackie DP, van Hertum WAJ, Schumburg T, et al: *J Trauma* 32:570–575, 1992.)

ceae (Fig 3–4). Gram-negative organisms were also less frequent in both urine and gastric aspirates. Respiratory infection occurred in 6.5% of SDD-treated patients and in 27% of control patients. Only 1 patient treated by SDD became septicemic, compared to 8 control patients. There was 1 death in the SDD-treated group; 7 control patients died.

*Conclusion.*—Selective decontamination may be advantageous in the management of patients with severe burn injuries. Use of a regimen that prevents colonization by gram-negative organisms is recommended.

▶ Where do the bugs come from? The answer in some patients appears to be the gut. The concept that, under certain clinically relevant circumstances, bacteria can escape from the gut and spread systemically has been firmly established experimentally, and this phenomenon has been termed "bacterial translocation."

Based on the recognition that the gut can be a reservoir for systemic infections, significant attention has focused on ways to prevent gut-origin sepsis. Selective gut decontamination (SDD) is one approach that has resulted from these studies.

The concept of SDD, which has evolved in the past 20 years, is based on several fundamental observations: First, most bacterial infections in the critically ill patient are caused by the patient's own microflora, and colonization and infection of the lower airways, bladder, skin, and blood are almost always preceded by oropharyngeal and gastrointestinal colonization by the infecting bacteria. Second, the ability of the host to be colonized by these potential pathogenic organisms is increased when the normal bacteria inhabiting the various body areas are eradicated (e.g., by broad-spectrum antibiotics), or when normal host antibacterial defenses are impaired (e.g., by neutralization of gastric acid by antacids).

The preceding 2 studies (Abstracts 3–16 and 3–17), although compared against previously treated patients, indicate that by controlling bacterial growth within the intestinal tract, the incidence and rate of burn wound colonization can be reduced significantly. As such, these studies support the concepts of SDD and bacterial translocation.—E.A. Deitch, M.D.

---

**Decreased Pulmonary Barotrauma With the Use of Volumetric Diffusive Respiration in Pediatric Patients With Burns**
Rodeberg DA, Maschinot NE, Housinger TA, Warden GD (Shriners Burns Inst, Cincinnati, Ohio)
*J Burn Care Rehabil* 13:506–511, 1992                                    3–18

---

*Purpose.*—In children undergoing mechanical ventilation, pulmonary barotrauma is a common and life-threatening complication. Adequate gas exchange can be achieved at lower airway pressures by means of the volumetric diffusive respiration ventilator, which uses a high-frequency progressive accumulation of subtidal volume breaths in a pressure-limited format with a percussive waveform. This might effectively decrease the incidence of pulmonary barotrauma occurring with conventional mechanical ventilation. The incidence of barotrauma was compared in children with burn injuries who received volumetric diffusive respiration or conventional ventilation.

*Methods.*—The analysis included 39 patients younger than 2 years admitted to a burns institute. Twenty-four patients received only conventional ventilation and 15 received only volumetric diffusive respiration. The 2 groups were compared for the incidence of barotrauma, which was defined as pneumothorax, pneumomediastinum, pneumopericardium, or pneumoperitoneum.

*Results.*—The 2 groups were not significantly different with regard to percent of total body surface burned, 46% vs. 55%; proportions with inhalation injury, 40% vs. 60%; or days of mechanical ventilation required,

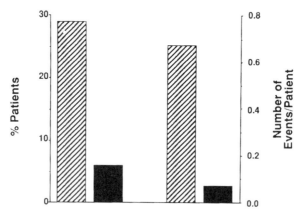

**Fig 3–5.**—Percent of patriots who experienced PB and incidence of PB events per patient. (Courtesy of Rodeberg DA, Maschinot NE, Housinger TA, et al: *J Burn Care Rehabil* 13:506–511, 1992.)

18 vs. 22. The incidence of barotrauma was 29% in the group receiving conventional ventilation and 6% in the group treated with volumetric diffusive respiration. Patients receiving conventional ventilation experienced 16 incidents of barotrauma, compared with only 2 in the group given volumetric diffusive respiration (Fig 3-5). Compared to the patients given conventional ventilation, the patients treated with volumetric diffusive respiration had significant reductions in peak inspiratory pressure, 60 cm $H_2O$ vs. 32 cm $H_2O$; mandatory respiratory rate, 33 breaths per minute vs. 11 breaths per minute; and fraction of inspired oxygen, .72 vs. .53.

*Conclusions.*—The use of volumetric diffusive respiration in burn patients younger than 2 years of age can decrease the incidence of barotrauma compared with conventional ventilation. This is a result of reductions in peak inspiratory pressure, mandatory respiratory rate, and fraction of inspired oxygen. The pressure-limited volumetric diffusive respiration ventilator operates in a mode similar to that of intermittent mandatory ventilation, which allows spontaneous breathing without asynchrony.

▶ The complications associated with high levels of postive end-exatory pressure and high $FIO_2$ (oxygen toxicity) are well recognized, and the pros and cons of their use have been debated for years. More recently, it has become increasingly recognized that high levels of peak inspiratory pressure (PIP) may result in significant barotrauma. For this reason, several strategies have been used to keep PIP levels less than 40–50 cm $H_2O$. One such encouraging option is described in this report. Others include variations of jet ventilation and, most recently, pressure-controlled inverse ventilation. Thus technical improvements in ventilator design have resulted in increased physiologic flexibility and given us the option of controlling more and more variables.

Based on my personal experience with some of these newer modes of ventilatory support, especially pressure-controlled inverse ventilation, I believe that we are now salvaging patients who would otherwise have died. Thus I believe it is worth the effort to learn the increasing complex options in ventilatory management techniques so that we can more exactly match the ventilator technique to the patient's physiologic state.—E.A. Deitch, M.D.

### Incidence of HIV Seroconversion in Paediatric Burn Patients

Rutan RL, Bjarnason DL, Desai MH, Herndon DN (Shriners Burns Inst, Galveston, Tex; Univ of Texas Med Branch, Galveston)
*Burns* 18:216–219, 1992                                       3–19

*Introduction.*—Reports of HIV infection first appeared in the United States in 1980, 5 years before a reliable test for HIV contamination of the blood supply was available.

*Methods.*—Medical records were reviewed to assess blood and blood product use between 1978 and May 1985. Patient data were grouped for the risk of HIV infection. Patients treated during the acute postburn period became part of a longitudinal follow-up study and were informed of the HIV testing in which an enzyme-linked immunosorbent assay (ELISA) was used, and the reason for the study.

*Results.*—Of the 1,524 pediatric burn patients, 582 received at least 1 unit of blood products and survived the burn injury. Among these, the risk of HIV infection was low in 42%, moderate in 35%, and high in 23%. Seropositivity for HIV was found in 214 patients (37%). In 5 patients, the ELISA yielded a positive result, which was confirmed by Western blot testing in 4. These 4 patients, aged 3–15 years, had been exposed to an average of 133 donors. Of the HIV-positive patients, 1 had active symptoms and was receiving zidovudine treatment, 1 died of AIDS-related sepsis, 1 was classed P-2, and 1 was asymptomatic.

*Conclusion.*—In this study, the incidence of HIV seroconversion was 1.9%. Other patient populations with a higher HIV positive rating included those individuals under treatment for chronic conditions such as renal failure or leukemia.

▶ The importance of this study is self-evident and suggests that burn patients receiving multiple transfusions should be screened for HIV seroconversion.—E.A. Deitch, M.D.

---

**Predictors of Posttraumatic Stress Disorder After Burn Injury**
Perry S, Difede J, Musngi G, Frances AJ, Jacobsberg L (Cornell Univ, New York City; Columbia Univ, New York City)
*Am J Psychiatry* 149:931–935, 1992                                    3–20

---

*Introduction.*—The scarcity of prospective data on posttraumatic stress disorder (PTSD) is one reason for the inconsistency in diagnostic criteria for this condition. To explore the subjective and objective predictors of PTSD, a representative sample of burn patients was followed to assess its development.

*Methods.*—Evaluations were made in adult patients hospitalized in a burn unit within 1 week of the injury. Assessment included both objective predictors (e.g., percentage of area burned and facial disfigurement) and subjective predictors, including emotional distress and perceived social support. Patients were followed for up to 1 year and assessed again for the development of PTSD. Fifty-one patients were available for follow-up at 2 months, 40 patients at 6 months, and 31 patients at 1 year.

*Results.*—Criteria for PTSD were met by 35% of the patients at 2 months, 40% at 6 months, and 45% at 1 year. Less perceived social support was a predictor of PTSD at all 3 follow-up assessments, but more severe injury was not. In fact, acute PTSD was more likely in patients with smaller burns. The severity of emotional distress and intrusive and avoidant thoughts were all significantly associated with concurrent PTSD.

*Conclusions.*—This prospective study suggests that subjective factors should be considered in assessing the severity of the stressor in PTSD, whereas the *DSM-III-R* diagnosis relies on an objective evaluation. The condition appears to occur in at least one third of burn patients in the year after injury, and they may not seek treatment for the emotional impact of their injuries. It is difficult to predict PTSD while the patient is in the acute stage after trauma and its treatment.

▶ As anyone who has treated any number of burn patients knows, the emotional response to a burn injury can be both severe and unpredictable. In many patients it is the psychological rather than the physiologic consequences of their burns that limit their ability to return to work and adjust to society. Although recognized in the abstract, little objective information is available on the incidence or natural history of this major problem. Consequently, studies directed at identifying patients at increased risk of having emotional difficulties after thermal injury are important. Thus the value of this study and another recent study (1) on postburn psychological problems is that they begin to quantitate the problem and clearly document that the risk of emotional problems developing after burn injury is not simply related to the size of the burn.—E.A. Deitch, M.D.

*Reference*

1. Williams EE, et al: *Burns* 17:478, 1991.

# 4 Trauma

## Introduction

Few would disagree that optimal care of the trauma patient is based on the combination of good clinical judgment, technical expertise, and an in-depth understanding of the host's response to injury. However, the best clinical approach to certain injuries remains controversial. One such controversy concerns the optimal operative management approach to venous injuries of the pelvis and lower extremities. Consequently, two sound clinical papers taking opposite opinions on the subject were selected; taken together, they provide a rational basis for the operative management of a wide spectrum of patients with venous injuries. Another area of emerging controversy is the potential role of diagnostic laparoscopy in patients with abdominal trauma. In some clinical scenarios, diagnostic laparoscopy is likely to be helpful, such as in determining whether or not peritoneal penetration has occurred. However, in other circumstances, such as in patients with small bowel injuries, its accuracy is poor. Consequently, only as further data are generated, clearly defining the strengths and weaknesses of this technique, will it be possible to know when diagnostic laparoscopy should be encouraged and when it should be avoided.

Inability to close the abdomen because of massive visceral edema is one of the most frustrating ways to end a stressful operation. Using all of one's talents and tricks to achieve an excessively tight closure clearly is emotionally unappealing to the surgeon. But, more importantly, all of this work does not benefit the patient, because the resultant increased intra-abdominal pressure has deleterious effects on pulmonary function and abdominal visceral blood flow. A second frustrating problem is what to do in the massively injured patient who becomes hypothermic, and acidotic, and has coagulopathy. Two articles are reviewed; one dealing with alternative approaches to abdominal wound closure (Abstract 4-4), and a second that addresses the role of an initial abbreviated laparotomy followed by a planned reoperation in selected critically injured patients (Abstract 4-6). Two other technical tricks in care of the injured have been included. One report describes the use of angiographically placed balloon catheters to control arterial hemorrhage (Abstract 4-7), and the second illustrates how tissue expanders can be used in secondary reconstruction of the abdominal wall (Abstract 4-8).

Increased appreciation of the substantial risks associated with nonautologous blood transfusion is clearly altering our clinical management practice patterns. For example, autotransfusion is being used more often, the hemoglobin threshold for transfusion is being reduced, and the risk-benefit ratio of nonoperative versus operative management of isolated splenic injuries is being evaluated. On the other hand, recognition that up to 24% of patients seen in the emergency rooms of inner city hospitals have evidence of hepatitis B, hepatitis C, or HIV-1 infections highlights the need for universal precautions (Abstract 4–11).

Other areas of interest that continue to receive attention include the optimal use of antibiotics, the beneficial effects of enteral versus parenteral nutrition, immunomodulator therapy, and the use of hypertonic saline in the resuscitation of patients with shock or head injuries.

Algorithims for the management of trauma victims continue to be developed to aid in optimizing rapid decision making with the hope that this approach will improve survival. The results of one such study documented that deviations from established protocols was associated with decreased survival in patients with blunt and penetrating thoracic and abdominal injuries (Abstract 4–17). A similar study was reported indicating that optimization of resuscitation can improve survival even in an established trauma center (Abstract 4–18). Quality assessment programs in trauma continue to occupy the attention of both trauma centers and the federal government. One widely proposed method for assessing both quality of care and cost control is utilization of professional review organizations (PRO). The inherently flawed nature of PRO programs as a means of quantifying quality of care and identifying preventable trauma care was the focus of one recent study (Abstract 4–19). This important study clearly illustrates the weakness of post-hoc peer review systems, as well as their potential sociologic dangers. A more rational approach to assessment of quality of care is presented in a prospective study directed at evaluation of provider-related as opposed to disease-related morbidity (Abstract 4–20).

Edwin A. Deitch, M.D.

---

**Long-Term Results of Venous Reconstruction After Vascular Trauma in Civilian Practice**
Nypaver TJ, Schuler JJ, McDonnell P, Ellenby MI, Montalvo J, Baraniewski H, Piano G (Univ of Illinois, College of Medicine, Chicago)
*J Vasc Surg* 16:762–768, 1992                                    4–1

---

*Objective.*—Many major trauma centers have adopted a more aggressive approach to the treatment of venous injuries, emphasizing repair rather than ligation. Some aspects of venous reconstruction remain controversial, however, and issues of patency and clinical outcome after vascular trauma remain to be documented. A long-term follow-up study was undertaken to define the physiologic results and patency of venous repair of the extremities.

Comparison of Early vs. Late Patency by Type of Repair

| Type of repair | Early patency (venography) | | | | Late patency (CFDS) | | | |
|---|---|---|---|---|---|---|---|---|
| | Patent (no.) | Occluded (no.) | Total | Patent (%) | Patent (no.) | Occluded (no.) | Total | Patent (%) |
| Lateral suture | 3 | 4 | 7 | 43 | 6 | 1 | 7 | 86 |
| Vein patch repair | 2 | 2 | 4 | 50 | 4 | 0 | 4 | 100 |
| End-to-end repair | 2 | 0 | 2 | 100 | 2 | 0 | 2 | 100 |
| Interposition vein graft | 1 | 3 | 4 | 25 | 4 | 0 | 4 | 100 |
| Total | 8 | 9 | 17 | 47 | 16 | 1 | 17 | 94 |

(Courtesy of Nypaver TJ, Schuler JJ. McDonnell P, et al: *J Vasc Surg* 16:762–768, 1992.)

*Patients.*—The study sample comprised 32 patients who underwent venous reconstruction after a vascular injury to the upper or lower extremity and were available for long-term follow-up. All but 1 were male, and the mean age was 29 years. Most injuries (81%) were in the lower extremity, and 88% resulted from gunshot or laceration/stab wound. More than half of the injuries (56%) were managed by lateral venorrhaphy, 22% by interposition grafting, 12.5% by patch repair, and 9.5% by end-to-end repair. The mean follow-up was 49 months and included noninvasive venous evaluation consisting of Doppler ultrasonography, impedance plethysmography, photoplethysmography, and color-flow duplex scanning (CFDS).

*Results.*—Of 17 patients who underwent postoperative venography, 8 had documentation of patency and 9 of thrombosis. At follow-up there were only 2 instances of significant clinical edema. Venous refilling time, assessed by photoplethysmography, was 35 seconds in the injured extremity and 37 seconds on the uninjured side. Almost all of the venous reconstructions (90%) were patent on standard color-flow ultronic duplex scanning (CFDS). All 8 repairs that appeared patent on venography remained patent, and 8 of 9 of those with early thrombosis were patent on CFDS (table).

*Conclusions.*—Reconstruction of venous injuries to the extremities appears to give good long-term results. Morbidity is minimal, long-term patency is good, and venous competence is maintained. The natural history of these repairs appears to consist of local thrombus absorption and recanalization.

## Venous Injuries of the Lower Extremities and Pelvis: Repair Versus Ligation

Yelon JA, Scalea TM (Kings County Hosp Ctr, Brooklyn, NY; State Univ of New York, Brooklyn)
*J Trauma* 33:532–538, 1992     4–2

| | Outcomes | | | |
| --- | --- | --- | --- | --- |
| | Ligation (n = 44) | | Repair (n = 30) | |
| Edema | Hospital Day 4 | Discharge | Hospital Day 4 | Discharge |
| 0 | 31 | 38 | 24 | 24 |
| Trace | 0 | 0 | 1 | 1 |
| + | 8 | 6 | 3 | 3 |
| ++ | 5 | 0 | 1 | 1 |
| +++ | 0 | 0 | 1 | 1 |
| Vascular complications | | | | |
|   Arterial thrombosis | 1 | | 2 | |
|   Deep venous thrombosis | 0 | | 1 | |
|   Pulmonary embolus | 0 | | 1 | |
|   Amputation | 1 | | 1 | |

(Courtesy of Yelon JA and Scalea TM: *J Trauma* 33:532–538, 1992.)

*Introduction.*—Disagreement remains as to the best management of venous injuries in the pelvis and lower extremities. Some surgeons recommend venous repair whenever possible; others suggest that venous ligation may not be as dangerous as previously thought. The policy of using ligation for venous injuries was evaluated.

*Patients and Methods.*—Seventy-nine venous injuries in the lower extremity or pelvis were treated in 74 patients seen in a 4.5-year period. All but 6 patients were men (mean age, 29 years). Sixty-one had gunshot wounds, 11 had been stabbed, 1 had a shotgun wound, and 1 had sustained blunt trauma. Treatment was by ligation in 48 injuries and repair in 31. Surgical techniques in the latter group included 16 venorrhaphies, 8 end-to-end repairs, 5 vein patches, and 2 interposition grafts. The 2 groups were not significantly different in age, mechanism and location of injury, severity and number of associated injuries, and incidence of arterial injury.

*Outcomes.*—The 2 groups had identical rates of postoperative morbidity. About one fourth of each group required fasciotomy. At discharge, 86% of patients treated by ligation were completely free of edema, and the rest had only mild edema that did not interfere with their daily activities (table).

*Conclusions.*—This experience demonstrates the safety of venous ligation as an alternative to repair in patients with venous injuries to the pelvis or lower extremity. Ligation is not associated with an increase in postoperative morbidity, need for fasciotomy, or leg edema. The risks of a problem resulting from venous ligation must be balanced against those of increased operative time and further blood and heat loss.

▶ Venous injuries: When do you ligate? When do you repair? Is there a difference? As illustrated by these 2 articles (Abstracts 4–1 and 4–2), these are some of the questions that continue to be debated.

In spite of the controversy, there are some points that I think are clear. First, lateral venorrhaphy for simple well-localized injuries is clearly indicated in essentially all patients. Second, in hemodynamically unstable patients with other life-threatening injuries, the routine use of complex and time-consuming venous reconstructive procedures seems ill advised. Third, venous repair should be attempted whenever possible in patients with combined arterial and venous injuries. This approach to combined injuries is based primarily, but not exclusively, on the military experience emphasizing the importance of venous reconstruction in optimizing lower limb salvage in patients with combined arterial and venous injuries. Nonetheless, before undertaking venous repair rather than ligation, the caveat "Life before limb" should always be kept in mind.—E.A. Deitch, M.D.

---

**Laparoscopy in the Evaluation of the Intrathoracic Abdomen After Penetrating Injury**
Ivatury RR, Simon RJ, Weksler B, Bayard V, Stahl WM (New York Med College, Bronx)
*J Trauma* 33:101–109, 1992                                                          4–3

---

*Background.*—It is difficult to evaluate the intrathoracic abdomen, especially the diaphragm, after penetrating trauma. The use of laparoscopy in assessment of stable patients with thoracoabdominal penetrating trauma was evaluated.

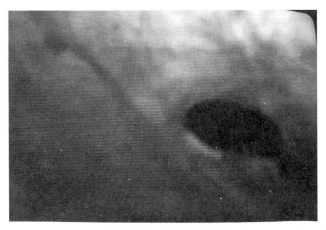

Fig 4–1.—Laparoscopic view of a diaphragmatic laceration. The diaphragmatic surface of the spleen can be seen in the **lower part.** (Courtesy of Ivatury RR, Simon RJ, Weksler B, et al: *J Trauma* 33:101–109, 1992.)

*Methods and Results.*—Forty stable patients (34 stab wounds, 6 gunshot injuries) with upper abdominal or lower thoracic injuries were evaluated by laparoscopy. In 20 of these patients, laparoscopy documented that the abdominal cavity was not penetrated. Of the remaining 20 patients with penetrating wounds to the lower chest and upper abdomen, 8 clinically unsuspected diaphragmatic lacerations were detected in 7 patients. Six of those were directly visualized by laparoscopy (Fig 4–1). All 20 patients who had evidence of a hemoperitoneum detected laparoscopically were explored surgically, and in 10, laparotomy was therapeutic.

*Conclusions.*—After preliminary evaluation, laparoscopy appears to be an excellent method for the detection of isolated injuries to the intrathoracic region and especially the diaphragm.

▶ The authors conclusion that laparoscopy is likely to be a valuable technique for identifying clinically occult diaphragmatic injuries appears valid. However, the overall accuracy of laparoscopy as a diagnostic test in patients with abdominal trauma is far from established. This is especially true in patients with penetrating injuries, because laparoscopic visualization of small bowel injuries is poor. The greatest value of this technique is likely to be in patients with penetrating trauma in whom there is a question of peritoneal penetration, as well as in selected patients with blunt trauma (e.g., nonbleeding liver injuries). Although laparoscopy is fun to do, in my opinion, at the current time, diagnostic laparoscopy is more recreational than educational. However, based on the results of ongoing studies at many trauma centers, we should soon know whether diagnostic laparoscopy is of significant value in trauma victims or whether this fad, too, will pass.—E.A. Deitch, M.D.

## Alternative Approaches to Abdominal Wound Closure in Severely Injured Patients With Massive Visceral Edema

Smith PC, Tweddell JS, Bessey PQ (Washington Univ, St Louis, Mo)
*J Trauma* 32:16–20, 1992                                                                 4–4

*Introduction.*—During operation for severe abdominal trauma, massive visceral edema may develop, leading to excessive tension at the abdominal excision line. Such tension can lead to fascial necrosis and wound sepsis. To evaluate the methods used to circumvent this problem, results in 13 patients treated in a 26-month period were reviewed.

*Subjects.*—Thirteen male patients with severe abdominal trauma had midline incisions that could not be closed primarily without excessive tension because of visceral edema. In 5 patients synthetic mesh was used to bridge the fascial defect, and in 8 patients only the skin was closed with towel clips (Fig 4–2).

*Outcome.*—Of the 5 patients with mesh closures, 4 survived the early postoperative period. All had large, open, midline wounds that required

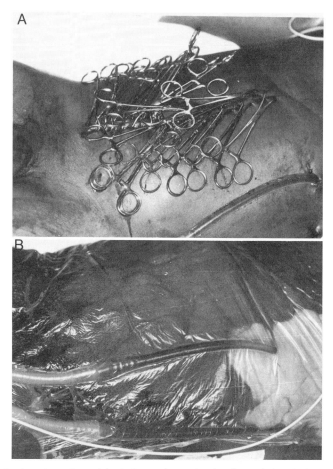

**Fig 4–2.**—**A,** patient whose abdominal wound was closed with towel clips 24 hours previously. Close spacing of the clips and the direction of the handles should be noted. Much of the distention from the visceral edema has already resolved. **B,** clips are covered with a towel, and a plastic adhesive drape is applied over the entire abdomen. (Courtesy of Smith PC, Tweddell JS, Bessey PQ: *J Trauma* 32:16–20, 1992.)

additional procedures. Two of those patients were left with large abdominal wall hernias. In the group having towel clip closure, 6 of the 8 patients survived the initial period. When they were reexamined after 48–96 hours, acute hemorrhage was halted, edema was resolved, and the fascia could be closed without excessive tension. All of those wounds healed satisfactorily.

*Conclusions.*—When visceral edema results in excessive tension that prevents primary closure of abdominal fascia, closure of the skin over the visceral area promotes resolution of the edema and allows satisfactory primary closure within a few days. This is the preferred method.

Synthetic mesh closure should be used only in patients with loss of abdominal wall or wound sepsis.

▶ The technique of towel clip closure of the skin has proved helpful to me on multiple occasions. The rapidity with which intestinal edema and distention resolve is frequently unbelievable. Not uncommonly, within hours the abdomen has become noticeably softer, and the patient can be returned to the operating room for definitive wound closure the next day. A second advantage of this technique is that it does not compromise pulmonary function and makes the ventilatory management of these patients easier.—E.A. Deitch, M.D.

---

**Effect of Increased Intra-Abdominal Pressure on Hepatic Arterial, Portal Venous, and Hepatic Microcirculatory Blood Flow**
Diebel LN, Wilson RF, Dulchavsky SA, Saxe J (Detroit Receiving Hosp, Detroit, Mich; Wayne State Univ, Detroit)
*J Trauma* 33:279–283, 1992                                                         4–5

---

*Objective.*—The adverse effects of increased intra-abdominal pressure (IAP) on cardiopulmonary and renal function are well known, but much less is known of the acute effects of IAP on hepatic perfusion in the normal state. Elevated IAP was investigated in anesthetized pigs.

*Methods.*—Intra-abdominal pressure was raised in 10-mm Hg increments up to 40 mm Hg by infusing warm Ringer's lactate intraperitoneally. Doppler flow probes were used to estimate hepatic artery and portal venous blood flows, and laser Doppler flowmetry was used to observe changes in hepatic microvascular blood flow.

*Findings.*—Both hepatic arterial and microvascular flow declined significantly at 10 mm Hg of IAP. Arterial flow was less than half of the baseline value at 20 mm Hg, whereas microvascular flow was 71% of baseline. Intra-abdominal pressure correlated strongly and inversely with changes in hepatic arterial, portal venous, and microvascular blood flow (table).

Correlation Coefficient Between Changes in IAP and Changes in Hepatic, Portal, and Liver Parenchymal Blood Flow, Cardiac Output, and Portal Venous Pressure

| IAP | ▲ HABF | ▲ PVBF | ▲ HMBF | ▲ CO | POVP |
|-----|--------|--------|--------|------|------|
| r | −0.80* | −0.69* | −0.85* | −0.20 | 0.96* |

*Abbreviations: HABF,* hepatic artery blood flow; *PVBF,* portal venous blood flow; *HMBF,* hepatic microcirculatory blood flow; *CO,* cardiac output; *POVP,* portal venous pressure.
° $P < .01$.
(Courtesy of Diebel LN, Wilson RF, Dulchavsky SA, et al: *J Trauma* 33:279–283, 1992.)

*Conclusion.*—In normal pigs, a modest rise in IAP can significantly compromise perfusion of the liver even though blood pressure and cardiac output remain normal.

▶ The importance of this ingenuous experimental study is its documentation that increased intra-abdominal pressure significantly reduces blood flow to the liver. Because impaired liver blood flow can lead to impaired liver function, and impaired liver function is clearly associated with increased mortality in the critically ill and injured, this study provides another physiologic reason for avoiding excessively tight abdominal wound closures.—E.A. Deitch, M.D.

---

**Abbreviated Laparotomy and Planned Reoperation for Critically Injured Patients**
Burch JM, Ortiz VB, Richardson RJ, Martin RR, Mattox KL, Jordan GL Jr (Baylor College of Medicine, Houston, Tex; Tripler Army Med Ctr, Honolulu, Hawaii)
*Ann Surg* 215:476–484, 1992                                              4–6

---

*Introduction.*—Two hundred critically injured patients, seen in a 7.5-year period, had initial laparotomy terminated by a variety of means with the intention of completing the procedure as a planned reoperation. Penetrating injuries were present in 85% of the patients.

*Management.*—Nearly one third of the patients underwent resuscitative thoracotomy. About 22 units of blood were given to control bleeding. Many different methods were used to end the operation. Enteric injuries were ligated in 34 patients. Vascular clamps were retained in 13 others, and in 4 temporary intravascular shunts were used. Diffusely bleeding surfaces were packed in the majority of patients. Multiple towel clips frequently served to close only the skin of the abdominal wall. Patients then were taken to the surgical intensive care unit for aggressive treatment of coagulopathy and metabolic disorders.

*Results.*—Ninety-eight of the 200 patients lived to have planned reoperation after a mean delay of 48 hours. Two thirds of these patients were discharged from the hospital. Two-thirds of the deaths occurring before reoperation took place within 2 hours of initial surgery. Both the rate of red blood cell transfusion and the pH appeared helpful in deciding when to consider abbreviated laparotomy.

*Conclusion.*—Critically injured patients with acidosis, coagulopathy, and hypothermia are at high risk of dying. They often are best managed by ending laparotomy when bleeding is controlled so that resuscitative measures may be undertaken.

▶ This very important paper stresses that once the clinical triad of hypothermia, acidosis, and coagulopathy has developed, death rapidly ensues unless this vicious cycle can be interrupted. The clinical approach the authors have used in an attempt to break this cycle and thereby improve survival consists of rapidly terminating the operation to prevent further heat loss and transferring the patient to the intensive care unit for rewarming and correction of the coagulopathy and acidosis. However, as stressed by these authors, a major consequence of the need to abruptly terminate the operation is that there may not be sufficient time to treat all of the injuries. Their solution to this problem in 200 severely injured patients was to use unorthodox surgical techniques to rapidly terminate the operation. These include ligation of enteric injuries to limit contamination and the use of packs and/or retained vascular clamps to temporarily control bleeding.

This approach of abbreviated laparotomy and planned reoperation after metabolic stabilization appears valid and effective. The overall survival rate of 33% is commendable, and the fact that two thirds of all of the early deaths occurred within the first 2 hours of the initial laparotomy highlights the critical state these patients were in. Although the use of the various unorthodox temporizing techniques described in this report seems drastic, in occasional well-selected patients this approach may be life-saving. Thus the value of this paper is that it provides evidence supporting a staged approach to the definitive surgical treatment of intra-abdominal injuries in the severely metabolically stressed patient.—E.A. Deitch, M.D.

---

**Angiographically Placed Balloons for Arterial Control: A Description of a Technique**
Scalea TM, Sclafani SJA (Kings County Hosp, Brooklyn, NY; State Univ of New York, Brooklyn)
*J Trauma* 31:1671–1677, 1991                                        4–7

---

*Purpose.*—In patients who have sustained arterial injuries, it is vital to obtain proximal and distal control in the course of repair. This may be difficult or pose problems with blood loss or exposure because of the location of the injury. A technique of percutaneous balloon placement was developed as an aid to vascular control.

*Technique.*—Arterial injuries are identified by angiography. Fluoroscopic guidance is used to place a balloon, which is then deflated. When vascular control is needed intraoperatively, the balloon is inflated. This technique has been used to manage very proximal injuries of the subclavian artery, as well as injuries of the internal carotid artery and external iliac artery, and injuries causing massive bleeding in the angiography suite.

*Case Report.*—Man, 26, with a gunshot wound to zone I of the neck had a pulsating hematoma of the proximal left subclavian artery adjacent to the thyrocervical trunk as identified on "proximity" angiography. Proximal control was achieved by placement of an occlusion balloon in the proximal subclavian artery (Fig 4–3). At surgery the proximal clavicle was resected and distal vascular control was obtained through a supraclavicular incision. The balloon was inflated,

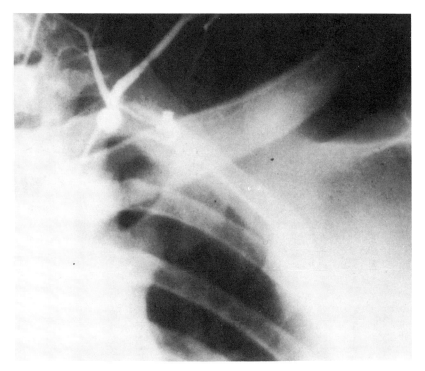

**Fig 4–3.**—Fluoroscopic confirmation of placement of percutaneous balloon for proximal control of the left subclavian artery. (Courtesy of Scalea TM, Sclafani SJA: *J Trauma* 31:1671–1677, 1991.)

the hematoma was unroofed, and revascularization was achieved with a saphenous vein interposition graft.

*Discussion.*—This technique greatly limits blood loss and permits repair through a limited incision. It can be used in patients with angiographically identified arterial injuries in whom operative exposure would be difficult, result in serious blood loss, or require an extensive incision and dissection.

▶ This report of 13 patients in whom percutaneously placed balloon catheters were used to aid in the surgical repair of selected vascular injuries is self-explanatory. The limitation of this approach is that it requires the on-site presence of a skilled radiologist. Nonetheless, this technique can be helpful in certain high-risk and difficult to treat vascular injuries.—E.A. Deitch, M.D.

### Tissue Expanders for Abdominal Wall Reconstruction Following Severe Trauma: Technical Note and Case Reports

Livingston DH, Sharma PK, Glantz AI (UMD-New Jersey Med School, Newark)
J Trauma 32:82–86, 1992                                    4–8

*Background.*—Temporary closure of the abdominal wall with prosthetic material may be necessary in trauma patients because of massive tissue loss or intestinal distention related to resuscitative measures. An alternative to using prosthetic material or myocutaneous flaps is to place tissue expanders well in advance of abdominal reconstruction.

*Technique.*—Usually, at least 6 months elapse between grafting and reconstruction. Tissue expanders are placed on either side of the ventral defect about 6 weeks before planned reconstruction and inflated at weekly intervals. At reconstruction, the skin graft covering the ventral defect is denuded of its dermal elements and then sutured to the existing rectus fascia. The fascial graft is covered with full-thickness skin using local advancement flaps.

*Experience.*—Two patients underwent this procedure, 1 in conjunction with closure of a colostomy and the other in association with closure of an enterocutaneous fistula. The wounds in both patients healed without infection. Follow-up after 1 year showed no evidence of hernia.

*Advantages.*—With the new procedure, the ventral defect is closed at completion of laparotomy. Tissue expansion produces a fibrous reaction that interposes an additional layer on the anterior abdominal wall. The width may be adjusted to allow for tension-free closure.

▶ This paper deals with an infrequent, but not uncommon, difficult problem in trauma victims as well as in other patient populations. In this report, the authors describe the use of tissue expanders to aid in definitive wound closure in 2 patients who had skin graft closure of their abdominal cavities. The authors stress that this technique avoids the need for prosthetic material or the use of myocutaneous flaps. Although I have never used this technique, it appears conceptually attractive, especially in those patients who have lost significant amounts of abdominal wall, either through injury or infection. On the other hand, in my experience, if a significant portion of the abdominal wall has not been lost, it is usually possible to achieve primary wound closure after removal of the skin graft and moderate to extensive lateral dissection of the abdominal wall.—E.A. Deitch, M.D.

### Updating the Management of Salvageable Splenic Injury

Witte CL, Esser MJ, Rappaport WD (Univ of Arizona, Tucson)
Ann Surg 215:261–265, 1992                               4–9

*Introduction.*—Today, at least half of all injured spleens can be salvaged by repair or partial splenectomy, minimizing the risk of overwhelming sepsis and other sequelae. Two recent developments suggest the need to reassess the management of patients with salvageable spleen injuries. One is increasing concern about transmitting HIV infection and viral hepatitis, and the other is the availability of automated "cell savers" to reinfuse shed intra-abdominal blood.

*Recent Experience.*—In a 6-month period, 20 patients were treated for blunt trauma and splenic injury. Nine patients with relatively minor lacerations were managed effectively without surgery. The other 11 patients had continued bleeding or associated visceral injury, which made laparotomy necessary. Two of the latter patients who had life-threatening accompanying injuries underwent total splenectomy. In 8 of the remaining 9 patients the spleens were salvaged. The patients lost a mean of 1,250 mL of blood and had an average of nearly 800 mL reinfused through the cell saver. Three patients received homologous blood in addition. When the hilus was lacerated, it was helpful to occlude the splenic pedicle temporarily and suture torn polar branches through the site of laceration.

*Recommendations.*—Early laparotomy with reinfusion of shed autologous blood is recommended for both children and adults with major splenic injury. In most patients, the spleen, or a large part of it, can be salvaged. Homologous blood transfusion often can be avoided, eliminating the risk of transmitting disease.

▶ The major point of this report is that it is possible to both salvage the spleen and avoid homologous transfusions with their respective potential risks.

However, the question remains: Which patients with splenic injuries should be managed operatively and which expectantly? Because patients with other associated visceral injuries almost always require laparotomy, this question centers on the management of patients, especially children, with isolated splenic injuries in whom nonoperative management is frequently effective. The answer to this question is beginning to change as the risks of nonautologous blood transfusions become better defined. Blood transfusions are not only associated with the risk of transmission of viral infections, but they are also immunosuppressive and are associated with an increased incidence of bacterial infectious complications. Thus, at the current time, a nonoperative approach is reasonable in hemodynamically stable patients with isolated splenic injuries in whom blood transfusions are not likely to be necessary. However, if blood transfusions (especially if more than 2 units) will be required, then operative repair becomes a more attractive option.—E.A. Deitch, M.D.

### Autotransfusion of Potentially Culture-Positive Blood (CPB) in Abdominal Trauma: Preliminary Data From a Prospective Study

Ozmen V, McSwain NE Jr, Nichols RL, Smith J, Flint LM (Tulane Univ, New Orleans)

J Trauma 32:36–39, 1992 4–10

*Background.*—The increased use of autotransfusion for trauma-induced bleeding may decrease the amounts of banked blood needed for severe injuries. Although autotransfusion is standard for traumatic hemothorax, its use has been limited in patients with abdominal injuries. The use of autotransfusion of potentially culture-positive blood in patients with abdominal injuries was examined in a prospective study.

*Methods.*—Microbiological data on 152 patients with intestinal injuries were used. When blood loss was anticipated to be more than 1,000 mL, blood from the peritoneal cavity was cultured, washed, concentrated, and recultured for reinfusion. The Penetrating Abdominal Trauma Index (PATI) was used to stratify infection rates. The results in 50 patients with a PATI exceeding 20 who received a mean of 1,800 mL of banked blood were compared with results in 20 patients who received a mean of 3,900 mL of autotransfused, potentially culture-positive blood.

*Outcomes.*—Wound infection occurred in 25% of patients in both groups. When severity of injury was stratified according to the PATI, there were no significant increases in site-specific infection risk. Bacteria cultured from autotransfused blood did not cause bacteremia, or pulmonary or urinary infections.

*Conclusions.*—Autotransfusion of blood aspirated from the peritoneal cavity is feasible and has the potential to reduce the need for banked blood in trauma victims. Blood washing removes bacteria from most of the units, and infusion of culture-positive blood does not increase the risk of subsequent infection in seriously injured patients. Further research is needed to assess the use of this technique in larger groups of patients.

▶ Although autotransfusion is commonly used in certain elective procedures and in patients with traumatic hemothorax, its use in patients with multiple intra-abdominal injuries has been limited. To some extent, this limitation is based on the potential risks of autotransfusing blood contaminated with bowel contents and bacteria. Thus this prospective study comparing the incidence of infectious complications in patients with intestinal injuries who did or did not receive autotransfusions is of value. Basically, the results indicate that the incidence of site-specific infections was not different between the groups. However, the overall incidence of infections was higher in the auto-transfused group, as was the septic mortality rate. This study, as well as a large retrospective study of autotransfusion in patients with intestinal injuries (1), thus has not resolved the controversy.—E.A. Deitch, M.D.

*Reference*

1. Horst, et al: *J Trauma* 32:646, 1992.

**Hepatitis B and Hepatitis C in Emergency Department Patients**
Kelen GD, Green GB, Purcell RH, Chan DW, Qaqish BF, Sivertson KT, Quinn TC (Johns Hopkins Univ, Baltimore, Md; Univ of North Carolina, Chapel Hill; Natl Inst of Allergy and Infectious Diseases, Bethesda, Md)
*N Engl J Med* 326:1399–1404, 1992                                    4–11

*Introduction.*—Although hepatitis B virus (HBV), hepatitis C virus (HCV), and HIV-1 share modes of transmission and similar prevalence rates, their relative seroprevalence and possible interrelationship has not been investigated. The seroprevalence of HBV and HCV and related HIV-1 infectivity was investigated in more than 2,500 patients treated in an emergency department.

*Methods.*—For 6 consecutive weeks from June through August 1988, excess serum was obtained from all patients treated at the Johns Hopkins Hospital emergency department. Demographic and other data also were collected. The excess serum underwent analysis for HIV-1, HCV, and hepatitis B surface antigen (HBsAg) using an enzyme-linked immunosorbent assay.

*Results.*—There were 5,229 patient visits, and 2,523 patients participated in the study. The seroprevalence for viral markers demonstrated that 24% were seropositive for at least 1 viral marker, 18% were seropositive for HCV, 5% were positive for HbsAg, and 6% were positive for HIV-1. The mean age overall was 43 years; those seropositive for the viruses had a mean age of 41 years. In 91 samples there was evidence of HCV and HIV-1 infection, and 17 samples had evidence of HIV-1 and HBsAg infection. Statistical analysis showed that the 2 concomitant infections were related and were not a result of independent distributions. Routine testing for HIV-1 alone would have missed 80% of the HCV and 87% of the HBsAg infections.

*Conclusion.*—A high percentage of patients infected with HCV and HBV in this series also had a high prevalence of HIV-1 infection. Sexual transmission of HCV may occur more frequently than previously thought. Routine screening methods for HIV-1 do not identify most individuals positive for the virus, and health care providers must use universal precautions rigorously.

▶ The importance of this study is that it documents both the high incidence of potentially transmissible viral diseases in this patient population as well as the limitations of focusing purely on HIV-1 screening. Screening only for HIV-1 would have missed 73% of the patients with HBV and HCV infections. In fact, almost a third of the patients who went directly from the emergency department to the operating suite were found to have at least 1 viral infection, and the vast majority of these patients (79%) would not have been identified by routine screening for HIV-1 alone. The high seroprevalence rates of these 3 viral diseases mandates compliance with universal precautions policies, especially during the initial emergency room trauma triage and resuscitation period.—E.A. Deitch, M.D.

---

### Duration of Antibiotic Therapy for Penetrating Abdominal Trauma: A Prospective Trial

Fabian TC, Croce MA, Payne LW, Minard G, Pritchard FE, Kudsk KA (Univ of Tennessee, Memphis; Presley Regional Trauma Ctr, Memphis)
Surgery 112:788–795, 1992                                                    4–12

---

*Background.*—The optimal duration of antibiotic therapy in penetrating abdominal trauma is still unclear. Whereas antibiotic treatment for up to 24 hours is sufficient in patients with mild to moderate injuries, it may not be adequate in those with a severe injury or a colon injury. A prospective, double-blind study was undertaken to compare the efficacy of 24-hour antibiotic therapy with that of a 5-day course in patients at high risk for major abdominal infection.

*Methods.*—During a 34-month period, 515 patients aged 18–88 years were treated for penetrating injuries; 235 (46%) had hollow viscus injuries and 280 (54%) did not. Patients without hollow viscus injuries were randomly allocated to receive cefoxitin or cefotetan intravenously for 24 hours. Patients with hollow viscus injuries were randomly allocated to receive a 24-hour or a 5-day antibiotic regimen and were further randomized within each group to receive either cefoxitin or cefotetan intravenously. Major abdominal infection was defined as the presence of an abscess, necrotizing fasciitis, or diffuse peritonitis.

*Results.*—A major abdominal infection developed in 22 patients, 8% in patients treated with antibiotics for 24 hours and 10% in those treated for 5 days. All patients with a major abdominal infection had hollow viscus injuries, and no major abdominal infections developed in patients without such injuries. Twenty-two patients had abdominal abscesses, 2 had necrotizing fasciitis, and 2 had diffuse suppurative peritonitis. When analyzed by type of antibiotic used, the infection rates were 9% for both cefotetan and cefoxitin. When analyzed by duration of treatment, the infection rates were 8% after the 24-hour course and 10% after the 5-day course. The difference was not statistically significant. The incidence of major abdominal infection was highest among patients with colon wounds and an abdominal trauma index of more than 25, but it was not reduced by treating the patients with 5 days of antibiotics.

*Conclusions.*—The use of a single-agent, second-generation cephalosporin antibiotic for 5 days to reduce the risk of major abdominal infection among high-risk patients with penetrating abdominal trauma offers no advantage over a 24-hour treatment course.

▶ Not only can the choice of prophylactic (perioperative) antibiotics be confusing in trauma patients, but how long to use them continues to be debated. The concept espoused in this study of using a single second-generation antibiotic for a short period of time (24 hours) fits my bias. This is what I do and what I teach. Not only is it cost effective, it makes sense and is easy to remember.—E.A. Deitch, M.D.

---

**Enteral Versus Parenteral Feeding: Effects on Septic Morbidity After Blunt and Penetrating Abdominal Trauma**
Kudsk KA, Croce MA, Fabian TC, Minard G, Tolley EA, Poret HA, Kuhl MR, Brown RO (Presley Mem Trauma Ctr, Memphis, Tenn; Univ of Tennessee, Memphis)
*Ann Surg* 215:503–513, 1992                                        4–13

---

*Objective.*—There is substantial evidence that the route of nutrient administration influences the response to injury. A prospective study was undertaken to compare the effects of early enteral and parenteral feeding on the outcomes in 98 adults with intraabdominal injuries requiring laparotomy. All patients had an abdominal trauma index of 15 or higher.

*Management.*—Patients were randomly assigned to enteral or parenteral feeding within 24 hours of injury. The formulas contained nearly identical amounts of fat, carbohydrate, and protein. The goal was to administer 1.5–2 g of protein/amino acids and 30–35 kcal of nonprotein calories per kilogram daily.

*Observations.*—There were no significant differences in blood requirements, days on a ventilator, extent of antibiotic treatment, or nitrogen balance between the enterally and parenterally fed patients. Those

| Sepsis | Septic Morbidity | | |
|---|---|---|---|
| | ENT | TPN | p |
| Pneumonia | 6/51 (11.8%) | 14/45 (31%) | <.02 |
| Intra-abdominal abscess | 1/51 (1.9%) | 6/45 (13.3%) | <.04 |
| Empyema | 1/51 (1.9%) | 4/45 (9%) | NS |
| Line sepsis | 1/51 (1.9%) | 6/45 (13.3%) | <.05 |
| Fasciitis/dehiscence | 3/51 (5.9%) | 4/45 (8.9%) | NS |
| Abscesses (intra-abdominal and/or empyema) | 2/51 (3.9%) | 8/45 (17.8%) | <.03 |
| Pneumonia and/or abscesses | 8/51 (13.7%) | 17/45 (37.8%) | <.02 |
| Pneumonia, abscesses, and/or line sepsis | 9/51 (15.7%) | 18/45 (40%) | <.02 |

*Abbreviations:* ENT, enteral; TPN, total parenteral nutrition.
(Courtesy of Kudsk KA, Croce MA, Fabian TC, et al: *Ann Surg* 215:503–513, 1992.)

assigned to enteral nutrition had significantly less septic morbidity than those assigned to parenteral nutrition (table). The major difference was in patients with relatively high injury severity scores and abdominal trauma indexes and in those with penetrating injury. Diarrhea was more frequent in enterally fed patients.

*Conclusion.*—Enteral access should be gained at the time of surgery so that nutrients may be delivered enterally. This technique may be most advantageous in those patients with the most severe abdominal injuries.

▶ That enterally fed trauma victims have fewer infectious complications than parenterally fed patients now seems firmly established. Because this study by Kudsk et al. is the fourth such clinical study documenting the benefits of enteral feeding in trauma patients, the preferential use of parenteral alimentation in trauma victims can no longer be supported. Although in this study the patients were fed through operatively placed jejunostomy tubes, nasoenteric tubes are an acceptable alternative, especially in those patients who do not require a laparotomy.

The exact physiologic reasons why enteral feedings are so beneficial remain to be determined. However, there is increasing experimental evidence documenting that enteral alimentation maintains intestinal barrier function better than parenteral alimentation and thereby limits the leak of intestinal contents (including bacteria) from the gut into systemic tissues. Thus this clinical study adds further support to the concepts that the gut can be a reservoir for bacteria that cause systemic infections, and that attempts to maintain intestinal barrier function may reduce the incidence of infectious complications.—E.A. Deitch, M.D.

---

**A Randomized Prospective Clinical Trial to Determine the Efficacy of Interferon-γ in Severely Injured Patients**
Polk HC Jr, Cheadle WG, Livingston DH, Rodriguez JL, Starko KM, Izu AE, Jaffe HS, Sonnenfeld G (Univ of Louisville, Louisville, Ky; Univ of Medicine and Dentistry of New Jersey, Newark; State Univ of New York, Buffalo; Genentech Inc, South San Francisco)
*Am J Surg* 163:191–196, 1992                                4–14

---

*Background.*—Infection represents one of the most common and most serious threats to survival in trauma victims who survive their acute injuries. Research into the basic host defense processes against microbial sepsis has led to the clinical emergence of nonantibiotic methods for the prevention and/or treatment of infection. Reduced monocyte human leukocyte antigen-DR (HLA-DR) levels in trauma patients correlate with poorer clinical outcome. A pilot study of recombinant interferon-γ (rIFN-γ) showed that it can restore depressed HLA-DR levels to normal after major injury. A prospective, multicenter, randomized, double-blind study was undertaken as an extension of the pilot study.

*Patients.*—Of 213 trauma patients at high risk of infection, 108 received 100 μg of rIFN-γ/day subcutaneously for 10 days, or until discharge or death if this occurred before 10 days; 105 patients were given placebo.

*Results.*—Twenty patients were subsequently excluded from the efficacy analysis. Of the 193 evaluable patients, 97 (mean age, 34 years) were treated with rIFN-γ and 96 (mean age, 31 years) received placebo. The mean injury severity score was 33 in both groups. On day 3 after admission, patients treated with rIFN-γ had significantly higher monocyte HLA-DR antigen levels and significantly better outcome predictive scores than the placebo-treated patients. There were 9 deaths in the group given rIFN-γ and 12 deaths among those given placebo. Both groups had similar major and minor infection rates; 17 rIFN-γ-treated patients and 22 placebo-treated patients had major infections that warranted reoperation for drainage or CT-guided needle aspiration and drainage or débridement. Furthermore, rIFN-γ-treated patients had fewer serious renal complications than placebo-treated patients. But, 93% of the rIFN-γ-treated patients had fever compared with 83% of the placebo-treated patients, and the fever level was higher in those treated with rIFN-γ.

*Conclusions.*—Fewer infections requiring surgery developed in rIFN-γ-treated trauma patients than in placebo-treated patients. There was no difference in the overall rates of minor or major infections between the 2 groups, however.

▶ Although rINF-γ was not effective in reducing infectious complications in this study, the article was selected because it represents the wave of the future. As more information accrues on the basic biology of infection, inflammation, and injury, the use of various compounds to modulate the host's immune response will increase. Therefore, it is increasingly important for all practicing surgeons to become familiar with the basic biology of inflammation and to add the cytokine jargon to their everyday language. I believe that just as adjuvant chemotherapy has become an integral component of cancer therapy, so too will drug therapy directed at the host's inflammatory and metabolic responses become part of standard trauma and critical care therapy.—E.A. Deitch, M.D.

---

**Hypertonic Saline Treatment of Uncontrolled Hemorrhagic Shock at Different Periods From Bleeding**
Krausz MM, Landau EH, Klin B, Gross D (Hadassah Univ Hosp, Jerusalem, Israel)
*Arch Surg* 127:93–96, 1992                                                 4–15

---

*Background.*—Hypertonic saline (HTS) has been recommended in the treatment of hemorrhagic shock. In all previous studies, HTS was administered 5 minutes after the hemorrhagic injury. The effects of giv-

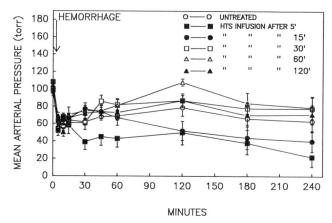

**Fig 4–4.**—Change in mean arterial pressure in animals in uncontrolled hemorrhagic shock treated with 7.5% HTS, 5 mL/kg, administered at different periods after hemorrhagic shock. (Courtesy of Krausz MM, Landau, EH, Klin B, et al: *Arch Surg* 127:93-96, 1992.)

ing HTS at several different periods during the first 2 hours after injury were investigated.

*Methods.*—Six groups of rats were studied. Group 1 animals had uncontrolled hemorrhagic shock, induced by tail resection, and no HTS. Hypertonic saline was administered to group 2 at 5 minutes after shock was induced, to group 3 at 15 minutes, to group 4 at 30 minutes, to group 5 at 60 minutes, and to group 6 at 120 minutes. Blood loss was measured over a 4-hour observation period.

*Results.*—Group 1 animals lost a mean of 2.7 mL of blood in 5 minutes. The mean arterial pressure dropped from 95 mm Hg to 63 mm Hg

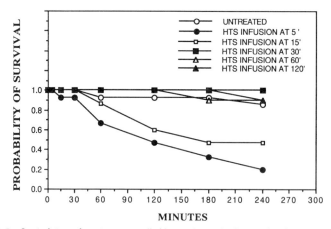

**Fig 4–5.**—Survival time of rats in uncontrolled hemorrhagic shock treated with 7.5% HTS, 5 mL/kg, administered at different periods after hemorrhagic insult. (Courtesy of Krausz MM, Landau EH, Klin B, et al: *Arch Surg* 127:93-96, 1992.)

(Fig 4-4). When HTS was given at 5 minutes and 15 minutes, additional bleeding of 6.3 mL and 3.8 mL, respectively, occurred, and the mean arterial pressure decreased to 36 mm Hg and 56 mm Hg respectively. Eighty percent of animals in group 2 and 53% of those in group 3 died during the observation period. In groups 4 and 5, HTS infusion increased bleeding only minimally and did not affect mean arterial pressure or survival. The 4-hour survival of the 6 groups is shown in Figure 4-5.

*Conclusions.*—Animal experiments suggest that infusion of HTS within 15 minutes after hemorrhagic insult results in increased bleeding, hypotension, and early death, whereas infusion after 30 minutes or 60 minutes does not alter bleeding, mean arterial pressure, or survival. Early infusion of HTS may be dangerous in human trauma victims. Ongoing clinical studies are needed to critically evaluate the timing of HTS infusions.

▶ This experimental study was chosen to illustrate one of the potential dangers of HTS resuscitation in the treatment of hemorrhagic shock. It clearly documents that the mortality rate and amount of blood loss are increased when HTS is used to raise the blood pressure when the source of bleeding is not controlled. The results of this study of "uncontrolled" shock thus differ markedly from the results observed in "controlled" hemorrhagic shock models in which blood is withdrawn through an arterial catheter. In these controlled shock models, HTS restored blood pressure and improved survival.

Although HTS improves survival in controlled shock models, because it actually can decrease survival in uncontrolled shock models, and hemorrhagic shock in trauma patients is uncontrolled, HTS therapy before surgical control of the bleeding sites may be dangerous. However, because of the potential benefits of HTS, especially when combined with dextran in head-injured patients, HTS may have a role in the treatment of selected patients. Nonetheless, at the current time, HTS resuscitation of trauma patients must be considered investigational.—E.A. Deitch, M.D.

---

**Focal Brain Injury Results in Severe Cerebral Ischemia Despite Maintenance of Cerebral Perfusion Pressure**

Zhuang J, Schmoker JD, Shackford SR, Pietropaoli JA (Univ of Vermont, Burlington)
*J Trauma* 33:83–88, 1992                                                4–16

*Introduction.*—Brain injury frequently is associated with increased intracranial pressure and decreased cerebral blood flow and cerebral oxygen delivery. The result is secondary ischemic brain injury. Increased intracranial pressure is considered to be the main cause of this secondary brain injury, because it reduces cerebral perfusion pressure (CPP). Therefore, it is possible that maintenance of CPP would provide adequate oxygen and prevent cerebral ischemia. This hypothesis was tested in a porcine model of cryogenic brain injury.

*Methods.*—Fifteen mature swine were randomized to either an experimental group, which received a brain lesion, or to the control group, which received only instruments. Cerebral perfussion pressure, intracranial pressure, cerebral blood flow, cerebral oxygen delivery, cerebral oxygen extraction ratio, and cortical water content were studied for 24 hours.

*Results.*—In the experimental group, cryogenic injury significantly increased the intracranial pressure and decreased cerebral blood flow and cerebral oxygen delivery compared with the control group. Cerebral perfusion pressure was maintained above the ischemic threshold in both groups for the duration of measurements, and there was no significant difference in CPP between the 2 groups. The cerebral oxygen extraction ratio increased significantly in the first 3 hours after brain injury, but decreased after 12 hours to a level that was not significantly different from control levels. Cortical water content was significantly increased in the injured region.

*Conclusions.*—Despite normal CPP, focal brain injury resulted in persistent ischemia in this porcine model. This result suggests that a significant increase in cerebral vascular resistance occurs after brain injury. Therefore, in addition to the maintenance of CPP, intervention to reduce cerebral vascular resistance may be necessary to improve cerebral blood flow and oxygen delivery and to prevent secondary ischemic brain injury.

▶ Head injury, either alone or in combination with hemorrhage, is responsible for more than a third of trauma deaths. Furthermore, more than two thirds of patients dying of head injury have evidence of secondary ischemic brain damage. Because the injured brain is very vulnerable to a decrease in oxygen delivery, studies clarifying the pathophysiology of secondary ischemic brain injury are important in order to develop new and effective therapy. The significance of this experimental study is that it refutes the hypothesis that by maintaining CPP it will be possible to maintain cerebral oxygen delivery, thus directing our attention in other therapeutic directions.

Cerebral blood flow (CBF) is determined by CPP divided by cerebral vascular resistance (CVR) as shown in this equation: CBF = CPP/CVR. Based on this equation and the authors' observation that CBF was decreased even when the CPP was not, the conclusion that the decrease in CBF resulted primarily from an increase in CVR appears valid. These results also support their conclusion that medical interventions to reduce CVR in addition to the maintenance of CPP will be required to improve CBF and oxygen delivery and thereby prevent secondary ischemic brain injury. One such therapy that appears to be effective in improving CBF is the use of hypertonic sodium solutions (1). The mechanism by which hypertonic fluids appear to increase CBF is by reducing endothelial edema and thus CVR. This study thus illustrates how clinically relevant basic physiologic studies can provide the information necessary to develop and evaluate new therapeutic options.—E.A. Deitch, M.D.

*Reference*

1. Schmoker JD, et. al: *J Trauma* 31:1607, 1991.

## Evaluation of a Comprehensive Algorithm for Blunt and Penetrating Thoracic and Abdominal Trauma

Bishop M, Shoemaker WC, Avakian S, James E, Jackson G, Williams D, Meade P, Fleming A (King-Drew Med Ctr, Los Angeles, Calif)
*Am Surg* 57:737–746, 1991                                                    4–17

*Introduction.*—Severely injured patients must be expeditiously evaluated and treated. Critical management decisions must be made rapidly. Most poor outcomes when the patient is salvageable reflect errors made during initial resuscitation and treatment.

*Objective.*—A single branched-chain decision tree, applicable to patients with either blunt or penetrating thoracic and abdominal trauma, was developed. An algorithm consisting of 14 patient management loops and 31 decision nodes was applied to 434 trauma patients seen prospectively during a 4-month period.

*Results.*—The 400 patients with signs of life on arriving at the emergency department had a mean Injury Severity Score of 21 and a mean Trauma Score of 13. The mortality rate was 17% overall; it was 61% in patients with major deviations from the algorithm and 6% in patients managed according to the algorithm. In 3% of the 64 patients who died, there were major deviations from the algorithm. These deviations contributed directly to 21 deaths and probably contributed to 14 others. Compliance with the algorithm was especially important for patients with Injury Severity Scores of 20–50.

*Conclusion.*—Compliance with specific management criteria can substantially improve the survival of patients with blunt or penetrating thoracic or abdominal injuries.

▶ The optimal care of the trauma patient frequently requires rapid decisions to be made during periods of stress. Because there is little time for indecision, one approach to optimizing care has been the development of therapeutic algorithms to guide the initial care of these patients. The results of this study clearly indicate that when the algorithm was ignored or major deviations were made, mortality was greatly increased. Thus there is a heavy penalty to be paid for not obeying the rules.

Consequently, the placement and ready access to algorithms in emergency department areas are likely to decrease the incidence of management errors and improve outcome. In this regard, I strongly urge the placement and use of these or similar algorithms in the emergency rooms of all hospitals where trauma patients are treated.—E.A. Deitch, M.D.

## Improvement in Outcome From Trauma Center Care
Champion HR, Sacco WJ, Copes WS (Washington Hosp Ctr, Washington, DC)
*Arch Surg* 127:333–338, 1992                                          4–18

*Objective.*—Although many studies have confirmed reductions in mortality with establishment of trauma centers and systems of care for trauma victims, no study has documented the ongoing efficacy of in-hospital trauma center care in a diverse group of seriously injured patients.

*Methods.*—The outcomes of blunt trauma victims managed at a 907-bed urban teaching hospital were examined over a 6-year period during which a resuscitation facility with integrated operating rooms was established.

*Observations.*—Patient survival improved during the period under review when the mix of injury severity was controlled. Survival improved the most after the trauma resuscitation facility opened and was most notable for the more severely injured patients. Among patients whose Injury Severity Scores exceeded 15, there were an average of 13.4 more survivors per 100 patients treated per year in the last 2 years than in the first 2 years.

*Implications.*—Impressive savings of further lives might well be expected were all seriously injured patients managed at improved trauma centers. Current cost constraints make it doubtful, however, that the development of trauma centers will continue at the present rate.

▶ That the establishment of trauma centers and trauma systems of care improve survival is well recognized. However, the importance of this study is that it clearly shows that even in level I trauma centers, further improvements in the survival of significantly injured patients can be attained by increasing an institution's commitment to trauma care.

Because trauma care is expensive, and the survival and growth of trauma centers and systems are ultimately dependent on institutional, local government, and federal financial support, studies such as this one documenting a relationship between resource commitment and improved outcome are important. Basically, it is necessary for both the public and the government to remember that there is no free lunch.—E. A. Deitch, M.D.

## Identification of Preventable Trauma Deaths: Confounded Inquiries?
Wilson DS, McElligott J, Fielding LP (St Mary's Hosp, Waterbury, Conn; Yale

Univ, New Haven, Conn; Tennessee Ctr for Internal Medicine, Knoxville)
*J Trauma* 32:45–51, 1992                                              4–19

*Background.*—The medical profession's response to increased public awareness and regulation of clinical practice has included a number of programs generically called quality assessment. Concurrently, federal and professional organizations have instituted measures for cost containment. In recent years, quality assessment and cost containment have become intertwined in many programs. One tool of quality assessment aimed at identifying avoidable mortality is the professional review organization (PRO). A PRO reviews cases or charts in the expectation that, if avoidable mortality and morbidity can be identified, an educational process can follow, leading to improved standards of care. A study was done to explore the assumption that peer review has the intrinsic capability to make these judgments. To investigate the reliability of published methods for identifying preventable trauma deaths, 3 consensus systems were compared.

*Methods.*—Separate 5-member general review panels assessed 20 non–CNS fatalities. Panel A assessed cases based on independent judgment; panel B, on discussion of all cases preceding individual judgments; and panel C, on independent judgments followed by discussion and equivocal case reassignment.

*Results.*—The kappa concordance index was low for all methods. Although 11 deaths were judged preventable by at least 1 panel, only 1 death was judged preventable by all 3 panels. Different consensus methods yielded different results. Consensus agreement, based on 4 of 5 assessors, was 20% for panel A, 45% for panel B, and 10% for panel C. In panel C, discussion had a significant impact on judgment, the rate of equivocal case designation changing from 30% before to 5% after discussion.

*Conclusion.*—The consensus methods used to identify preventable trauma death appear to be flawed because of the high degree of subjectivity involved. It was recommended that more objective methods based on patient population outcome data replace individual case reviews as a measure of institutional quality of care. One such objective method is the PROFILE system, which combines the admission Glasgow Coma Scale score, systolic blood pressure, respiratory rate, and anatomical injury scores.

▶ The basic importance of this study is that it documents the inherently flawed nature of the subjective PRO process. It also calls into question the basic tool of the current PRO approach, which is the individual case (chart) review system. Because of the widespread utilization of the PRO approach, the results of this study transcend trauma care and speak to every practicing surgeon. Consequently, we must all strive to prevent Monday morning quarterbacks from developing next week's medical game plan and insure that decisions are based on objective data and not on post-hoc "in my opinion" statements. Otherwise, we face more and potentially less effective institutional and government regulation.

Similar results on the lack of interrater reliability was recently reported by MacKenzie et al. (1).—E.A. Deitch, M.D.

*Reference*

1. MacKenzie , et al: *J Trauma* 33:292, 1992.

---

### An Evaluation of Provider-Related and Disease-Related Morbidity in a Level I University Trauma Service: Directions for Quality Improvement

Hoyt DB, Hollingsworth-Fridlund P, Fortlage D, Davis JW, Mackersie RC (Univ of California, San Diego)
*J Trauma* 33:586–601, 1992                                                          4–20

*Introduction.*—The system of regionalized trauma care units has dramatically reduced the incidence of preventable death after injury to 1% to 2%, a rate that has remained stable for 5 years. Therefore, if further reductions in preventable trauma-related mortality are to be made, quality improvement must occur in a new way. A study was conducted to identify the incidence and type of complications that occur in an intensive care unit (ICU) and to distinguish between those that are provider related and those that are disease related.

*Study Design.*—All trauma patients who died, who were admitted to the ICU or operating room, who were hospitalized for more than 3 days, or who were interfacility transfers to an academic trauma unit were evaluated concurrently for 1 year. All complications were defined, reviewed, and classified, and then subdivided into provider-specific and disease-specific complications. Provider-related complications were classified as justified or unjustified to identify areas in which improvement could occur.

*Findings.*—Of the 1,108 patients reviewed, 97 died. There were 3 potentially preventable deaths, 857 complications, and 285 provider-related complications. There was potential for improvement in 59 events. Disease-specific morbidity was primarily related to infection, especially pneumonia.

*Summary.*—Review of the number and types of complications occurring during 1 year on a trauma service indicated that there was a significant potential for improvement in 21% of all provider-related events. This analysis of the levels of disease-related and provider-related morbidity in a trauma system can be used as a guide for a continuous improvement process.

▶ Of the many articles appearing on quality assurance during the past year, this is one of the best. This unique approach to identifying and analyzing surgical complications should be considered by all those involved in trauma care. For other excellent articles in this area, please see the articles by Davis et al. (1), Milzman et al. (2), and Karmy-Jones et al. (3).

*References*

1. Davis JW, et al: *J Trauma* 32:660, 1992.
2. Milzman, et al: *J Trauma* 32:236, 1992.
3. Karmy-Jones, et al: *J Trauma* 32:196, 1992.

# 5 Infections

## Introduction

Operative treatment continues to be the mainstay in management of most surgical infections. The first three articles reviewed here deal with surgical techniques to treat serious intra-abdominal infections. The article by Schein (Abstract 5–1) proposes open management in reoperation for treatment of peritonitis and other critical intra-abdominal infections. The problem is defining which patients are good candidates for this type of management and precisely what the indications are. Two articles appeared that deal with the treatment of pancreatic infections. One (Abstract 5–2) discusses the retroperitoneal approach to pancreatic abscess. The other (Abstract 5–3) proposes operating on patients with pancreatic necrosis rather than waiting until it becomes infected, because pancreatic necrosis per se results in such high mortality. The increasingly aggressive operative approach toward patients with intraperitoneal infections is warranted, because operation is the main method of treating these problems. Antibiotic therapy is only an adjunctive measure.

Antibiotics and other adjunctive therapies are nevertheless important. The article by Mosdell et al. (Abstract 5–4) discusses antibiotic therapy for patients with surgical infections. Patients who had no cultures taken did as well as those who did have cultures taken. Broad-spectrum coverage is warranted in patients with intra-abdominal infections despite the culture results because we know that anaerobes and aerobes are both recovered from intra-abdominal infections, and that with good culture techniques, multiple organisms are usually found. Culture data were usually ignored even when obtained. A trial of immunoglobulin for preventing infections in high-risk surgical patients was undertaken by Cometta and colleagues (Abstract 5–5). Surprisingly, patients treated with immunoglobulin selected for a high antibody titer to core-lipopolysaccharide (LPS) did not fare as well as those treated with standard immunoglobulin. The reasons for this are unclear. Walsh et al. (Abstract 5–6) describe the prophylactic treatment of animals with anti-TNF-$\alpha$ monoclonal antibody and demonstrate that it can protect them against subsequent intravenous infusions with *Pseudomonas*. Immunoglobulin and antibody to TNF-$\alpha$, or antibodies to other mediators or endotoxin, are probably too expensive to be used prophylactically in surgical patients because of the small decrease in infections that can be expected. Studies are needed that test these biological agents in the treatment of established infections. At least two studies examining the effect of antibody to LPS (HA-1A and E5) have appeared. These antibodies showed some efficacy, and further studies of E5 are currently taking place. A study of HA-1A was recently stopped, however, because of a high mortality rate.

Blood cultures were not effective in reducing morbidity and mortality when obtained perioperatively in patients who had no evidence of sepsis except for fever. Blood cultures are frequently obtained in any patient who has a fever. The article by Theuer et al. (Abstract 5-7) challenges that concept.

Bacterial translocation is a phenomenon currently looking for its appropriate place in clinical medicine. This is easy to demonstrate in animals subjected to experimental conditions, but its true role in clinical disease is unclear. Certainly, there are some diseases and specific types of bacteria for which translocation is an important method of pathogenesis, but it is still hard to prove that it is of clinical significance in most diseases.

The article by Calligaro et al. (Abstract 5-10) provides guidelines for preserving infected arterial grafts. The authors developed an algorithm that allows salvage of some infected "smooth-walled" grafts made of vein or polytetrafluoroethylene. Many surgeons think that infection of the graft means it must be removed. These authors show that such is not always the case.

Tuberculosis and other mycobacterial infections are having a resurgence in patients with AIDS and can be transmitted from these patients to health care workers. Mycobacterial infection may be the disease of the 1990s, whereas HIV and hepatitis were the diseases of the 1980s. Of particular concern is the drug resistance of many strains of mycobacteria. Surgeons may have to relearn surgical lessons of the past in order to successfully treat patients with tuberculosis. There is great concern that health care workers be infected by these patients because the disease is spread by aerosolized particles. Other conditions that may lead to its spread include the crowding that occurs in large cities where these patients tend to reside. We will probably hear more about tuberculosis in the 1990s.

Richard J. Howard, M.D.

---

**Planned Reoperations and Open Management in Critical Intra-Abdominal Infections: Prospective Experience in 52 Cases**
Schein M (Univ of the Witwatersrand, Johannesburg, South Africa)
*World J Surg* 15:537–545, 1991                                     5–1

---

*Introduction.*—The outcome of an intraabdominal infection depends on the patient's systemic and peritoneal defenses and the degree and duration of contamination. Planned reoperations and open management have been used aggressively in selected patients with severe intra-abdominal infections since 1985.

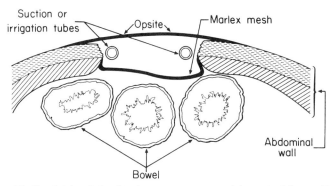

**Fig 5–1.**—The "sandwich technique" in the open management of the septic abdomen. (From Schein M; *World J Surg* 15:537–545, 1991. Courtesy of Schein M, Saadia R, Jamieson J, et al: *Br J Surg* 73:369, 1986.)

*Methods.*—From January 1985 to July 1989, 52 patients aged 23–84 years underwent treatment with this aggressive therapy protocol. Group I included 29 individuals with diffuse postoperative peritonitis, group II included 14 patients with diffuse fecal peritonitis, and group III included 9 individuals with infected pancreatic necrosis. The surgical protocol began with the usual clearing of the contamination source. Planned relaparotomies were done every 2–3 days under general anesthesia irrespective of the patient's clinical status. The use of open management was determined at laparotomy and depended on the patient's build, amount of abdominal distention, degree of parietal inflammation, necrosis, and predicted number of reoperations. Figure 5–1 shows the sandwich technique used in open management of the septic abdomen.

*Results.*—The mortality rates in groups I, II, and III were 55%, 14%, and 56%, respectively. There were 154 relaparotomies, an average of 3 procedures in each patient. Twenty-one patients had the abdomen closed, an average of 1.7 relaparotomies, and a 24% death rate. In 41 patients, gastrointestinal fistulas developed, and 21 (51%) in this group died. Two patients experienced intra-abdominal hemorrhage requiring surgery. Thirteen patients treated with open management survived.

*Conclusions.*—Planned relaparotomies can benefit patients who have severe intra-abdominal infections such as fecal peritonitis. Because multiple organ failure caused 20 of the 23 deaths, it appears that even the most aggressive treatment of intra-abdominal infection cannot reverse this complication.

▶ A problem with approaches such as this is selecting which patients have intra-abdominal infection severe enough to warrant reoperation and/or open management. Many studies of patients with intra-abdominal infection report mortality rates similar to those presented here using more conventional operative treatments without relaparotomy or open management. It is difficult to compare patients between centers, and even within a center, because they differ so markedly from one another. Even scoring systems such as the Acute Physiology and Chronic Health Evaluation II have not proved to be reliable enough for strict patient comparability. It is extremely difficult for any one center to randomize enough patients to comprise groups large enough to allow statistically valid comparisons. Multicenter studies of these techniques would be required. Even then, stratification of patients might still result in groups too small to permit significant statistical comparisons. Despite these shortcomings, it is important to continue to study innovative operative treatments for patients with severe intra-abdominal infections that will decrease the current high mortality rate.—R.J. Howard, M.D.

---

### Retroperitoneal Drainage in the Management of the Septic Phase of Severe Acute Pancreatitis

Villazón SA, Villazón DO, Terrazas EF, Raña GR (Hosp Español, Mexico City)
*World J Surg* 15:103–108, 1991                                                      5–2

---

*Background.*—Severe sepsis is a major complication of acute pancreatitis in patients who have survived its early systemic deleterious effects. Experience with retroperitoneal drainage in the management of the septic phase of severe acute pancreatitis was reviewed.

*Treatment.*—Between 1980 and 1987, 18 consecutive patients with sepsis caused by surgically confirmed peripancreatic necrosis that extended diffusely into the retroperitoneal fat underwent early retroperitoneal débridement of necrotic tissue and drainage through lumbar incisions. Based on the location and extent of the necrosis, the peritoneum was approached from a right, left, or bilateral lumbar incision. Necrotic tissue was removed manually, followed by abundant pressure lavage with saline solution. Two Silastic tubes were placed on each side to provide continuous lavage and drainage. All patients were fed through a feeding jejunostomy for 3–8 days after the first surgery.

*Results.*—Forty reoperations were performed, for an average of 2.6 per patient. There were 32 major complications, including respiratory failure in 17 cases, renal failure in 4, gastrointestinal bleeding in 4, retroperitoneal bleeding in 1, and gastrointestinal fistulas in 6. Four patients died, for a mortality of 22%, compared with 100% mortality before 1980 when patients were treated with different management techniques. The major cause of death was multiple organ failure secondary to sepsis.

*Conclusion.*—Retroperitoneal débridement and drainage substantially reduce the mortality associated with peripancreatic necrosis. Recognition of the necrotic stages of acute pancreatitis with modern imaging techniques will allow for prompt and better management of these patients.

▶ This novel approach to patients with pancreatic necrosis obviated the need to enter the peritoneal cavity. Nevertheless, the mortality rate (22%)

was comparable to that of series using the standard transperitoneal approach to the pancreas. Avoiding peritoneal contamination has some attraction, but it does not seem to affect overall results.—R.J. Howard, M.D.

---

**Early Surgical Débridement of Symptomatic Pancreatic Necrosis Is Beneficial Irrespective of Infection**
Rattner DW, Legermate DA, Lee MJ, Mueller PR, Warshaw AL (Massachusetts Gen Hosp, Boston; Harvard Med School, Boston)
*Am J Surg* 163:105–110, 1992 5–3

---

*Introduction.*—Recent studies indicate that infection is the primary determinant of outcome in pancreatitis complicated by the development of necrosis. Thus nonoperative management has been advocated for cases of sterile necrosis. The recent trend of minimally invasive therapy in patients with symptomatic necrotizing pancreatitis was assessed.

*Methods.*—During a 5-year period, 253 patients were admitted with a primary or secondary diagnosis of acute pancreatitis; 73 had significant pancreatic necrosis or abscess. The records of these patients were examined for 82 variables.

*Results.*—The median age was 60 years, and most patients (73%) were men. The etiology of pancreatitis was gallstone related in 34% and ethanol abuse related in 19%. Nearly all patients were symptomatic. The overall mortality rate was 25%. Preintervention variables associated with mortality were an Acute Physiology and Chronic Health Evaluation (APACHE) II score greater than 15, preintervention blood transfusion, respiratory failure, and shock. Almost all deaths (17 of 18) occurred in patients with recurrent sepsis after the initial intervention. Recurrent sepsis was correlated with the APACHE II score. The presence of infection had little impact on the patients' clinical course. Percutaneous drainage was associated with a longer hospital stay, more days in intensive care, and more days of total parenteral nutrition.

*Conclusion.*—Contrary to recommendations in some previous studies, the presence of infection should not determine the need for intervention in patients with pancreatic necrosis. Whereas infection is an absolute indication for débridement and drainage, the converse is not true. Symptomatic collections should be drained regardless of the bacteriologic status.

▶ These authors suggest that infection is not the indication to operate on patients with necrosis; rather, necrosis per se is associated with a high mortality rate if not treated surgically. Attempts at percutaneous drainage only delay appropriate surgical intervention and increase the likelihood of death. This report represents another important step in the increasingly aggressive approach to pancreatic necrosis that is necessary because the mortality rate associated with this complication of pancreatitis continues to be high.—R.J. Howard, M.D.

---

### Antibiotic Treatment for Surgical Peritonitis

Mosdell DM, Morris DM, Voltura A, Pitcher DE, Twiest MW, Milne RL, Miscall BG, Fry DE (Univ of New Mexico, Albuquerque; Albuquerque VA Med Ctr)
*Ann Surg* 214:543–549, 1991                                              5–4

---

*Background.*—Intraoperative cultures were long assumed necessary to determine proper postoperative therapy in patients with acute abdominal infections. But with the common use of broad-spectrum antibiotics in patients with peritonitis, the routine collection of culture material during surgery has been questioned. To examine this issue further, the charts of patients with secondary bacterial peritonitis, were reviewed.

*Methods.*—The target population consisted of patients with acute onset of peritonitis requiring operative therapy. During a 3-year period, 480 patients met the study criteria. Hospital records were evaluated in detail and patients divided into categories based on empiric antibiotic treatment. The antibiotics used were compared with the culture and sensitivity data obtained at surgery.

*Results.*—The patients included 300 males and 180 females whose average age was 44 years. More than half (281) of the infections were secondary to perforation of the appendix. Perforated colonic lesions accounted for 130 cases. The mortality rate was 6% and the intra-abdominal abscess rate, 10%. Intraoperative cultures were taken in 326 patients. The most common of the 781 bacterial isolates cultured were *Escherichia coli* and *Bacteroides fragilis.* In most cases (63%), a single antibiotic was the empiric choice; 19% were treated with 3 drugs and 17% with 2 drugs. Patients treated with a single broad-spectrum antibiotic had a better outcome than patients receiving multiple-drug treatment. Patients treated for anticipated organisms with no cultures taken did as well as patients who had cultures taken.

*Conclusion.*—The findings support the effectiveness of single-drug therapy in peritonitis. Killing normal bowel flora may be detrimental. Culture data rarely contribute in a useful way to the postoperative outcome and are often ignored by the surgeon.

▶ This retrospective review of 480 patients with peritonitis found that the main factor associated with poor outcome was the use of inadequate empiric antibiotics. Interestingly, patients who had no culture taken did as well as those who had cultures taken. Furthermore, culture data were usually ignored after operation. Although most discussed, antibiotic therapy is probably far less important than the adequacy of surgical treatment and the status of the patient's host defenses in treatment of secondary peritonitis. But because we can as yet do little about host defenses, surgical therapy has become rather standard, thus most discussion centers around antibiotic therapy. This study does not compare antibiotics, so one cannot say anything about one antibiotic possibly being better than another. In fact, even in prospective, randomized, comparative studies, usually no clear superiority of one antibiotic over another is found.—R.J. Howard, M.D.

**Prophylactic Intravenous Administration of Standard Immune Globulin as Compared With Core-Lipopolysaccharide Immune Globulin in Patients at High Risk of Postsurgical Infection**
Cometta A, for the Intravenous Immunoglobulin Collaborative Study Group (Centre Hospitalier Universitaire Vaudois, Lausanne, Switzerland)
*N Engl J Med* 327:234–240, 1992                                      5–5

*Introduction.*—Infections caused by gram-negative bacteria remain a major source of morbidity and mortality among patients in intensive care units. Preliminary data have suggested that antiserum from patients immunized with *Escherichia coli* J5 could lower mortality, as could antibodies against R595 lipopolysaccharide. A placebo-controlled, double-blind, randomized trial was conducted to determine whether standard immune globulin and core-lipopolysaccharide hyperimmune globulin could prevent postsurgical infections in high-risk patients.

*Methods.*—Patients who had undergone 1 of 7 types of surgery were stratified according to the type of operation for randomization. The core-lipopolysaccharide intravenous immune globulin was extracted from the plasma of 290 selected donors, and levels of IgG and anti-R595 lipopolysaccharide IgG antibody were measured.

*Results.*—The study population included 329 patients. All patients averaged about 1.5 infusions throughout the study. After randomization, patients receiving standard immune globulin had a significantly lower incidence of infections (e.g., pneumonia) than patients given placebo. The standard immune globulin groups also had a lower rate of acquired focal infections per 100 patient-days. The incidence of shock remained the same in all 3 comparative study groups. The mortality rate and hospital duration were lower in those receiving standard immune globulin, but the differences did not reach statistical significance.

*Conclusions.*—Prophylactic use of standard immune globulin significantly reduced infections and pneumonia after surgery compared with placebo. Overall, core-lipopolysaccharide hyperimmune globulin does not prevent gram-negative infections or accompanying complications.

▶ Interest has been renewed lately in treating bacterial infection with biological agents. Two reports of antibodies to endotoxin, HA-1A and E5, appeared recently (1, 2). Neither of these products is yet approved and both are undergoing further testing, although a clinical trial of HA-1A was stopped because of an unexpected high mortality rate. These authors examine whether or not prophylactic immunoglobulin can prevent infections in high-risk surgical patients. Surprisingly, immunoglobulin selected for a high antibody titer to core-lipopolysaccharide (C-LPS) did not lower the postoperative infection rate. Only standard immunoglobulin did. This lower infection rate resulted almost entirely from a decreased rate of pneumonia. There was also a statistically significant difference in focal infections after esophageal surgery but not other types of operations. There was no difference among any of the 3 groups for other types of infections. Furthermore, there was no decrease in sepsis or septic shock. In their discussion, the authors provide reasons for the surprising finding that treatment with C-LPS immune globulin resulted in no lower infection rate than placebo, whereas standard immune globulin did so. One would have thought that C-LPS immune globulin would at least be as good as standard immune globulin. The difference may have resulted from a type II statistical error.—R.J. Howard, M.D.

*References*

1. Greenman RL, et al: *JAMA* 266:1097, 1991.
2. Zeigler EJ, et al: *N Engl J Med* 324:429, 1991.

---

**Monoclonal Antibody to Tumor Necrosis Factor α Attenuates Cardiopulmonary Dysfunction in Porcine Gram-Negative Sepsis**
Walsh CJ, Sugerman HJ, Mullen PG, Carey PD, Leeper-Woodford SK, Jesmok GJ, Ellis EF, Fowler AA (Virginia Commonwealth Univ, Richmond; Cutter Biological Miles Inc, Berkeley, Calif)
*Arch Surg* 127:138–145, 1992                                    5–6

---

*Introduction.*—Antibiotic therapy and other new treatment modalities have not eliminated septic shock from patients in intensive care units, but new therapies are not under study. Recently developed therapeutic agents have focused on the biochemical and physiologic effects of bacteria and the release of its endotoxin into the human host. The outcome of the administration of antitumor necrosis factor-alpha (TNF-α) monoclonal antibody as pretreatment for gram-negative sepsis was evaluated in pigs.

*Methods.*—The IgG1 anti-TNF-α monoclonal antibody was purified to a 99% purity from a murine hybridoma cell culture. It was given to Yorkshire pigs 48 hours after they received penicillin G benzethine and penicillin G procaine. The animals then were ventilated and received a 5-F lung-water catheter. Both TNF and plasma thromboxane $B_2$ activity were measured in 3 study groups: group 1 received live *Pseudomonas aeruginosa*, group 2 received anti-TNF-α monoclonal antibody treatment, and group 3 received a saline control solution.

*Results.*—*Pseudomonas* infusion caused significant rises in plasma TNF levels within 30 minutes after initiation of the procedure; these lev-

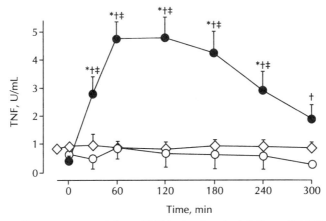

**Fig 5–2.**—Plasma tumor necrosis factor (TNF) levels, where 1 unit indicates 50% L929 cytotoxicity. *Open circles* represent saline-treated control animals ($n = 5$); *filled circles*, septic animals ($n = 7$) *squares*, anti-TNFα monoclonal antibody ($n = 6$); *asterisks*, $P < .05$ vs. baseline; *daggers*, $P < .05$ vs. saline-treated controls; and *double daggers*, $P < .05$ vs. anti-TNFα monoclonal antibody. (Courtesy of Walsh CJ, Sugerman HJ, Mullen PG, et al: *Arch Surg* 127:138–145, 1992.)

els remained high for up to 240 minutes (Fig 5–2). Pretreatment with anti-TNF-α monoclonal antibody eliminated the TNF increase. Plasma thromboxane levels rose markedly after the beginning of the *Pseudomonas* infusion and also peaked at 30 minutes, but were not reduced by anti-TNF-α monoclonal antibody pretreatment. Pulmonary artery occlusion and systemic arterial hypertension increased sharply during early sepsis, whereas arterial oxygen tension decreased markedly in both the septic and antibody-treated animals. Extravascular lung water increased significantly in the septic animals but not in the group given anti-TNF-α antibody.

*Conclusions.*—These findings indicate that the anti-TNF-α monoclonal antibody treatment significantly protected the animals against sepsis. The outcome of this trial does not eliminate the possibility of other mediators playing a role in early changes observed in the pig model.

▶ Antibiotics have been a great addition to the treatment of infectious diseases, but one wonders how much additional refinement of antibiotic therapy can improve the outcome of surgical infections. New therapies with biological agents such as antibodies to endotoxin (HA-1A and E5) or to mediators of infections such as antibody to TNF are currently undergoing clinical evaluation. The experimental study demonstrates that anti-TNF-α monoclonal antibody protected animals against a subsequent intravenous infusion with *Pseudomonas*. Although this treatment was effective when given before infection, it is critical to evaluate it when given after infection has already occurred, because that is what the clinician faces with patients. Clinical studies of anti-TNF antibody, in fact, are currently underway.—R.J. Howard, M.D.

### Are Blood Cultures Effective in the Evaluation of Fever in Perioperative Patients?

Theuer CP, Bongard FS, Klein SR (Harbor-UCLA Med Ctr, Torrance, Calif)
*Am J Surg* 162:615–619, 1991                                                          5–7

*Objective.*—The value of blood culture in the perioperative period was examined by reviewing all cultures performed on adult surgical services in a 5-week period.

*Methods.*—The 364 cultures examined represented 108 febrile events (temperature of 101.5°F or higher) in 72 patients without evidence of sepsis.

*Findings.*—All but 11% of the patients had undergone surgery before fever developed. Organisms were isolated in cultures from 9 patients, and cultures from 5 of these patients contained pathogens. Two of the 5 patients with positive cultures had an identifiable source of bacteremia. The cost of identifying each of these 5 patients was $2,800. Neither peak temperatures nor leukocyte counts predicted positive cultures, but immune depression, the day on which blood was drawn (table), and the presence of an indwelling device were predictive. In no instance did a positive result lessen morbidity or the risk of death.

*Conclusion.*—Blood cultures are not likely to be helpful in febrile adult perioperative patients who have no signs of sepsis.

▶ The results of this study question the value of doing routine blood cultures in febrile perioperative patients who have no other evidence of sepsis, something that could result in a great cost saving and might be unnecessary. Even in the 5 of 72 patients who had true positive blood cultures there was no measurable effect of the positive culture in reducing morbidity and mortality, even though the patients received antibiotic therapy. We must always be

Proportions of Positive Blood Culture Vials and Positive
Culture Events by Day of Collection

|  | Pre-operative | Post-operative Days 0–3 | Post-operative Days 4–7 | Post-operative Days 8–10 | Post-operative Days >10 |
|---|---|---|---|---|---|
| Number + vials/vials submitted | 0/38 | 0/85 | 5/100 | 6/36 | 0/97 |
| Number + cultures/febrile events | 0/12 | 0/26 | 4/30 | 2/10 | 0/29 |

(Courtesy of Theuer CP, Bongard FS, Klein SR: *Am J Surg* 162:615–619, 1991.)

ready to challenge our closely held, but unsubstantiated, assumptions.—R.J. Howard, M.D.

---

**Postinjury Shock and Early Bacteremia: A Lethal Combination**
Moore FA, Moore EE, Poggetti RS, Read RA (Denver Gen Hosp, Denver, Colo)
*Arch Surg* 127:893–898, 1992                                              5–8

---

*Background.*—There is expeimental evidence for the hypothesis that bacterial translocation or the transmural migration of viable indigenous organisms from the gastrointestinal tract has a pivotal role in irreversible postinjury shock. Clinical evidence fot this phenomenon, however, remains elusive. The incidence of early bacteremia in trauma patients at risk for hemorrhagic shock was determined and the association between bacteremia and mortality examined.

*Patients.*—During a 14-month period, blood cultures were obtained in the emergency department (ED) from 132 patients who required urgent laparotomy for acute abdominal traumatic injuries. The mechanism of injury was blunt trauma in 40 patients, gunshot wounds in 42, and stab wounds in 50. Shock was defined as 2 systolic blood pressure (SBP) recordings in the ED of less than 90 mm Hg. In 38 patients, mesenteric lymph nodes and a liver biopsy specimen were also obtained and cultured.

*Results.*—Twenty-two of the 132 patients (17%) had positive blood culture results. Ten of 94 patients (11%) with ED SBPs of 90 mm Hg or greater and 12 of 38 patients (32%) with shock had positive blood culture results. Eight of the 12 bacteremic patients with shock died, including all 7 of those with enteric bacteremias (table). In contrast, coagulase-negative staphylococci were isolated in 5 bacteremic patients with shock

Mortality by Emergency Department Shock and
Culture Results

| | Mortality, No. (%) |
|---|---|
| No shock, no bacteremia | 1/72 (1) |
| No shock, bacteremia | 0/10 (0) |
| Shock, no bacteremia | 7/27 (26) |
| Shock plus bacteremia | 8/12 (75)* |
| Shock plus enteric bacteremia | 7/7 (100) |

Note: Shock was defined as 2 emergency department systolic blood pressure recordings less than 90 mm Hg.
* Significantly different (P < .05) from shock, no bacteremia; no shock, bacteremia; and no shock, no bacteremia.
(Courtesy of Moore FA, Moore EE, Poggetti RS, et al: *Arch Surg* 127:893–898, 1992.)

but only 1 of those 5 patients died of late multiple organ failure; the other 4 recovered uneventfully. None of the 10 bacteremic patients with ED SBPs of 90 mm Hg or higher died. Four of the 38 patients (11%) from whom liver biopsy specimens were obtained had positive cultures. Three of those 4 patients had coagulase-negative staphylococcal cultures and all 3 survived. The fourth patient had *Enterobacter* bacteremia and died.

*Conclusions.*—Enteric bacteremia was found only in moribund trauma patients with hemorrhagic shock. Whether the early enteric bacteremias contributed to their early death or were simply an epiphenomenon of the severe shock remains to be determined.

▶ These authors seek evidence that bacterial translocation occurs more commonly in patients with shock than in patients without shock, as is found in experimental animals. As is pointed out in the discussion, however, these blood cultures were drawn in the emergency room and may not be very reliable because of the high rate of contamination and because a single blood culture that grows coagulase-negative staphylococci may not be reliable. Most of the bacteria (73%) were gram-positive isolates, whereas one would suspect gram-negative intestinal bacteria to predominate if translocation were a truly important cause of bacteremia.

Unfortunately, the authors included patients who had perforation of a hollow viscus, and one cannot prove that bacteremia occurred only from translocation and not from absorption of spilled intestinal contents in the peritoneal cavity. The authors do not set apart this group of patients. It also would have been interesting to culture the portal vein for bacteria or to measure endotoxin levels.

The question of the role of bacterial translocation in enteric bacteremia remains, with the exception of a small number of diseases and a specific type of bacteria that translocates. One is still hard pressed to prove it is of clinical importance for most diseases. Yet, the doubters must hypothesize another route that allows entrance of bacteria from the gastrointestinal tract into the bloodstream if it does not occur by translocation.—R.J. Howard, M.D.

---

**Clostridial Bacteremia: Implications for the Surgeon**
de Virgilio C, Klein S, Chang L, Klassen M, Bongard F (Harbor-UCLA Med Ctr, Torrance, Calif)
*Ann Surg* 57:388–393, 1991                                              5–9

---

*Introduction.*—Clostridial bacteremia is a rare event, but its associated mortality rate is as high as 50% to 70%. Indications vary from a lack of symptoms to septic shock. Experience with clostridial bacteremia was reviewed to better understand its predisposing conditions and the prognostic factors associated with survival.

*Patients.*—The study group included 29 men and 18 women whose average age was 49 years. These patients had a variety of underlying disorders, including ethanol abuse (18), severe atherosclerotic disease (12), liver disease (9), and malignancy (7). Common signs and symptoms included gastrointestinal bleeding (38%), abdominal pain (28%), hyperthermia (40%), hypotension (40%), and altered mental status (43%). Leukocytosis was found in 55% of the patients.

*Findings.*—Predisposing factors included systemic immunosuppression (53%), locally decreased oxidation reduction potential (Eh) (43%), and a site of epithelial barrier disruption. The gastrointestinal tract was the site of clostridial invasion in 22 patients; sites in the other patients were pulmonary (7), cutaneous (7), female genital tract (4), and undetermined (7). Histotoxic species (*Clostridium perfringens* and *Clostridium septicum*) accounted for 79% of blood culture isolates. Mortality was 47% and was associated with advanced age, underlying illness, and presence of a histotoxic species.

*Conclusion.*—Though clostridia are normally found in the gastrointestinal and female genital tracts, clostridial sepsis is a rare event. Clostridia proliferate only when the Eh is reduced. Another predisposing factor is disruption of an epithelial barrier that allows access of the organism into the bloodstream. Prompt intervention should include high-dose intravenous penicillin and surgical removal of the focus of infection.

▶ Clostridial bacteremia, a rare event, is associated with a high mortality rate. Yet, the true role of clostridial bacteremia in the patients described in this study is difficult to evaluate. Although 23 patients died, the authors do not indicate which deaths they thought were caused by clostridial bacteremia or what role the clostridia had in the patients' demise. Many patients were sick from other diseases such as pancreatic abscess that were potentially lethal. The clostridial bacteremia may have occurred in the terminal phases of a process that was lethal anyway. We also do not get a sense of what the underlying diseases of these patients were and how sick they were. The most common organisms identified, *C. perfringens* and *C. septicum,* can cause rapidly lethal necrotizing soft tissue infections. When these organisms are cultured only from the blood, it can be difficult to evaluate what role they have in causing actual disease.—R.J. Howard, M.D.

**Infrainguinal Anastomotic Arterial Graft Infections Treated by Selective Graft Preservation**
Calligaro KD, Westcott CJ, Buckley RM, Savarese RP, DeLaurentis DA (Pennsylvania Hosp, Philadelphia)
*Ann Surg* 216:74–79, 1992                                                   5–10

*Introduction.*—Patients with infections involving an arterial graft anastomosis are usually treated by removing the graft. This approach, however, is associated with a high mortality rate. These complications could

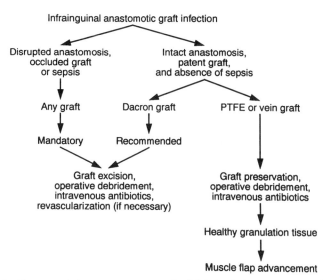

**Fig 5–3.**—Recommended management protocol of infrainguinal anastomotic graft infections. (Courtesy of Calligaro KD, Westcott CJ, Buckley RM, et al: *Ann Surg* 216:74–79, 1992.)

be avoided in aseptic patients by preserving those grafts that are patent and have intact anastomosis. A study was undertaken to determine whether "smooth-walled" polytetrafluoroethylene (PTFE) or autologous vein grafts are more easily sterilized post infection, or are more resistant to infection than knitted or woven Dacron grafts. An analysis was made of the records of 35 patients of both sexes aged 48–85 years who had anastomotic infections involving a common femoral or distal artery.

*Results.*—Fourteen patients had Dacron grafts. Immediate graft excision was necessary in 9 patients because of anastomotic bleeding, systemic sepsis, or graft occlusion. An attempt was made to preserve the graft in the remaining 5 patients, but delayed excision was necessary in 3 because of nonhealing wounds. Thus, of the original 14 patients, preservation was possible in only 2 (14%). In contrast, of the 21 patients with smooth-walled grafts, including 14 with PTFE grafts, only 10 required immediate excision. Eight of these 10 patients had PTFE grafts. Also, a single patient with a PTFE graft required a delayed excision. Ultimately, graft preservation was successful in 10 patients (48%) with smooth-walled grafts.

*Conclusions.*—The results support earlier work indicating the difficulty of eradicating bacteria from Dacron graft interstices. Excision of Dacron grafts is recommended when it is determined that the anastomosis is infected. In contrast, the prognosis for preservation of smooth-walled grafts is good after operative débridement and treatment with antibiotics intravenously (Fig 5–3).

▶ Attempts to save infected synthetic arterial grafts almost always lead to failure, especially if the anastomotic line is involved. These authors almost uniformly failed to save Dacron grafts, which had interstices in which bacteria might "hide" from phagocytic cells. They were able to save just under half of "smooth-walled" grafts made of vein or PTFE in patients who had intact anastomoses and absence of sepsis. Critical to their treatment was repeated aggressive operative excision of infected soft tissue, including removal of exudate on the graft or artery. Once healthy granulation tissue was present, myocutaneous flaps were used to cover the graft. They also found that grafts could be saved only when gram-positive organisms were cultured from the graft. They failed when gram-negative organisms were cultured. These infections are uncommon but can be disasters when they occur. Physicians who follow the authors' algorithm may be able to preserve some infected "smooth-walled" arterial grafts.—R.J. Howard, M.D.

## Tuberculosis and the Surgeon

Langdale LA, Meissner M, Nolan C, Ashbaugh DG (Univ of Washington, Seattle; King County Health Dept, Seattle)
*Am J Surg* 163:505–509, 1992                5–11

*Introduction.*—Surgery was a mainstay in the treatment of tuberculosis (TB) during the early part of the century. With the introduction of antibiotics and effective screening programs, the United States experienced a steady decline in the number of reported TB infections. Tuberculosis has returned, however, as a significant threat to public health. The current role of surgery in the diagnosis and treatment of tuberculosis was assessed.

*Methods.*—During a 5-year period, 121 of 357 patients who received care for TB required invasive procedures during their workup. Their records were examined for demographics, mycobacterium type, treatment regimen, and associated illnesses.

*Results.*—The mean age was 48 years; the male to female ratio was 4.3:1. Alcoholism (55%) and smoking (64%) were common risk factors in the patients requiring invasive procedures. Chronic obstructive pulmonary disease was documented in 23% of the patients; 11% were HIV positive. *Mycobacterium tuberculosis* was cultured in 68% of patients and atypical mycobacteria in 19%. The 121 patients underwent a total of 189 invasive procedures, 88% of which were performed to establish diagnosis or treat a complication of known disease. Nineteen of the 93 patients with pulmonary evidence of TB required operative intervention.

*Conclusion.*—The findings confirm that the resurgence of TB is not explained solely by the rise in AIDS. Surgeons may be called upon with increasing frequency to treat the thoracic complications of the disease.

▶ Until the 1950s, TB was the cause of much surgical disease. Thoracic surgeons were educated to operate on patients with pulmonary TB. Better nutrition and effective chemotherapy greatly decreased the prevalence of the disease. Tuberculosis is making a resurgence, especially in individuals who are HIV positive. The prevalence of TB is rapidly increasing in this population, and it may spread to other individuals as well. This and other articles document the resurgence of TB as a cause of surgical disease. Many lessons of the past will have to be relearned by surgeons who currently have never seen or operated on a patient with TB. Tuberculosis and other mycobacterial infections in patients with AIDS are particularly worrisome because they are frequently not treatable by current chemotherapeutic agents, and the mortality rate is extremely high.—R.J. Howard, M.D.

---

**Nosocomial Transmission of Multidrug-Resistant *Mycobacterium tuberculosis:* A Risk to Patients and Health Care Workers**
Pearson ML, Jereb JA, Frieden TR, Crawford JT, Davis BJ, Dooley SW, Jarvis WR (Ctrs for Disease Control, Atlanta, Ga)
*Ann Intern Med* 117:191–196, 1992                                     5–12

---

*Introduction.*—Tuberculosis (TB) has again become a major public health problem in the United States, with nearly 26,000 cases documented in 1990. Whereas drug-resistant TB used to occur mainly in previously treated TB patients and in immigrants from countries in which drug-resistant TB is prevalent, it has now become an important problem outside those 2 high-risk groups. A retrospective case-control study was undertaken to identify risk factors for the acquisition of multidrug-resistant TB and to investigate the possibility of nosocomial transmission in an inner-city hospital.

*Patients.*—From January 1989 through March 1991, 17 men and 6 women (median age, 34 years) had a diagnosis of active TB. Their *Mycobacterium tuberculosis* isolates were resistant to at least isoniazid and rifampin. Nineteen men and 4 women (median age, 42 years) who had a diagnosis of active TB during the same period and whose isolates were susceptible to all drugs tested served as controls. All *M. tuberculosis* isolates were typed by restriction fragment length polymorphism (RFLP) analysis. Tuberculin skin test conversion rates were compared for health care workers assigned to wards where patients with TB were either frequently or rarely admitted.

*Results.*—Twenty-one cases (91%) and 11 controls (48%) were HIV seropostive. Nineteen cases (83%) and 5 controls (22%) had a previous admission to the study institution within 7 months before onset of TB. Thus patients with HIV infection and previous exposure to multidrug-resistant TB at this hospital were identified as being at increased risk for multidrug-resistant TB. Eleven of 32 health care workers assigned to wards housing cases had tuberculin skin test conversions, compared with only 1 of 47 health care workers assigned to other wards. Fourteen of the 16 multidrug-resistant isolates available for RFLP analysis had identical banding patterns, whereas all control isolates had unique banding patterns. Only 6 of the 23 cases had been placed in acid-fast bacilli isolation, and none of the rooms had negative pressure when tested.

*Conclusions.*—Nosocomial transmission of multidrug-resistant TB occurs from patient to patient, and from patient to health care worker. Better policies for isolating patients infected with M. *tuberculosis* are urgently needed.

▶ Whereas viral diseases transmitted by blood and body fluids (e.g., HIV and hepatitis) were the diseases of the 1980s, TB may be the disease of the 1990s for health care workers. This study shows the increased risk of health care workers for tuberculin skin test conversions (and presumably TB as well) if they are on a ward housing patients with TB compared to health care workers assigned to other wards. Tuberculosis occurring in AIDS patients is of great concern because it is resistant to most currently available drugs and because it is transmitted by aerosols. In the hospital setting, one can theoretically completely avoid transmission of HIV and hepatitis by avoiding direct contact with patients' blood and body fluids. Transmission of these diseases to health care workers from patients is sporadic. On the other hand, patients with TB can spread the infection both to health care workers and other patients. Proposals by the National Institute for Occupational Safety and Health call for health care workers visiting the rooms of patients with TB to wear a self-contained breathing apparatus much like a scuba diving gear. This device, if required, will be expensive and may compromise care of the patient. No doubt we will hear much more about hospital-acquired TB during the 1990s.—R.J. Howard, M.D.

---

**Value of Lymph Node Biopsy in the Treatment of Patients With the Human Immunodeficiency Virus**
Wong R, Rappaport W, Gorman S, Darragh M, Hunter G, Witzke D (Univ of Arizona, Tucson)
*Am J Surg* 162:590–593, 1991                                              5–13

---

*Purpose.*—Although lymphadenopathy is a common finding in patients with AIDS or AIDS-related complex (ARC), the value of lymph node biopsy in HIV-infected individuals has not been established. In a retrospective chart review of 24 patients with AIDS or ARC who underwent lymph node biopsy, indications for biopsy were identified and the impact of this procedure on treatment was evaluated.

*Methods and Patients.*—Data analyzed included demographics, biopsy site and complications, findings and resultant treatment, and T cell subsets. The 22 men and 2 women had a mean age of 36 years. They underwent 29 lymph node biopsy procedures, 9 under local anesthesia and 20 under general anesthesia.

*Results.*—Sixteen of the biopsies were performed because of symptoms suggestive of B type lymphoma. The most common diagnosis was atypical follicular hyperplasia. Results of 19 biopsy procedures resulted in initiation or change of treatment. Patients who received treatment based on biopsy results had lower absolute T helper cell counts than those who were not treated 140 vs. 320 cells/$\mu$L). During a mean follow-up of 16 months, 12 patients died of complications of AIDS. Survivors had lymph node biopsy performed sooner after the onset of adenopathy than did the patients who died (7 months vs. 24 months).

*Conclusion.*—Lymph node biopsy can significantly alter therapy in certain subsets of HIV-infected patients. Indications for biopsy include new or worsening symptoms in patients with known adenopathy of uncertain etiology, a single disproportionately large or enlarging lymph node in a patient with generalized adenopathy, and a need to rule out further concomitant disease. General anesthesia is recommended to avoid the risk of accidental needlesticks. Complications in this series were few and minor.

▶ These authors found that lymph node biopsy in patients with AIDS and ARC is helpful in alternating or initiating therapy. Lymph node biopsy was commonly performed early in the era of AIDS to look for a treatable cause of fever or treatable diseases or for diagnosis before serologic testing was available. Our own experience is that lymph node biopsy is rarely, if ever, helpful in either of these circumstances and does not change the ultimate outcome of the disease. Many centers do not perform lymph node biopsy but, rather, rely on fine-needle aspiration cytology or core needle biopsy. The authors state that they perform all biopsies under general anesthesia to avoid needlestick injuries when local anesthesia is used. The CDC's Universal Precautions provide that all patients should be regarded as if they have a potentially infectious disease (e.g., HIV, hepatitis B or C), thus all patients should be treated the same. The authors' use of general anesthesia to perform lymph node biopsy demonstrates, in fact, that human behavior dictates that individuals who are known to be infectious are treated differently from those who are only potentially infectious.—R.J. Howard, M.D.

# 6 Transplantation

## Introduction

In recent years, the development of better transplantation techniques, new immunosuppressive regimens, extension to more organs, and an increased number of transplant centers have greatly increased the indications for transplantation and the number of suitable potential recipients. These factors have combined to accentuate the shortage of organs available for transplantation. The first three articles reviewed here deal with problems related to the waiting time of graft recipients and the shortage of organs. The first article by Sanfilippo et al. (Abstract 6-1) discusses factors that lead to a long time on the waiting list for cadaveric kidneys. Articles by Evans et al. (Abstract 6-2) and Roth et al. (Abstract 6-3) discuss the efficiency of obtaining potential cadaveric donors and suitability for transplantation of organs from donors positive for antibody to hepatitis C.

The results of kidney transplantation continued to improve. Two articles discuss the improving results of transplantation and provide data against which individual transplantation programs can compare their own results. The first is from the United Network for Organ Sharing (Abstract 6-4), and the second is from the University of Minnesota (Abstract 6-5). Patients previously thought to be marginal transplant candidates—the very young and older patients—can experience graft survival comparable to that seen in individuals who historically are thought to be more suitable candidates.

Liver transplantation continues to progress as well. The most common technical complication of liver transplantation remains problems relating to the biliary tract. Two articles discuss biliary tract complications and possible methods of prevention and treatment (Abstracts 6-9 and 6-10). Indications for liver transplantation are also continuing to widen. Alcoholic cirrhosis was formerly thought to be a contraindication to transplantation. It still is if the patients continue to use alcohol and do not have good social support networks. However, patients with cirrhosis caused by alcohol abuse apparently do as well as those who have liver disease from other causes. Patients with clotted portal veins or previous portacaval shunts also were regarded as having contraindications to liver transplantation. Transplantation can now be done successfully in individuals with these conditions. The recurrence rate of carcinoma of the liver or bile ducts is high. Many centers are still reluctant to perform transplant procedures in individuals with these conditions, but reasonable survival rates can be achieved in selected patients with hepatocellular cancer and cholangiocarcinoma.

An article from the Pittsburgh transplant group demonstrated donor cells in liver transplant recipients outside of the transplant organ. Finding these cells is taken as evidence that, because systemic chimerism is achieved, tolerance has been achieved. Whether this will lead to a reduction or possible elimination of the necessity for immunosuppression remains to be seen.

A remarkable article on small bile transplantation for short gut syndrome reports success in 16 patients, with 12 patients completely off total parenteral nutrition. This article and one on lung transplantation, a procedure that is rapidly gaining acceptance at many transplant centers, provide further evidence for the continued expansion of transplantation into new organs.

Richard J. Howard, M.D.

---

### Factors Affecting the Waiting Time of Cadaveric Kidney Transplant Candidates in the United States

Sanfilippo FP, Vaughn WK, Peters TG, Shield CF III, Adams PL, Lorber MI, Williams GM (Duke Univ, Durham, NC; United Network for Organ Sharing, Richmond, Va; Methodist Med Ctr, Jacksonville, Fla; St Francis Regional Med Ctr, Wichita, Kan; Bowman Gray School of Medicine, Winston-Salem, NC; et al)
*JAMA* 267:247–252, 1992                                                    6–1

---

*Background.*—Equitable access to donor organs is a subject of some controversy. Reports have suggested that blacks have a longer waiting period than whites, and foreign nationals appear to have received preferential treatment at certain centers. The relative impact of factors that might account for differences in waiting time of cadaveric kidney transplant candidates was examined.

*Methods.*—Patient data were obtained from the Organ Procurement and Transplantation Network (OPTN) of the United States. All United States transplant centers and organ procurement organizations are required to be members of the OPTN. Multivariate analyses were used to identify associations between 36 patient, donor, and center factors with waiting time for the 23,468 cadaveric renal transplant candidates listed between October 1, 1987 and June 30, 1990.

*Results.*—Immunologic factors had the greatest effect on waiting time for a cadaveric kidney. Among these factors were presensitization to HLA antigens, O or B blood type, candidacy for a repeat transplantation, and expression of rare HLA-A or HLA-B antigen phenotypes. Waiting times were significantly shorter for younger patients and those listed at multiple centers. The mean waiting times were 11.9 months for whites and 15.4 months for blacks. Patients whose local center had a small number of transplantation candidates and those who lived in areas with a high kidney organ recovery rate had shorter waiting times.

*Conclusion.*—Although immunologic factors are most important in determining the waiting time for a cadaveric kidney, other variables result in a longer wait for blacks. Increased organ donation from blacks should help to shorten this time. Further, the OPTN should consider whether it is fair for patients who can afford it to be listed at multiple centers. This practice discriminates against socioeconomically disadvantaged recipients.

▶ Data from the UNOS are used to evaluate those parameters that affect time on the waiting list for cadaveric kidney transplant candidates. As might be expected, presensitization to HLAs and having O or B blood types are the most important factors. Despite the desire for "fairness" and to allow patients equal access to cadaveric kidneys, this paper shows that certain patient characteristics contribute to longer waiting times. The current system of organ sharing awards points to patients who have high levels of panel reactive antibody and have been on the waiting list a long time to facilitate transplantation in these individuals. Patients who have 6 antigen matches with the donor are given top priority. Strategies for organ sharing other than those currently used by the UNOS can also be applied but might be less "fair" to certain groups of patients.—R.J. Howard, M.D.

---

## The Potential Supply of Organ Donors: An Assessment of the Efficiency of Organ Procurement Efforts in the United States

Evans RW, Orians CE, Ascher NL (Battelle-Seattle Research Ctr, Seattle, Wash; Univ of California, San Francisco)
*JAMA* 267:239–246, 1992                6–2

*Background.*—As of May 1991, more than 23,000 persons in the United States were awaiting transplant procedures. The number of available donors remained virtually unchanged from 1986 to 1989, despite efforts to increase the supply. In 1990 the donor supply increased modestly by 9%. Surveys show that the general public is well aware of the need for donor organs, but people remain reluctant to have their own organs donated or to consent to donation by relatives.

*Study Plan.*—The potential organ supply was estimated from cause-of-death and sociodemographic data collected by the National Center for Health Statistics. Estimates were based on deaths involving significant head trauma only and on deaths involving head trauma or incidents in which brain death was less likely.

*Findings.*—As many as 10,700 potential donors are available annually, meaning that current organ procurement efforts are 37% to 59% efficient. The efficiency varies widely by state and by organ procurement organization.

*Implications.*—Many more organ donors are available than are being accessed. It may be feasible to increase the numbers of available donors by 80%. The demand will, however, continue to increase.

▶ Despite the thousands of persons in the United States awaiting transplant operations, the number of donors for transplantation has remained relatively constant since 1986. The authors estimate the number of potential donors could be increased by 172% to 267%. They discuss reasons for the lack of efficiency in donor procurement and methods to increase the organ retrieval rate. A controversial method to increase the number of organ donors currently undergoing discussion is financial reimbursement to families of donors. What role it will have in increasing the donor supply, if it is ever adopted, remains to be seen.—R.J. Howard, M.D.

---

### Detection of Hepatitis C Virus Infection Among Cadaver Organ Donors: Evidence for Low Transmission of Disease
Roth D, Fernandez JA, Babischkin S, De Mattos A, Buck BE, Quan S, Olson L, Burke GW, Nery JR, Esquenazi V, Schiff ER, Miller J (Miami, Fla; Div of Transplantation, Miami; Tissue Bank, Miami; Chiron Corp, Emeryville, Calif)
*Ann Intern Med* 117:470–475, 1992                                          6–3

---

*Background.*—The safety of organs obtained from donors seropositive for antihepatitis C virus (HCV) for use in transplantation remains controversial because the clinical consequences are still unknown and

Clinical Characteristics of HCV-Seronegative Recipients of a Kidney from an
Anti-HCV–Seropositive or Anti-HCV–Seronegative Donor

| Variable | Donor Anti-HCV Status | | *P* Value |
|---|---|---|---|
| | Positive | Negative | |
| Patients, *n* | 15 | 120 | > 0.2 |
| Men/women, *n/n* | 9/6 | 75/45 | > 0.2 |
| Age (± SD), *y* | 43.1 ± 9.1 | 44.8 ± 11.4 | > 0.2 |
| Follow-up (± SD), *mo* | 60.4 ± 13.8 | 54.6 ± 20.1 | > 0.2 |
| Blood transfusions, *n†* | 7.0 ± 3.9 | 7.6 ± 6.2 | > 0.2 |
| ALG, mg‡ | 5650 ± 6470 | 6973 ± 4588 | > 0.2 |
| Post-transplant liver disease, *n/N(%)* | 4 of 15 (26) | 19 of 120 (16) | > 0.2 |
| Five-year survival (95% CI), %§ | | | |
|   Patient | 78 (57 to 99) | 83 (76 to 90) | > 0.2 |
|   Graft | 65 (41 to 89) | 61 (52 to 70) | > 0.2 |

*Abbreviation:* ALG, antilymphoblast globulin.
† Units of blood transfused pretransplant.
‡ Total antilymphoblast globulin administered for induction therapy.
§ Actuarial survival; numbers in parentheses are 95% confidence intervals.
(Courtesy of Roth D, Fernandez JA, Babischkin S, et al: *Ann Intern Med* 117:470–475, 1992.)

because the reliability of the anti-C100 enzyme-linked immunosorbent assay (ELISA) to detect HCV is uncertain. The prevalence of antibodies to HCV (anti-HCV) and HCV RNA was determined in cadaver organ donors, and the clinical consequences of infection with HCV were assessed.

*Methods.*—During a 12-year period, 1,096 cadaver organ donors were retrieved by an organ procurement program; stored serum samples were available for 484 cadavers. Fresh serum samples were obtained from 28 of 46 renal allograft recipients of organs harvested from donors with positive recombinant immunoblot assay (RIBA) results. Serum samples were analyzed for anti-HCV using the anti-C100 ELISA. Seropositive samples were retested with a second-generation RIBA. Hepatitis C viral RNA in serum was detected using the polymerase chain reaction (PCR). Liver biopsy specimens obtained from organ donors were analyzed by a pathologist who was blinded to the clinical data.

*Results.*—Of the 484 cadaver serum samples, 89 were seropositive for HCV by ELISA, but only 33 of these were RIBA seropositive. Serum samples from 30 RIBA-positive donors were tested for HCV RNA by PCR, and HCV RNA sequences were detected in 15 (50%) of these. Sixteen of 24 available liver tissue samples from RIBA-positive donors had evidence of chronic active hepatitis, 2 indicated chronic persistent hepatitis, and 6 were normal. In 13 (28%) of the 46 recipients of a kidney from a RIBA-positive donor posttransplant liver disease developed, but 6 of these 13 remained HCV seronegative at follow-up. Of the 46 kidney recipients of a kidney from a RIBA-positive donor, 29 still had a functioning graft after a mean follow-up of 40.5 months, 10 returned to dialysis, and 7 died. None of the deaths was attributable to liver disease. When compared with 120 HCV-seronegative renal allograft recipients who received a kidney from an anti-HCV-negative donor, the outcome in those who received a kidney from an anti-HCV-positive donor was not significantly different (table).

*Conclusions.*—Transmission of HCV by organ transplantation is infrequent, and the consequences of infection are small. The use of an organ from an anti-HCV-seropositive donor should be considered in seriously ill potential recipients who have exhausted other viable options.

▶ With the current great shortage of cadaveric donors, one is reluctant to discard any organ that can be transplanted safely. Most surgeons are currently not willing to transplant HCV-seropositive organs, although some transplant these organs into HCV-seropositive recipients. (There is still the risk that various serotypes of HCV exist, and that even an HCV-seropositive recipient could be infected with a different strain of HCV.) This paper provides evidence that organs from HCV-seropositive donors did not seem to have a measurable effect on the development of liver disease or mortality rate in recipients during a 12-year period. Hepatitis C virus is indolent, however, and a longer follow-up may be required to detect adverse effects of receiving HCV-positive kidneys.—R.J. Howard, M.D.

## Analyses of the UNOS Scientific Renal Transplant Registry at Three Years: Early Events Affecting Transplant Success

Cecka JM, Cho YW, Terasaki PI (Univ of California, Los Angeles)
Transplantation 53:59–64, 1992 6–4

*Introduction.*—The success of cadaver kidney transplantation in the first posttransplant year depends to a considerable extent on events occurring during the patient's hospitalization. Data concerning 19,525 cadaver renal transplants performed since late 1987 at more than 200 centers nationwide and reported to the United Network for Organ Sharing Scientific Renal Transplant Registry were reviewed.

*Findings.*—The overall 1-year graft survival for recipients of primary cadaver grafts was 78%, and for patients undergoing retransplantation, 69%. Rates were better in both groups if the graft produced urine on the first posttransplant day. If the graft functioned adequately for the first week and dialysis was not required, the 1-year graft survival rate was 83% in primary transplant recipients and 80% in those with repeat transplants. Lack of rejection through the time of discharge also was associated with a relatively good outcome. A well-functioning graft or a discharge serum creatinine level of less than 2.6 mg/dL was the strongest single predictor of graft survival at 1 year.

*Donor and Treatment Factors.*—A cold ischemia time exceeding 48 hours disposed to early nonfunction, as did a donor age greater than 50 years and a donor history of stroke. The only comparably important recipient factor was pretransplant blood transfusion. Administration of antilymphocyte globulin or OKT3 was not a prominent factor in the 1-year outcome. Prophylactic use of antibody in patients with retransplants did significantly (but modestly) improve graft survival at 1 year.

*Implication.*—If a cadaver kidney recipient is discharged with a well-functioning transplant, the risk of failure in the first year is lowered to 1 in 10, whether or not a previous graft has failed.

▶ This large series of transplant recipients from the United Network for Organ Sharing Scientific Renal Transplant Registry provides a standard against which individual programs can be measured. The authors describe survival of cadaveric graft recipients and discuss various parameters that led to improved graft survival.—R.J. Howard, M.D.

## Causes of Renal Allograft Loss: Progress in the 1980s, Challenges for the 1990s

Schweitzer EJ, Matas AJ, Gillingham KJ, Payne WD, Gores PF, Dunn DL, Sutherland DER, Najarian JS (Univ of Minnesota, Minneapolis)
Ann Surg 214:679–688, 1991 6–5

*Introduction.*—The management of kidney transplant recipients has undergone a number of refinements during the past decade. To assess the impact of changes in operative techniques, immunosuppressive drugs, anesthesia, and intensive care, the rate and causes of graft loss during 2 time periods were compared.

*Methods.*—During the first period (1970–1979), 1,012 primary kidney transplants were performed; the second period (1980–1989) included 1,384 patients. There were proportionately more cadaver donors and diabetic recipients in the 1980s, but the mean age and sex distribution were similar in the 2 periods. On October 23, 1990, actuarial patient and graft survival rates were calculated by cause of graft loss and decade of transplantation.

*Results.*—Differences in actuarial graft survival rates and actuarial patient survival rates were highly significant for the 2 periods. At 10 years, the actuarial graft survival was 43% in the 1970s and 52% in the 1980s; the actuarial patient survival at 10 years was 57% in the 1970s and 68% in the 1980s. The overall improvement in graft survival rates in the 1980s was principally the result of fewer cases of acute rejection and fewer deaths from infection. In both decades, death with function accounted for 48% of grafts losses; 24% of graft losses were caused by chronic rejection, and 18% by cardiovascular events.

*Conclusion.*—Cardiovascular causes of death and chronic rejection, which showed little improvement over the years, should be the focus of research efforts. Graft survival and patient survival have improved significantly for kidney transplant recipients, however.

▶ This retrospective review comparing the decade of the 1970s and the decade of the 1980s from a large transplant center, the University of Minnesota, discusses the continued improvement in results of kidney transplantation despite accepting higher-risk patients for transplantation. Although chronic rejection was the main immunologic cause of graft loss, death with function accounted for almost half of all graft losses. Cardiovascular disease was the most common cause of death and showed little improvement over the years. As the authors stress, further improvement in kidney transplant results requires a focus on these 2 difficult problems.—R.J. Howard, M.D.

---

**Renal Transplantation in Children: A Report of the North American Pediatric Renal Transplant Cooperative Study**

McEnery PT, Stablein DM, Arbus G, Tejani A (Children's Hosp Med Ctr, Cincinnati, Ohio; EMMES Corp, Potomac, Md; Hosp for Sick Children, Toronto, Ont, Canada; State Univ of New York, Brooklyn)
*N Engl J Med* 326:1727–1732, 1992                                          6–6

---

*Objective.*—Many studies of pediatric renal transplantation have addressed the survival of both grafts and patients. There are few data, how-

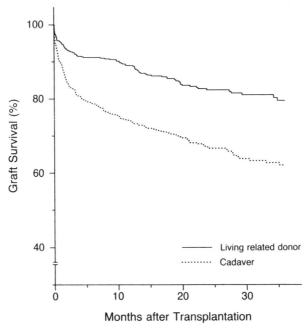

**Fig 6–1.**—Graft survival according to source. (Courtesy of McEnery PT, Stablein DM, Arbus G, et al: N *Engl J Med* 326:1727-1732, 1992.)

ever, on the causes of kidney disease in children, the sources of the transplanted organ, or the children's growth after the operation. The North American Pediatric Renal Transplant Cooperative Study identified diseases that require transplantation in children and examined factors affecting its success.

*Methods.*—The analysis included data from 73 pediatric transplant centers obtained from 1987 through 1990. Demographic characteristics, data on graft function, and the therapy administered 1 month postoperatively and every 6 months thereafter were reviewed.

*Findings.*—In all, 1,667 kidney allografts were given to 1,550 children, 31% of whom were age 5 years or younger. Most of the grafts (57%) were cadaveric, with the rest coming from a living related donor. Congenital malformations of the kidney and urinary tract were the most common causes of renal disease leading to transplantation (42% of the patients), with focal segmental glomerulosclerosis the next most common (12%). The 3-year graft survival rates were 80% in children receiving a kidney from a living related donor and 62% in those receiving cadaveric kidneys (Fig 6-1). Patients aged 5 years or younger at the time of operation had the best growth after transplantation. Overall, 79 patients died, and cancer developed in 12 during the follow-up period.

*Conclusions.*—This systematic study of renal transplantation in children found that congenital malformations and focal segmental glomerulosclerosis are the most common conditions leading to the need for transplantation. Graft survival is better with living related than with cadaveric donors. In children, the use of multiple immunosuppressive drugs appears to increase the risk of cancer as well as infection.

▶ This large multicenter review of the results of renal transplantation in children showed that graft survival in pediatric recipients of both living related and cadaveric kidneys is comparable to that seen in adults. Many centers are still reluctant to perform transplantation in children younger than 2 years because of concern about the increased risk of technical problems and the perceived increased likelihood of rejection in these very young recipients. The authors do not separate out the graft survival in this very young age group. The increased growth rate of young children receiving cadaveric transplants is gratifying.—R.J. Howard, M.D.

---

## Cadaveric Renal Transplantation in Elderly Recipients: Is It Worthwhile?

Morris GE, Jamieson NV, Small J, Evans DB, Calne SR (Addenbrooke's Hosp, Cambridge, England)
*Nephrol Dial Transplant* 6:887–892, 1991                                  6–7

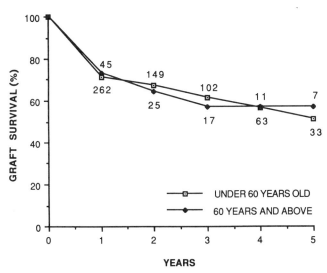

**Fig 6–2.**—The 5-year actuarial graft survival of 45 cadaveric renal transplants in 45 recipients aged 60 years and older compared with 262 transplants in 243 recipients aged younger than 60 years. The *figures by each point* indicate the number of grafts at risk at that point. (Courtesy of Morris GE, Jamieson NV, Small J, et al: *Nephrol Dial Transplant* 6:887–892, 1991.)

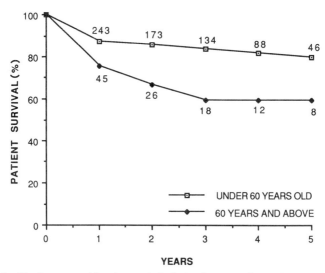

**Fig 6–3.**—The 5-year actuarial patient survival of 45 cadaveric renal transplant recipients aged 60 years and older compared with 243 recipients aged younger than 60 years. The *figures by each point* indicate the number of patients at risk at that point. (Courtesy of Morris GE, Jamieson NV, Small J, et al: *Nephrol Dial Transplant* 6:887–892, 1991.)

*Introduction.*—The number of patients waiting for renal transplants has increased significantly because of the success in treating end-stage renal failure with transplantation in the past 5 years. A study was conducted to determine whether old age alone significantly affects the result of patient and graft survival in cadaveric transplantation, and whether it should be a selection criterion for induction into transplant programs.

*Methods.*—From January 1983 to December 1987, 288 patients underwent 307 solitary cadaveric renal transplants. Among the patients younger than 60 years (mean age, 39 years), 243 received 262 kidneys; 45 patients older than 60 years (mean age, 64 years) received 45 kidneys. Initially cyclosporine A was given alone; after 1986 cyclosporine A, azathioprine, and prednisolone were administered as a triple therapy, which was maintained after transplantation.

*Results.*—At follow-up 18–66 months after surgery, graft survival was 61% and patient survival was 80%. Graft survival was 62% in older patients and 60% in patients younger than 60 years (Fig 6–2). Rejection was the cause of 4 of 17 graft losses in the older patient group compared with 83 of 104 graft losses in the younger group. This difference was significant. The overall irreversible rejection rate in the older group was also significantly lower. At the time of review, 64% of the older patients were alive compared with 83% of the younger patients (Fig 6–3).

*Conclusion.*—Patients older than 60 years may need less immunosuppression after receiving a cadaveric renal transplant. If a renal graft fails, however, the mortality rate in this patient group is very high. Cadaveric renal grafting in elderly patients should be considered carefully. Patients and their families should have full counseling about the risk of death from this procedure.

▶ As the results of solid organ transplantation continue to improve, potential recipients formerly believed not to be appropriate candidates are now receiving grafts. This and many other recent studies demonstrate that transplantation can be done safely in patients previously considered to be too old. Graft survival was not significantly different from that in younger patients in this and many other reports. These patients do have somewhat lower rates of survival, as would be expected, because older individuals die at a higher rate than younger ones. Careful patient selection is required to exclude older individuals with advanced cardiovascular disease.—R.J. Howard, M.D.

---

**Studies on the Afferent and Efferent Renal Nerves Following Autotransplantation of the Canine Kidney**
Sankari B, Stowe N, Gavin JP, Satoh S, Nally JV, Novick AC (Cleveland Clinic Found, Cleveland, Ohio)
*J Urol* 148:206–210, 1992                                                    6–8

---

*Objective.*—The abundant sympathetic nerve supply of the kidney comprises both postganglionic efferent and sensory afferent nerves. The presence of both afferent and efferent renal nerves after renal transplantation was studied in a canine autotransplant model.

*Methods.*—Experiments were carried out in adult female mongrel dogs. Eight animals underwent right nephrectomy only and were studied at 2 weeks postoperatively (group I, native innervated kidneys); 6 underwent autotransplantation of 1 kidney with contralateral nephrectomy and were studied 2-3 weeks postoperatively (group II, autotransplant kidneys, early); 8 animals were treated as in group II, but were studied 12-35 months after transplantation (group III, autotransplant kidneys, late). Afferent sensory renal nerves were examined by the systemic blood pressure response to renal arterial injection of capsaicin. The animals were then killed and the kidney removed. The glyoxylic acid method was used for histofluorescence demonstration of tissue adrenergic monoamine.

*Results.*—Intrarenal injection of capsaicin significantly increased systemic blood pressure in group I animals, a response that was equivalent to the blood pressure increase after injection of capsaicin into the mesenteric artery. The renal tissue histofluorescence grade in group I was 4. Group II animals had no increase in systemic blood pressure after the intrarenal injection of capsaicin; renal tissue histofluorescence was graded 0 in 3 dogs and 1 and 2 in 2 dogs. Group III animals showed a significant increase in systemic blood pressure with capsaicin and had renal tissue histofluorescence grades of 1-3.

*Conclusion.*—The findings confirm the normal distribution of the efferent nerves in the kidney along the arterial supply and surrounding the tubules. Afferent renal nerve activity was found late post transplant despite a lack of such activity early post transplant, suggesting possible regeneration. Thus the data support the presence of both afferent and efferent renal nerves in the kidney beyond a year after transplantation.

▶ A dictum of transplantation is that transplanted kidneys are not reinnervated. These authors provide experimental evidence using a canine model that autotransplanted kidneys are innervated when studied late (12 to 35 months) after autotransplantation using capsaicin as a centrally acting vasoconstrictor. Whether these findings apply to allotransplanted kidneys is not certain.—R.J. Howard, M.D.

---

### Ischemic-Type Biliary Complications After Orthotopic Liver Transplantation
Sanchez-Urdazpal L, Gores GJ, Ward EM, Maus TP, Wahlstrom HE, Moore SB, Wiesner RH, Krom RAF (Mayo Clinic and Found, Rochester, Minn)
*Hepatology* 16:49–53, 1992                    6–9

---

*Background.*—Problems with biliary reconstruction formerly accounted for 25% to 30% of deaths after orthotopic liver transplantation. Refinements in surgical technique significantly decreased the number of such complications, but a new difficulty involving nonanastomotic biliary strictures was observed. To determine the incidence of and risk factors for ischemic-type biliary complications (ITBCs) the orthotopic liver transplantation procedure was reviewed.

*Methods.*—Of 259 OLTs performed at the Mayo Clinic between March 1985 and July 1990, 188 were studied. Ninety-seven grafts were preserved with Euro-Collins solution and 91 were preserved with University of Wisconsin (UW) solution. Potential risk factors for ITBCs included total duration of graft ischemia, primary liver disease, type of biliary reconstruction, and the presence of cellular rejection before the development of ITBCs. Also, the cytomegalovirus serologic status of the donor, occurrence of posttransplantation cytomegalovirus infection before the development of ITBCs, and a positive lymphocytotoxic crossmatch between donor and recipient were evaluated.

*Results.*—Thirty-one grafts (16.5%) had ITBCs. The incidence of ITBCs was significantly higher in grafts ischemic for more than 11.5 hours (35%) than in grafts ischemic for less than 11.5 hours (2%); the incidence was even higher (52%) when ischemia was prolonged for more than 13 hours. The probability of ITBCs significantly increased as a function of cold ischemic storage time, whether the Euro-Collins or UW solution was used. Other potential risk factors were not associated with the development of ITBC.

*Conclusion.*—Some ITBCs occurred in the absence of the known risk factors of ductopenic rejection, ABO blood group incompatible grafts, and hepatic artery thrombosis. Use of the UW solution allowed liver grafts to be preserved twice as long as previously possible with the Euro-Collins solution. The total time of grafts in UW solution was limited to less than 13 hours with good results. In a later series of grafts, an ITBC developed in only 3% preserved for less than 13 hours.

▶ A large percentage of papers on liver transplantation deal with problems relating to the biliary tract. As noted by these authors, as surgical technique has improved, the number of complications related to the biliary anastomosis has decreased but the percentage attributable to other causes (e.g., ischemia and rejection) has increased. A large percentage of livers transplanted in patients with ischemic biliary complications had long preservation times. Some of the ischemic complications occurred in the absence of rejection. The "vanishing bile ducts syndrome," which is associated with rejection, has been seen less commonly in recent years. The ischemic complications may represent problems other than, or in addition to, rejection.—R.J. Howard, M.D.

---

**Management of Biliary Complications After Liver Transplantation**
Lopez RR, Benner KG, Ivancev K, Keeffe EB, Deveney CW, Pinson CW (Vanderbilt Univ, Nashville, Tenn; Oregon Health Sciences Univ, Portland)
*Am J Surg* 163:519–524, 1992                                                          6–10

---

*Introduction.*—Biliary tract complications often occur in liver transplant patients. To determine whether endoscopic and radiologic or operative methods provide the most effective treatment, data on biliary tract complications and the effectiveness of various treatment modalities were reviewed.

*Methods.*—Over a 3-year period, 62 transplants were performed in 55 adults. Biliary tract reconstruction was performed using choledochocholedochostomy (CC) in 84% of patients; Roux-en-Y choledochojejunostomy (RYJC) was used in the rest. In 16 patients, 17 biliary tract complications occurred, for an overall rate of 29%. Data on 4 patients with biliary tract complications who received their transplants at other centers were analyzed.

*Results.*—There was an equal incidence of complications in the CC and RYJC groups. Among the present patients, 47% of the complications occurred within the first month; surgery was necessary in 35% of patients. One patient died of a biliary tract complication; none of the other grafts was lost. Including the referral patients, 9 had bile leakage, 8 had bile duct stricture, 2 had Roux loop hemorrhage, 1 had choledocholithiasis, and 1 had ampullary dyskinesia. Placement of temporary or permanent stents was successful in 7 of 8 patients with strictures and 5 of 9 bile leaks were treated nonoperatively.

*Conclusion.*—For most patients with late bile leaks, biliary tract strictures, or choledocholithiasis occurring after liver transplantation, nonsurgical treatment is appropriate and must be individualized. Operative treatment or carefully placed catheter stents should be used for early strictures.

▶ There are probably more articles about hepatic artery thrombosis and biliary complications than any other surgical problems after liver transplantation. Early cholangiograms frequently show radiographic narrowing at the anastomosis that does not seem to be functionally important. Extrahepatic biliary problems are frequently the result of technical errors, a compromised vascular supply to the biliary duct, rejection, or stricture associated with healing. Intrahepatic biliary tract narrowing is usually caused by rejection, whereas that associated with the development of cystlike structures or dilations is commonly associated with arterial blood supply problems. Innovative radiologic techniques, including balloon dilation and stent placement, have obviated the need for surgical repair in the majority of patients. Nevertheless, 35% of those in this series did require surgical repair, usually in the first month. Late occurring strictures may occasionally require retransplantation.—R.J. Howard, M.D.

## Resource Utilization and Outcome of Liver Transplantation for Alcoholic Cirrhosis: A Case-Control Study

McCurry KR, Baliga P, Merion RM, Ham JM, Lucey MR, Beresford TP, Turcotte JG, Campbell DA Jr (Univ of Michigan, Ann Arbor)
*Arch Surg* 127:772–777, 1992
6–11

*Background.*—Liver transplantation in patients with alcohol-related liver disease remains controversial because of the perception that these patients have a potentially poor outcome and because of concerns about the high utilization of medical resources. Because the outcome after liver transplantation for alcohol-related liver disease has not been well studied, resource utilization and outcome were evaluated in alcoholic and nonalcoholic cirrhotic patients undergoing liver transplantation.

*Patients.*—The study sample consisted of 56 patients aged 27–61 years with end-stage alcohol-related liver disease and 56 nonalcoholic cirrhotic controls matched for age, sex, Child-Pugh class, and date of transplantation. Resource utilization variables examined included the number of transfused blood units, days of mechanical ventilation, days in the intensive care unit, days in the hospital, and number of readmissions during the first year after the transplant. The median follow-up was 1.41 years for alcoholic patients and 1.16 years for nonalcoholic controls.

*Results.*—There were no significant differences between alcoholic organ recipients and nonalcoholic controls with regard to resource utiliza-

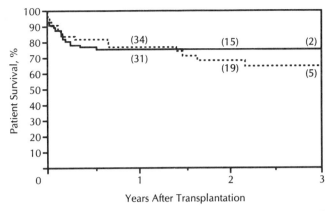

**Fig 6–4.**—Actuarial survival following orthotopic liver transplantation in patients with alcohol-related (*solid line*) and non–alcohol-related (*broken line*) cirrhosis. *Number in parentheses* are numbers of patients. (Courtesy of McCurry KR, Baliga P, Merion RM, et al: *Arch Surg* 127:772–777, 1992.)

tion variables or in terms of early graft function, sepsis or rejection rates, renal function, and retransplantation rates. The 1-year actuarial survival rate was 75% in alcoholic liver transplant recipients and 76% in nonalcoholic controls (Fig 6–4).

*Conclusion.*—Resource utilization and outcome among alcoholic liver transplant recipients is similar to that among nonalcoholic liver transplant recipients with a similar severity of illness.

▶ Individuals undergoing liver transplantation for alcoholic cirrhosis apparently do not differ either in immediate resource utilization or 1-year survival compared to patients undergoing liver transplantation for other causes. Critical in the decision to perform transplantation in alcoholic cirrhotic patients is the psychosocial evaulation, which includes (1) dependence on alcohol, (2) recognition of alcoholism by the patient and family, (3) abstinence prognosis, and (4) social stability. Using these criteria, less than 50% of alcoholic cirrhotic patients were acceptable for liver transplantation. The authors do not state how long the patients must have been free of alcohol, but most centers have some period during which the patient must have been alcohol free before being considered for transplantation.—R.J. Howard, M.D.

---

**Liver Transplantation in Patients With Portal Vein Thrombosis and Central Portacaval Shunts**
Shaked A, Busuttil RW (Univ of California, Los Angeles)
*Ann Surg* 214:696–702, 1991                                                              6–12

*Introduction.*—The pathology and possibly the morbidity and mortality of orthotopic liver transplantation (OLT) are considerably increased in patients with preexisting disease of the portal vein.

*Methods.*—To determine the effects of portal vein disease on the outcome of OLT, data were reviewed on 550 patients who received 676 OLTs. In each patient portal vein patency was determined by ultrasonograph or duplex sonography, and the need for portal vein reconstruction was documented. Celiac and superior mesenteric artery angiography was performed to determine possible portal vein occlusion or previous portosystemic shunt.

*Results.*—There was a high incidence of portal vein pathology in patients with chronic active hepatitis, hypercoagulation, trauma, previous porta hepatis dissection, and splenectomy. Portal vein thrombosis (PVT) was diagnosed in 23 patients, and a surgical central portosystemic shunt was seen in 10. These findings were documented by Doppler sonography or angiography in 26 cases and by operative observation in 10. In 24 patients thrombectomy and dismantling of the portacaval shunt (PCS) was successful. An interpositional vein graft to the superior mesenteric vein was needed in 9 patients. Patients had increased blood loss and coagulopathy. Compared with all liver transplants, the immediate postoperative complication rate was higher for primary nonfunction (33% vs. 8%). Patients with portal vein pathology also had a higher rate of reexploration for intraperitoneal bleeding and hematomas, and a higher rate of morbid infections. Rethrombosis occurred in 2 patients. The mortality rate was 35% in patients with PVT, 30% in those with PCS, and 12% in the other OLT patients.

*Conclusion.*—In patients undergoing OLT, the presence of preexisting portal vein pathology is associated with increased rates of perioperative complications and mortality. Results should improve with improved patient selection, surgical experience, and anticipation of complex postoperative courses. Neither PVT nor PCS is a contraindication to OLT.

▶ Portal vein thrombosis and central portacaval shunts were formerly contraindications to liver transplantation. With greater experience, surgeons have been performing transplant procedures in patients with these conditions. The authors document their experience with 24 of 33 of these patients in whom they dismantled the portacaval shunt or removed a portal vein thrombus. Although blood loss, immediate postoperative complications, and mortality rates are increased in these patients, the presence of PVT or a previously placed central portacaval shunt is no longer a contraindication to orthotopic transplantation. The results are expected to improve with continuing surgical experience.—R.J. Howard, M.D.

## Liver Transplantation for Primary Hepatic Cancer

Haug CE, Jenkins RL, Rohrer RJ, Auchincloss H, Delmonico FL, Freeman RB, Lewis WD, Cosimi AB (Massachusetts Gen Hosp, Boston; New England Dea-

coness Hosp, Boston; New England Med Ctr, Boston)
*Transplantation* 53:376–382, 1992                                6–13

*Introduction.*—Early survival after liver transplantation for hepatic cancer is excellent. The reported recurrence rates, however, have been high, discouraging the use of transplantation for patients with liver cancer.

*Methods.*—Data on liver transplantation performed in patients with primary hepatic malignancy over a 7-year period were reviewed to determine the factors associated with prolonged survival. Of 383 patients who received liver transplants, the indication was primary hepatic malignancy in 33 (9%). During the 7-year period, 56% of patients with cancer who were evaluated for liver transplantation were found to be unsuitable; 24 patients with hepatocellular carcinoma (HCCA) received 28 grafts, and 9 patients with cholangiocarcinoma (CHCA) received 9 grafts. The follow-up averaged 24 months for the patients with HCCA and 26 for patients with CHCA.

*Results.*—In the group with HCCA, the actuarial survival rate was 71% at 1 year, 56% at 2 years, and 42% at 3 years. In the group with CHCA, the actuarial survival rate was 89% at 6 months and 56% at 1, 2, and 3 years. There were recurrences in 56% of the patients with CHCA, although other complications were generally absent. The recurrence rate was 25% in patients with HCCA who survived for more than 3 months after transplantation; the other deaths in this group resulted from perioperative complications (17%), sepsis (8%), coronary artery disease (4%), or lymphoma (4%). The prognosis tended to be better in patients with primary tumors smaller than 3 cm and without associated cirrhosis.

*Conclusion.*—Of patients with primary liver cancer unresectable by conventional means, about half can experience long-term cure with orthotopic liver transplantation. Patients without cirrhosis or with smaller tumors reliably have excellent survival and low recurrence rates.

▶ The results of transplantation in the treatment of unresectable liver cancer, except for fibrolamellar carcinoma, have been discouraging because of the high recurrence rate. This paper shows that it is possible to achieve acceptable long-term results in carefully selected patients with HCCA and CHCA. The results of transplantation are substantially better than those of other treatment modalities. The authors maintain that, in carefully selected patients, transplantation may be the treatment of choice for CHCA and HCCA. Others would claim that a precious resource such as organs for transplantation should be reserved for individuals who would be more likely to experience greater long-term benefit.—R.J. Howard, M.D.

## The Results of Reduced-Size Liver Transplantation, Including Split Livers, in Patients With End-Stage Liver Disease

Langnas AN, Marujo WC, Inagaki M, Stratta RJ, Wood RP, Shaw BW Jr (Univ of Nebraska, Omaha)
*Transplantation* 53:387–391, 1992                            6–14

*Introduction.*—The shortage of donor organs continues to limit the use of organ transplantation for a host of disorders. The organ shortage particularly affects children awaiting transplantation, and many die because of the lack of an organ of appropriate size. The reduced-size liver transplant (RSLT) technique was developed to alleviate this problem in the pediatric population.

*Method.*—The reduction in organ size occurs after the donor organ arrives at the recipient location and before the start of recipient surgery. An extensive hilar dissection delineates the vascular supply of both liver halves before the hepatic division, allowing for correct blood vessel allocation (Fig 6–5). Orthotopic implantation of the liver is performed with the left lateral segment grafts revascularized without vascular grafts and the venous outflow comprising the left hepatic vein.

*Results.*—Data on patients who had RSLT between June 1988 and January 1991 were reviewed. In 29 patients (28 children, 1 adult), 30 RSLTs were performed. The mean age of the children was 2.2 years, and 21 children weighed less than 10 kg. Of the 30 RSLTs, 7 were retransplantations, 18 were left-lobe, 7 were left-lateral segment, and 5

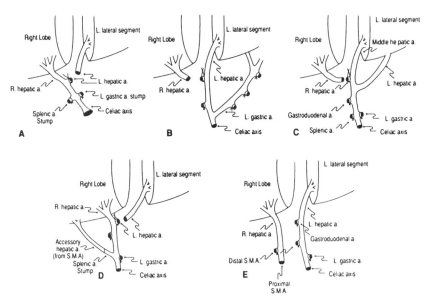

**Fig 6–5.**—Methods of arterial reconstruction used for split-liver transplantation. (Courtesy of Langnas AN, Marujo WC, Inagaki M, et al: *Transplantation* 53:387–391, 1992.)

were right-lobe grafts. No hepatic vein blockages occurred, but there were several complications. The 1-year actuarial patient and graft survival rates were 69% and 67%, respectively, based on a mean follow-up of nearly .1 months. Nine deaths occurred, 3 in patients with a primary nonfunctional liver.

*Conclusion.*—Reduced-size liver transplantation can be safe and effective in children critically ill with end-stage liver disease. The 1-year actuarial patient and graft survival rates primarily reflect the pretreatment condition of the young, critically ill patients.

▶ The use of reduced size livers for transplantation in pediatric patients with end-stage liver disease has meant that very few small children die for want of a size-matched whole liver. Technical complications were not significantly different from those in patients who had whole-organ transplants, and the 1-year survival of 69% in these very young children is excellent.—R.J. Howard, M.D.

---

**Systemic Chimerism in Human Female Recipients of Male Livers**
Starzl TE, Demetris AJ, Trucco M, Ramos H, Zeevi A, Rudert WA, Kocova M, Ricordi C, Ildstad S, Murase N (Univ of Pittsburgh, Pittsburgh, Pa)
*Lancet* 340:876–877, 1992                                    6–15

---

*Objective.*—In a previous study, it was suggested that organ tolerance after transplantation may depend on a state of host-graft balanced lymphodendritic cell chimerism. Studies were made in HLA-mismatched liver allograft recipients to gather data supporting this hypothesis.

*Methods.*—Nine women had received livers from ABO-identical but HLA-mismatched male donors, 10–19 years previously. All were receiving continuous azathioprine or cyclosporine treatment, except for 1 noncompliant patient. In the latter case the transplant failed after 12 years because of recurrent chronic viral hepatitis. Evidence of chimerism in liver biopsy specimens was sought by in situ hybridization and polymerase chain reaction.

*Findings.*—Chimerism was seen in allografts and extrahepatic tissues from all patients. All 8 women with good graft function had evidence of the Y chromosome in the skin, lymph nodes, and/or blood (table). In the patient with graft failure, chimerism was seen in the lymph nodes, skin, jejunum, and aorta at the time of retransplantation.

*Conclusions.*—Chimerism is found in a variety of tissues in long-term female survivors after liver transplantation with organs from HLA-mismatched male donors. Cell migration probably occurs in all types of transplantation—the privileged tolerogenicity of the liver most likely re-

Microchimerism According to Y Chromosome Detection With In Situ Hybridization or Polymerase Chain Reaction

| | Liver allograft | | Blood | Lymph node | | Skin | |
| | | | | Tissue distribution | | | |
| Date of (age at) transplant* | In-situ hybrid-isation | PCR | PCR | In-situ hybrid-isation | PCR | In-situ hybrid-isation | PCR |
|---|---|---|---|---|---|---|---|
| 1. 21/1/76(30) | + + + | + + + | + | + | – | + | + |
| 2. 26/2/78(5) | + + + | + + + | + | + | + | + | NT |
| 3. 9/3/80(29) | NT | + + + | – | NT | – | NT | + |
| 4. 4/1/78(2) | + + + | + + + | + | + | + | + | NT |
| 5. 21/3/80(34) | + + + | + + + | + | – | – | + | + |
| 6. 18/2/73(3) | + + + | + + + | – | – | + | + | + |
| 7. 28/2/82(45) | + + + | + + + | + | + | + | + | + |
| 8. 9/9/79(35) | + + + | + + + | + | + | + | + | + |
| 9. 29/8/80†(28) | + + + | + + + | NT | + | – | – | + |

* All postoperative studies completed in April-June, 1992.
† This patient also tested positive in intestine with in situ hybridization and polymerase chain reaction (PCR), and in the aorta with PCR.
(Courtesy of Starzl TE, Demetris AJ, Trucco M, et al: *Lancet* 340:876-877, 1992.)

sults from the large population of migratory cells in, and the extent of their seeding from, hepatic grafts.

► Specific immunologic tolerance, the "Holy Grail" of transplantation ever since Billingham, Brent, and Medawar (1) demonstrated its feasibility experimentally, has continued to elude transplant surgeons. This paper provides evidence that a degree of tolerance may occur in long-term female transplant patients who receive livers from HLA-mismatched male donors. Whether these long-term survivors who demonstrate chimerism can have the level of immunosuppression reduced or even eliminated entirely remains to be seen. Occasional reports of patients who have gone for prolonged periods without taking immunosuppressive drugs and yet have seemed to experience no ill consequences provide further clinical data suggesting that some degree of tolerance may occur.—R.J. Howard, M.D.

*Reference*

1. Billingham RE, et al: *Nature* 172:603, 1953.

### Intestinal Transplantation in Composite Visceral Grafts or Alone

Todo S, Tzakis AG, Abu-Elmagd K, Reyes J, Nakamura K, Casavilla A, Selby R, Nour BM, Wright H, Fung JJ, Demetris AJ, Van Thiel DH, Starzl TE (Univ of Pittsburgh, Pa; VA Med Ctr, Pittsburgh)
*Ann Surg* 216:223–234, 1992                6–16

*Background.*—Experimental studies have shown the difficulty of small intestinal transplantation and, until recently, intestinal transplants were considered relatively futile. A review was made of experience with small bowel transplantation and the use of the new immunosuppressive drug, FK 506.

*Patients and Methods.*—The study population consisted of 1 recipient of a full multivisceral graft containing a liver, stomach, and pancreas; 8 recipients of liver-intestine grafts; and 8 recipients of isolated small intestine grafts. Fifteen patients had short-gut syndrome. All patients had been maintained on total parenteral nutrition (TPN) for 1–132 months before transplantation, and all had experienced more than 1 episode of sepsis, liver damage, or other TPN-associated complication. Nine patients were children between 6 months and 4 years of age. Cadavers of similar or smaller size and ABO blood groups identical to those of recipients were selected as donors. Two recipients had antigraft cytotoxic antibodies. Conventional surgical techniques were used for reconstruction of the gastrointestinal tract (Figs 6–6 and 6–7). Intravenous infusion of FK 506 for immunosuppression was started immediately after graft

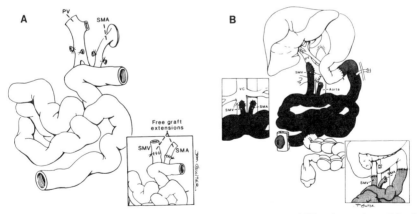

**Fig 6–6.**—Isolated small bowel transplantation. **A,** donor operation; full-length vascular pedicle of the superior mesenteric artery (SMA) (with Carrel patch) and the superior mesenteric vein (SMV). If both vessels are divided more distally, they can be lengthened on the back table with arterial and venous grafts (*insert*). **B,** recipient operations. Anastomosis of full-length SMA to the aorta and the angled end of the SMV to the portal vein. Alternative method with which the SMV is anastomosed to the recipient SMV inferior to the pancreas (*lower insert*). Option of SMV drainage into the inferior vena cava (**upper insert**). (Courtesy of Todo S, Tzakis AG, Abu-Elmagd K, et al: *Ann Surg* 216:223–234, 1992.)

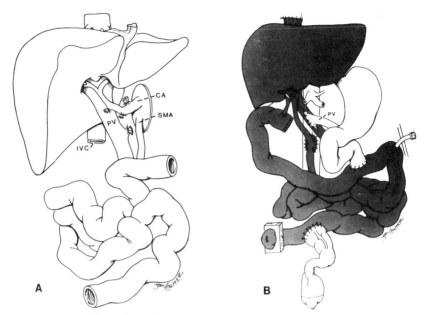

**Fig 6–7.—A,** small bowel–liver allograft. Note the continuity of donor portal vein. **B,** recipient operation. Carrel patch containing the origin of the superior mesenteric artery and the celiac axis is anastomosed to the aorta. Ideally, the venous return from residual splanchnic viscera of the recipient is routed by vascular anastomosis into the graft portal vein. (Courtesy of Todo S, Tzakis AG, Abu-Elmagd K, et al: *Ann Surg* 216:223-234, 1992.)

revascularization. The route of administration of FK 506 was changed to oral administration twice daily when enteral feeding was initiated. Methylprednisolone and prostaglandin $E_1$ were also given. Endoscopy with mucosal biopsy was performed when rejection was suspected on clinical grounds.

*Results.*—Fifteen of the 17 original grafts were still in place and 16 patients were alive after a follow-up of 1–23 months, including all 8 isolated small bowel recipients. One liver-intestine recipient died after an intestinal anastomotic leak, sepsis, and graft-vs.-host disease. One recipient of an isolated intestinal graft required graft resection and retransplantation 22 months after the first operation. This patient had experienced bouts of severe rejection, sepsis, and renal failure associated with drug noncompliance. The early convalescence of most of the recipients was prolonged and complicated, and 2 had irreversible renal failure requiring cadaver renal transplantation. Twelve patients are now TPN free. The convalescence of the 8 recipients of isolated intestinal grafts was faster and more trouble free than that of recipients of liver-intestine or multivisceral grafts.

*Conclusion.*—It would appear that FK 506 provides more potent immunosuppression than cyclosporine and opens up new options for the treatment of end-stage intestinal disease, with or without liver involvement.

▶ This initial report from Pittsburgh of a series of successful small bowel transplant procedures provides hope for individuals with short-gut syndrome. The immunologic challenges are formidable. Rejection must be diagnosed early, usually by endoscopic biopsy, if it is to be treated promptly so that graft failure does not occur. Twelve of the 16 patients had no need for total parenteral nutrition, indicating that the transplanted intestine functions even without normal lymphatic drainage.—R.J. Howard, M.D.

---

**Single Lung Transplantation for Severe Emphysema**
Marinelli WA, Hertz MI, Shumway SJ, Fox JMK, Henke CA, Harmon KR, Savik K, Bolman RM III (Univ of Minnesota, Minneapolis)
*J Heart Lung Transplant* 11:577–583, 1992                        6–17

---

*Introduction.*—Lung transplantation is being used with increasing frequency for patients with severe emphysema. The clinical outcome in 7 patients who underwent single-lung transplantation (SLT) at the University of Minnesota between August 1989 and September 1990 was assessed.

*Methods.*—All 7 patients had a forced expiratory volume in 1 second of less than 30% predicted and a deteriorating clinical course. The mean age was 48 years. All underwent SLT (left in 6 cases, right in 1) after posterolateral thoracotomy. Surveillance bronchoscopy was performed every 2 months for the first year after operation and every 3 months thereafter. Immunosuppressive therapy included orally administered cyclosporine and prednisone.

*Results.*—Pulmonary function improved markedly after SLT, achieving maximal values within 6 months. Studies of cardiac function revealed moderately reduced right ventricular function, moderately elevated pulmonary artery pressure, and normal left ventricular function. Coronary angiography was normal in all patients. One patient died 21 days after SLT when massive pulmonary embolization occurred. Three patients experienced episodes of acute rejection within the first 30 days after transplantation, but all responded to corticosteroid therapy. Six patients were alive at periods ranging from 6 months to 19 months after SLT.

*Conclusion.*—Lung transplantation can be an effective treatment for patients with severe emphysema and mild to moderate reduction in right ventricular function. There is a limited supply, however, of donor lungs. The advantages of SLT over heart-lung transplantation and double-lung transplantation include a shorter waiting time for a donor organ, better utilization of organs, and less frequent need for cardiopulmonary bypass.

▶ It was not so long ago that lung transplantation was uniformly unsuccessful. With better surgical technique and better immunosuppression, the results of lung transplantation have improved remarkably. More and more centers are beginning to do these procedures. This report from the University of Minnesota demonstrates success in 6 of 7 SLT recipients. The indications for lung transplantation are still being refined.—R.J. Howard, M.D.

# 7   Endocrine

## Introduction

There has been an increasing tendency to perform total thyroidectomy for thyroid cancer. The first three articles reviewed (Abstracts 7-1, 7-2, and 7-3) argue for total thyroidectomy in patients with thyroid cancer, even if the operation is performed after permanent sections have been done and another operation is needed. The basis for this argument is the high rate of residual disease in an apparently normal thyroid gland. Support for this argument is found in the study by Katoh et al. (Abstract 7-4) in which glands removed at completion thyroidectomy for thyroid cancer were examined. These authors found a high rate of neoplastic disease in the ipsilateral and contralateral thyroid lobes. The assumptions are that total thyroidectomy or completion thyroidectomy will lead to a better survival than thyroid lobectomy, and that the neoplastic tissue in the contralateral thyroid lobe will behave biologically like carcinoma at some time in the future and will metastasize. A study comparing patients who had unilateral thyroid resection as opposed to thyroidectomy with those who had bilateral thyroid resection for differentiated thyroid cancer found no difference in survival when patients were stratified by age-based risk, although it was not a randomized study.

Nevertheless, there is a tendency among experienced surgeons to perform total or near-total thyroidectomy. The latter procedure leaves a small rim of thyroid tissue around the parathyroid glands so as not to devascularize them. This is no small issue, because most surgeons do not perform large numbers of thyroidectomies. Performing total or near-total thyroidectomy is bound to lead to a higher complication rate than unilateral lobectomy. If it does not result in a better survival rate, then total thyroidectomy might produce only a higher rate of morbidity and provide no increase in survival. Experienced thyroid surgeons (the ones who write articles favoring total thyroidectomy) can perform total thyroidectomy with a low complication rate, but most thyroidectomies for cancer are not done by these individuals; rather, they are performed by community surgeons who do not specialize in thyroid surgery. The article by Harris (Abstract 7-6) discusses the two main complications of thyroid and parathyroid operations: recurrent laryngeal or superior laryngeal nerve injury and hypoparathyroidism. An article on thyroid cancer in children by Harness et al. (Abstract 7-7) shows that a large percentage of these children have had previous radiation to the head and neck, but also that, with more experience and training, modern surgeons should not have the same complication rate as surgeons who performed thyroidectomy in earlier years.

Two articles about parathyroid disease also discuss unilateral versus bilateral neck exploration. Arguments generally take the form of the higher risk of recurrent laryngeal nerve injury and longer operating time in patients who have bilateral neck exploration as opposed to the risk of missing a second parathyroid adenoma in patients who have only unilateral neck exploration. Both articles, however, have methodologic problems. The first article by Tibblin et al. (Abstract 7–10) excludes patients with more than one parathyroid adenoma, just the type of patient on whom you might want to do a bilateral neck dissection. The second article by Duh et al. (Abstract 7–11) uses a mathematical model that assumes all patients have localizing studies before operation. Because an experienced surgeon can locate a diseased parathyroid gland better than any currently available radiologic study, many surgeons do not do localizing studies before the initial neck exploration.

Parathyroid carcinoma, a rare disease, is not very susceptible to chemotherapy or radiation therapy, thus an aggressive surgical approach is warranted, as discussed by Wynne et al. (Abstract 7–13). The authors favor an aggressive surgical approach, especially in patients with recurrent disease.

Richard J. Howard, M.D.

---

### The Incidence of Bilateral Well-Differentiated Thyroid Cancer Found at Completion Thyroidectomy

Pasieka JL, Thompson NW, McLeod MK, Burney RE, Macha M (Univ of Michigan, Ann Arbor)
*World J Surg* 16:711–717, 1992                                                    7–1

---

*Introduction.*—Treatment of well-differentiated thyroid cancer (WDTC) has varied from unilateral lobectomy to total or near-total thyroidectomy. Although most would agree that all thyroid tissue containing thyroid cancer should be removed, there is disagreement on the need for reoperation when the diagnosis is not made until after a lobectomy. The outcome of completion thyroidectomy in patients with presumed unilateral WDTC was examined.

*Methods.*—At the University of Michigan Medical Center in Ann Arbor, 60 of 284 patients treated for WDTC between 1980 and 1991 underwent completion thyroidectomy. Forty-seven (group 1) had no evidence of regional recurrent or metastatic disease and underwent a prophylactic procedure. Of the 13 patients in group 2, 12 had regional recurrence and 1 had distant metastases. This group underwent either debulking or complete removal of regionally recurrent WDTC, along with completion thyroidectomy.

*Results.*—Twenty of the 47 group 1 patients were found to have WDTC in the contralateral thyroid lobe, and 5 had unsuspected positive cervical nodal disease. Two who had recurrent disease at 6 months and 12 months after completion thyroidectomy underwent a third operation. At a mean follow-up of 58 months, all group 1 patients were alive and disease free. At a mean of 72 months, 4 patients from group 2 were alive with evidence of thyroid cancer, and 4 were alive without evidence of thyroid cancer. Two patients died of extensive thyroid cancer, 1 died of an unrelated cause, and 2 were lost to follow-up.

*Conclusion.*—Because the diagnosis of WDTC cannot always be made intraoperatively, some patients require another procedure after lobectomy. Multifocal disease in the primary resected lobe was associated with a high incidence of contralateral thyroid cancer. Patients with regional recurrence also appear to have a high incidence of residual carcinoma in the remaining thyroid lobe. Completion thyroidectomy is recommended in such cases; the procedure resulted in few complications in this series.

▶ The argument for total thyroidectomy rather than lobectomy for well-differentiated thyroid cancer is made on the grounds of residual foci of neoplastic cells in the remaining lobe and the ability to detect and treat metastatic disease with radioactive iodine if the contralateral lobe is removed. Not all studies indicate increased survival in patients who have total or near-total thyroidectomy compared with those who have lobectomy. The morbidity is higher in patients who have total thyroidectomy than those who have lobectomy. The 2 serious complications are injury to the recurrent laryngeal nerve and the possibility of rendering the patient aparathyroid. Twenty of 47 patients who had no evidence of regional or metastatic disease who had completion thyroidectomy had well-differentiated thyroid cancer in the contralateral thyroid lobe, and 5 had unsuspected positive cervical nodal disease.

These data support the argument for completion thyroidectomy in patients who are found to have well-differentiated thyroid cancer, but they do not answer the question of whether this leads to better survival.—R.J. Howard, M.D.

---

**Necessity and Safety of Completion Thyroidectomy for Differentiated Thyroid Carcinoma**
De Jong SA, Demeter JG, Lawrence AM, Paloyan E (Loyola Univ, Maywood, Ill; Hines VA Hosp, Hines, Ill)
*Surgery* 112:734–739, 1992                                                    7–2

---

*Background.*—Thyroid carcinoma cannot always be identified in intraoperative frozen sections. The surgeon must limit initial thyroid resection to thyroid lobectomy in these situations. In such cases, the decision for complete thyroidectomy rests on the remaining malignant thyroid tissue discovered in subsequent histopathologic examinations. The timing, safety, and efficacy of this procedure were examined.

*Patients.*—Initial thyroid lobectomy was performed on 100 patients who did not have preoperative or intraoperative thyroid malignancies. After surgery, histopathologic examination of the lobectomy specimens revealed papillary carcinoma in 70 patients and follicular carcinoma in 30. Secondary completion thyroidectomy was performed several months later (mean, 6 months).

*Results.*—Papillary carcinoma was observed in completion thyroidectomy specimens from 33 of the initial 70 patients with papillary cancer and in 10 specimens from the 30 patients with follicular carcinoma. Overall, 43 patients had contralateral lobe thyroid carcinoma. After thyroidectomy completion surgery, 2 patients had transient recurrent nerve paresis; spontaneous resolution occurred within 6 weeks. Three patients had temporary hypoparathyroidism, and they were treated with calcium and vitamin D for 3–4 months.

*Conclusions.*—Most patients who undergo thyroid lobectomy for differentiated thyroid carcinoma should be considered for completion thyroidectomy because the occurrence of residual thyroid carcinoma may be as high as 47% (papillary tumors) and 33% (follicular tumors). If the procedure is to be beneficial, complications arising from it must be minimal. Therefore, an interval of 3–6 months between initial lobectomy and completion thyroidectomy is recommended.

▶ This is another paper discussing the necessity and safety of completion thyroidectomy after initial thyroidectomy when permanent sections show cancer. Overall, 43 of 100 patients (33 of 70 with papillary cancer, and 10 of 30 with follicular cancer) had residual thyroid cancer. Two patients had transient recurrent nerve paresis, and 3 had temporary hypoparathyroidism, thus demonstrating that completion thyroidectomy can be performed safely, and that a high percentage of patients have histologically abnormal tissue demonstrated in the contralateral thyroid gland. This article answers affirmatively the question of whether completion thyroidectomy can be performed safely. It does not answer the question, however, of whether it *should* be performed—that is, does total thyroidectomy lead to better survival rates than a lesser resection?—R.J. Howard, M.D.

---

**Completion Thyroidectomy in the Management of Well-Differentiated Thyroid Carcinoma**

Wax MK, Briant TDR (West Virginia Univ, Morgantown; St Michael's Hosp, Toronto, Ont, Canada)

*Otolaryngol Head Neck Surg* 107:63–68, 1992                7–3

---

*Introduction.*—The amount of thyroid tissue removed at surgery for well-differentiated carcinoma varies among centers. Total thyroidectomy is preferred at St. Michael's Hospital in Toronto. After lobectomy has been performed for a nodule first reported as benign, completion thyroidectomy is used in cases that later prove to be malignant. Experience with completion thyroidectomy was analyzed to determine the indications and complications of the procedure.

*Methods.*—Between 1982 and 1991, 32 of 244 patients with well-differentiated thyroid carcinoma underwent completion thyroidectomy. Twenty-five tumors had been misdiagnosed as follicular adenomas, 2 as Hürthle cell lesions, and 1 as a colloid nodule. All but 4 patients had a second procedure within 3 months after the initial surgery.

*Results.*—Completion thyroidectomy was a safe procedure, with no increased anesthetic morbidity or mortality at the time of the second procedure. Final histologic diagnoses included papillary carcinoma (47%), follicular carcinoma (50%), and medullary carcinoma (3%). Five patients had transient hypocalcemia after completion thyroidectomy, and 1 had transient vocal cord palsy. One patient required oral calcium and vitamin D supplementation to maintain normal calcemia.

*Conclusion.*—The rate of false negative frozen section diagnosis (approximately 10% in most series) does not warrant complete thyroidectomy as an initial procedure. Completion thyroidectomy can be safe, even when performed soon after the first operation, with little risk of laryngeal nerve paralysis or permanent hypocalcemia.

▶ This article also discusses the controversy of subtotal as opposed to near-total or total thyroidectomy in patients with thyroid cancer. The 32 patients reported in this article underwent lobectomy for a nodule that was reported to be benign on frozen section but later proved to be malignant on permanent section. These authors then went back and completed the thyroidectomy. This paper shows that the procedure can be performed safely, yet 5 patients had transient hypocalcemia and 1 had transient vocal cord palsy. One patient still requires oral calcium and vitamin D to maintain a normal level of calcium. Even though this procedure can be performed safely, that does not answer the question of whether it should be performed at all.—R.J. Howard, M.D.

---

**Multiple Thyroid Involvement (Intraglandular Metastasis) in Papillary Thyroid Carcinoma: A Clinicopathologic Study of 105 Consecutive Patients**
Katoh R, Sasaki J, Kurihara H, Suzuki K, Iida Y, Kawaoi A (Yamanashi Med College, Tamaho-cho, Japan; Iwate Med Univ, Morioka, Japan)
*Cancer* 70:1585–1590, 1992                                                7–4

---

*Background.*—It is still not known whether multiple thyroid involvement in papillary thyroid carcinoma is the result of multiple lesions arising de novo or of intraglandular dissemination. A histologic study was

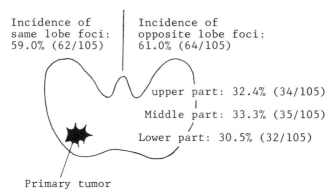

Incidence of                    Incidence of
same lobe foci:                 opposite lobe foci:
59.0% (62/105)                  61.0% (64/105)

upper part: 32.4% (34/105)

Middle part: 33.3% (35/105)

Lower part: 30.5% (32/105)

Primary tumor

**Fig 7–1.**—Distribution of intraglandular foci, other than the primary tumor, in papillary thyroid carcinomas. (Courtesy of Katoh R, Sasaki J, Kurihara H, et al: *Cancer* 70:1585–1590, 1992.)

performed to elucidate the biological nature and clinical significance of multiple thyroid involvement.

*Methods.*—Whole thyroid glands with papillary carcinoma removed from 105 patients during total thyroidectomy and regional lymph nodes removed from 97 of these 105 patients were studied. The diagnosis of papillary thyroid carcinoma had been confirmed by preoperative fine-needle aspiration cytology. The thyroid glands were sectioned sagittally at intervals of 2–3 mm, yielding to 15–50 slices each for histologic examination.

*Results.*—Multiple intraglandular cancer foci other than the primary focus were present in 82 of the 105 glands (78%). The foci were less than 4 mm in diameter and lacked sclerotic fibrous stroma or fibrous capsules. Sixty-two glands (59%) contained additional cancer foci in the same lobe as the primary lesion, and 63 glands (61%) contained cancer foci in the opposite lobe. When the opposite lobe was divided into upper, middle, and lower parts, 32% of the glands contained cancer foci in the upper part of the opposite lobe, 33% contained foci in the middle part, and 30.5% contained foci in the lower part of the opposite lobe (Fig 7–1). Sixteen glands contained cancer foci in 2 of the 3 parts of the opposite lobe, and 11 glands contained foci in all 3 parts of the opposite lobe. The mean number of cancer foci was highest in glands containing a primary tumor with a diameter greater than 30 mm. The mean number of foci was statistically correlated to age, presence of lymph node metastases, and presence of solid areas or psammoma bodies in the primary tumor. These findings support the suggestion that intraglandular metastases originate via the lymph vessels.

*Conclusion.*—The high probability of multiple thyroid involvement in papillary thyroid carcinoma is one of its most characteristic and important biological features.

▶ The rationale for doing total thyroidectomy for thyroid cancer is that the occult disease occurs in the apparently normal thyroid gland on the contralateral side. In this pathology study, thyroid glands were sectioned at frequent (2–3 mm) intervals for histologic examination. The authors found a high prevalence of neoplastic foci in the sides ipsilateral and contralateral to the dominate lesion, thus providing a histologic basis and rationale for total thyroidectomy. Experts still differ on the biological properties and metastatic potential of these foci.—R.J. Howard, M.D.

---

**Unilateral Versus Bilateral Thyroid Resection in Differentiated Thyroid Carcinoma**
Groot G, Colquhoun BPD, Murphy FA (Royal Univ Hosp, Saskatoon, Sask, Canada)
*Can J Surg* 35:517–520, 1992                                              7–5

---

*Introduction.*—Age-based risk groups have been defined to identify patients with a low risk of disease recurrence who can be treated conservatively. The validity of these groups, however, is open to question. The veracity of this method was evaluated relative to patients with differentiated thyroid carcinoma. The effect of the degree of surgical resection on patient survival in high- and low-risk groups was also examined.

*Patients and Methods.*—A total of 161 patients with differentiated thyroid carcinoma were studied retrospectively. Long-term follow-up (minimum, 25 years; maximum, 55 years) was undertaken. Low risk was defined as men 40 years of age or younger and women 50 years of age or younger.

*Results.*—Applying the age-based risk-group definition to the patients divided the cohort into 116 low-risk and 45 high-risk patients. Five patients (4%) in the low-risk group and 21 (44%) in the high-risk category died as a result of this disease. There was some survival benefit to high-risk patients from bilateral resection, but these differences were not significant. Survival in low-risk patients was also unaffected by the degree of resectioning.

*Conclusions.*—The age-based risk-group method is a valid tool to identify patients with aggressive disease. But, contrary to expectation, there does not appear to be a universal survival benefit resulting from bilateral thyroid resection.

▶ This paper was selected because it provides a comparison of unilateral versus bilateral thyroid resection for differentiated thyroid cancer, although it is not a randomized study. This retrospective analysis demonstrates an excellent survival rate for patients with thyroid cancer whether or not they had unilateral or bilateral thyroid resection. The age-based high-risk patients did have a significantly poorer rate of survival compared to low-risk patients, as might be expected. Based on this study, one can question whether subjecting the patient to total thyroidectomy really adds significantly to survival. In the hands of many surgeons, performing less than total thyroidectomy would result in outcomes comparable to those of total thyroidectomy and yet would not carry the risk of possible hypoparathyroidism or recurrent laryngeal nerve injury.—R.J. Howard, M.D.

---

### Thyroid and Parathyroid Surgical Complications

Harris SC (Madigan Army Med Ctr, Tacoma, Wash)
*Am J Surg* 163:476–478, 1992                                    7–6

---

*Background.*—Surgical intervention is still the primary treatment modality for many thyroid and parathyroid disorders. Some physicians are hesitant to refer patients for surgery, however, because of the reported potential for laryngeal nerve injury or permanent hypoparathyroidism. To examine whether this hesitancy is warranted, data on 114 thyroid and parathyroid operations performed during a 10-year period were reviewed to determine the rates of nerve injury and hypoparathyroidism.

*Patients and Methods.*—In all, 73 women and 22 men underwent thyroidectomy, and 16 women and 3 men underwent parathyroidectomy. Two patients underwent simultaneous thyroid and parathyroid resection for concomitant disease. Thirty-one patients had single lobectomies, 9 had bilateral subtotal lobectomies, and 55 had total thyroidectomies for malignant and benign disease. Only 1 patient underwent modified radical neck dissection. The same surgical technique was used for all thyroid resections. Patients were monitored after operation for clinical signs of hypocalcemia, and those who had undergone total thyroidectomy or parathyroidectomy also were monitored chemically for 2–3 days or until they were normocalcemic.

*Results.*—None of the patients died, and none had obvious injuries to the superior laryngeal nerve. Five of the 95 patients who underwent thyroid resection sustained unilateral injuries to the recurrent laryngeal nerve, but all injuries were recognized during operation. Only 1 nerve was transected, and it was immediately reanastomosed; the patient regained near-normal vocal cord function in 6 months. The other 4 patients recovered completely within 6 months. Three injuries occurred during lobectomy, 1 during total thyroidectomy, and 1 during completion thyroidectomy. None of the patients who underwent parathyroidectomy had an injury to the recurrent nerve, and none had permanent hypoparathyroidism.

*Conclusion.*—The 1% permanent laryngeal nerve injury rate, the 5% temporary nerve injury rate, and the 0% permanent hypoparathyroidism rate suggest that the benefits of early surgical therapy outweigh the risks of nerve or parathyroid injury.

▶ Certainly, the most feared surgical complications after thyroid and para-thyroid procedures are injury to the recurrent laryngeal or superior laryngeal nerve and permanent hypoparathyroidism. The rate of recurrent nerve injury is higher than previously reported in serveral large series. Carefully identify-ing the recurrent laryngeal nerve and dissecting its course completely from below the thyroid gland until its entrance into the laryngeal muscle remains the best way to prevent injury. I like to think of thyroidectomy as dissection of the recurrent laryngeal nerve. To dissect and see the recurrent laryngeal nerve clearly, one has to completely mobilize the thyroid gland, so that after the nerve dissection is done, the operation is virtually complete.—R.J. How-ard, M.D.

---

**Differentiated Thyroid Carcinoma in Children and Adolescents**
Harness JK, Thompson NW, McLeod MK, Pasieka JL, Fukuuchi A (Univ of Michigan, Ann Arbor)
*World J Surg* 16:547–554, 1992                                                7–7

---

*Introduction.*—In children with differentiated thyroid carcinoma (DTC), the rates of local and regional disease are high, but overall mor-tality remains low. The controversy about operative therapy for this tu-mor is even more intense regarding children than adults. A review was made of 54 years of experience with childhood DTC, focusing on surgi-cal management, local/regional disease control, and long-term results.

*Patients and Findings.*—The series included 72 girls and 17 boys aged 18 years or younger with DTC. The average age was 13 years. About a third of the children (34%) had previously received external head and neck irradiation, although there was only 1 patient so treated since 1971. Patients seen in the last 20 years of the study period had less-advanced disease. The rate of initial palpable cervical adenopathy decreased from 63% in the first part of the experience to 36% in the last 20 years. The incidence of local infiltration of primary cancer fell from 31% to 6%, and that of initial pulmonary metastases from 19% to 6%; the incidence of cervical node metastases remained stable at 88%. Almost all of the patients (93%) had papillary carcinoma or its follicular variant. Treat-ment was with total or completion total thyroidectomy in 89% of pa-tients, with management of lymphatic metastases ranging from regional excision to radical neck dissection.

*Outcome.*—There was a 4.5% rate of permanent accidental recurrent laryngeal nerve palsy and hypoparathyroidism, but these complications did not occur in any patient operated on in the last 25 years of the re-view. The rate of local/regional persistence or recurrence has been low since 1971. Although 21% of the patients had cervical nodal persistence, there were no thyroid recurrences. Radioactive treatment with io-dine-131 was given to 82% of the patients. The long-term mortality rate in the overall series was 2%, with no deaths among long-term survivors treated in the past 20 years.

*Conclusions.*—For children and adolescents with DTC, total thyroidectomy, cervical lymph node dissection, and postoperative iodine-131 therapy appears to be the best management. The authors intend to continue using this approach until some biological marker that identifies aggressive disease can be found.

▶ Thirty-four of the 89 children in this series had previous radiation to the head and neck, all but 1 before 1971. Children with thyroid cancer, even in the 33 patients identified from 1971 to 1990, had a high rate of metastatic disease. Total thyroidectomy resulted in a high rate (4.5%) of permanent recurrent nerve injury (5 patients) or permanent hypoparathyroidism (6 patients). These 11 patients were operated on before 1971. There has been no injury in the past 25 years, demonstrating that well-trained surgeons can perform total thyroidectomy safely. The 2 deaths of long-term survivors (if 2 early deaths in critically ill patients are excluded) occurred an average of 18.5 years after initial therapy. The long-term mortality rate was only 2.2%, and there have been no deaths in the past 20 years. Aggressive therapy with total thyroidectomy, removal of affected regional nodes, and treatment with radioactive iodine can result in good long-term results.—R.J. Howard, M.D.

---

**Efficacy of $^{131}$I Ablation Following Thyroidectomy in Patients With Invasive Follicular Thyroid Cancer**
Davis NL, Gordon M, Germann E, McGregor GI, Robins RE (Univ of British Columbia, Vancouver, BC, Canada; Vancouver Gen Hosp)
*Am J Surg* 163:472–475, 1992                                          7–8

---

*Background.*—The proper extent of surgical resection in patients with invasive follicular thyroid cancer remains controversial, although many researchers recommend near-total or total thyroidectomy. There is also ongoing debate over the benefit of adjuvant iodine-131 ($^{131}$I) ablative therapy. A study was done to determine the survival benefit of adjuvant $^{131}$I ablation in patients with follicular thyroid cancer, emphasizing the role of this therapy in patients with minimally invasive disease.

*Patients and Findings.*—During a 33-year period, 142 patients (mean age, 49 years) were treated for thyroid follicular cancer. Seventy-one patients (50%) had stage $T_2$ lesions, and 35 (24%) had $T_3$ nodules. Nineteen patients had positive lymph nodes at presentation, and in another 11 patients positive lymph nodes developed during follow-up. Fourteen patients had metastatic disease when first seen. Of 71 patients who had minimally invasive cancer and no evidence of extrathyroidal invasion, 17 received $^{131}$I ablation, 46 were treated with thyroid hormone suppression, and 8 received either no treatment, external beam radiotherapy, or another treatment combination. The average follow-up was 9 years.

*Outcome.*—Kaplan-Meier analysis showed no difference in overall survival or disease-free survival at 10, 20 or 30 years between patients receiving $^{131}$I ablation and those treated with thyroid hormone suppression.

The same results were obtained for the subset of patients who had minimal invasion and no extrathyroidal extension.

*Conclusions.*—Because [131]I ablation therapy did not improve overall survival or disease-free survival over thyroid hormone suppression alone, [131]I therapy is not recommended for patients with minimally invasive follicular thyroid cancer.

▶ Patients with follicular thyroid cancer were treated by [131]I ablation or suppression with thyroid hormone only. The authors do not stratify the patients according to whether or not they had subtotal or total thyroidectomy. They also fail to state on what basis the patients were treated with [131]I or hormone suppression. Of the 142 patients in the study, 90 were treated with hormone suppression and only 35 were treated with [131]I ablation. Women were more likely than men to have hormone suppression. Only patients treated with [131]I had bone scanning to exclude metastatic disease. Even if the groups are comparable, it is difficult to eliminate the likelihood of a type 2 error in these relatively small groups, because survival after the development of follicular cancer is not dismal, even if neither hormone suppression nor [131]I is used.—R.J. Howard, M.D.

---

**Hürthle Cell (Oxyphilic) Papillary Thyroid Carcinoma: A Variant With More Aggressive Biologic Behavior**
Herrera MF, Hay ID, Wu PS-C, Goellner JR, Ryan JJ, Ebersold JR, Bergstralh EJ, Grant CS (Mayo Clinic and Found, Rochester, Minn)
*World J Surg* 16:669–675, 1992                                           7–9

---

*Introduction.*—Papillary thyroid carcinoma, in the latest World Health Organization classification, is defined by its follicular cell differentiation and characteristic nuclear changes. But Hürthle cell (oxyphilic) papillary cancers have nuclei that resemble those of oxyphilic follicular carcinomas. Thus oxyphilic papillary tumors may be more aggressive and have a worse prognosis than typical papillary cancers. Twenty-two patients with rare oxyphilic papillary cancers were treated during a 32-year period.

*Methods.*—From an evaluation of 1,163 pathologic specimens (1,106 patients with papillary thyroid carcinoma and 57 with oxyphilic follicular cancer), 22 patients with oxyphilic papillary cancer were identified. All patients were followed for a mean period of 12.6 years. Those with oxyphilic papillary cancer were compared with the 1,084 patients with typical papillary cancers and the 57 with oxyphilic follicular cancer.

*Results.*—The 22 patients with oxyphilic papillary cancer had a median age at diagnosis of 51 years. Most (64%) had undergone near-total thyroidectomy; in all but 2 cases, the surgeon reported complete resection of the primary tumor without gross residual disease. The mean size of these tumors was 3.2 cm. Eighteen were histologically grade 1 and 4 were grade 2. Only 1 patient had neck nodal metastases. The mean follow-up for these 22 patients was 11 years. At latest follow-up, 4 had died of their cancer. Compared to patients with typical papillary tumors, the patients with oxyphilic papillary cancers had fewer neck nodal metastases at diagnosis (5% vs. 40%), and the tumors were more often DNA non-diploid (71% vs. 21%); they also had higher rates of tumor recurrence (28% vs. 11%) and cause-specific mortality (1.7% vs. 4%) at 10 years. Thus in 4 important respects, oxyphilic papillary cancers were closer to oxyphilic follicular tumors than to typical papillary tumors.

*Conclusion.*—A similarity between the 2 types of oxyphilic tumors was demonstrated. Future World Health Organization classifications should consider these characteristics and group oxyphilic papillary cancer with oxyphilic follicular cancer rather than with typical papillary carcinomas.

▶ The authors of this paper reviewed 22 patients with Hürthle cell papillary cancers from a large group of patients with thyroid cancer. The authors argue that these tumors histologically and biologically resemble oxyphilic follicular cancers more closely than they represent typical papillary neoplasms. Four of the 22 patients died after a mean follow-up of 11 years. At 10 years, the mortality rate of Hürthle cell cancer was 17% and the recurrence rate was 28%. Most patients had undergone near-total thyroidectomy. Thus Hürthle cell papillary tumors should be treated by aggressive surgical therapy, because they behave biologically like more advanced follicular tumors.—R.J. Howard, M.D.

---

### Primary Hyperparathyroidism Due to Solitary Adenoma: A Comparative Multicentre Study of Early and Long Term Results of Different Surgical Regimens

Tibblin S, Bizard JP, Bondeson A-G, Bonjer J, Bruining HA, Meier F, Proye C, Quievreux J-L, Rothmund M, Thompson NW, Udén P, Zielke A (Univ Hosp, Ann Arbor, Mich; Univ Hosp, Lille, France; Univ Hosp, Malmö, Sweden; Univ Hosp, Marburg, Germany; Univ Hosp, Rotterdam, The Netherlands)
*Eur J Surg* 157:511–515, 1991                                                  7–10

---

*Objective.*—There is controversy about the optimal surgical procedure for the treatment of solitary parathyroid adenoma. Previous reports of the diagnosis and treatment of this disorder are not comparable because of differences in study design. A multicenter study was done to compare the early and late results of 5 different operations for the treatment of solitary parathyroid adenoma under strict enrollment criteria.

*Patients and Treatment.*—The population consisted of 325 patients with solitary parathyroid adenomas operated on between September 1978 and August 1983. Only patients who underwent 1 of 5 specified operations were included. Fifty patients underwent unilateral parathyroidectomy after unilateral exploration, 44 had unilateral parathyroidectomy after bilateral exploration, 84 underwent bilateral exploration with removal of the enlarged gland and incisional biopsy of 1–2 normal-sized glands, 37 had the same procedure with incisional biopsy of 3 normal-sized glands, and 57 had bilateral exploration with removal of the enlarged gland without biopsy. Eight years after operation, 272 patients (84%) were available for follow-up examination.

*Results.*—Patients who underwent bilateral exploration had a significantly higher incidence of severe postoperative hypocalcemia than did those who had unilateral exploration. Severe postoperative hypocalcemia was also significantly more common in women than in men. Age and preoperative serum calcium level were not related to the severity of postoperative hypocalcemia. At follow-up, 96% of the patients who had undergone unilateral exploration and 89% of those who had bilateral exploration remained normocalcemic without additional treatment. Eight percent of patients who had undergone incisional biopsy of normal glands had hypercalcemia and 8% had hypocalcemia. Only 1% of those who had been operated on without biopsy or who had a whole normal gland removed without biopsy were hypercalcemic, and only 4% of them were hypocalcemic.

*Conclusions.*—Atraumatic handling of normal parathyroid glands can reduce the development of early and late hypocalcemia without increasing the risk of persistent or recurrent hypercalcemia.

▶ This multi-institutional, nonrandomized study of a large number of patients with primary hyperparathyroidism caused by a solitary adenoma concludes that patients who had unilateral neck exploration did as well as (in fact, slightly better than) those who had bilateral exploration. Only 50 of the 325 patients operated on underwent unilateral neck exploration. It is interesting that only in this group did none of the patients require vitamin D supplementation or have any voice changes indicating injury to the recurrent laryngeal nerve. The authors strongly suggest that even after bilateral neck exploration and identification of only 1 enlarged parathyroid gland, biopsy proof of a normal parathyroid is not required and may even be detrimental. By excluding patients who had more than 1 parathyroid adenoma, however, this study did not answer the question of whether finding an adenoma on the first side of the neck explored means that one can avoid disturbing the neck on the other side.—R.J. Howard, M.D.

---

**Unilateral Neck Exploration for Primary Hyperparathyroidism: Analysis of a Controversy Using a Mathematical Model**
Duh Q-Y, Udén P, Clark OH (VA Med Ctr, San Francisco, Calif; Univ of California, San Francisco)
*World J Surg* 16:654–662, 1992                                7–11

---

*Introduction.*—The choice of surgical approach in patients with primary hyperparathyroidism is controversial. Whereas some endocrine surgeons advocate the unilateral approach, others explore both sides of the neck to avoid missing a parathyroid tumor that may cause persistent problems. The strategy of the unilateral approach was analyzed using a mathematical model to determine the variables that influence the probability of missing a tumor on the unexplored side of the neck.

*Methods.*—A spread sheet program was used to create a mathematical model for the unilateral approach. Variables examined included the prevalence of multiple adenomas, the probability of missing a tumor on the side of the neck that is explored, and the sensitivity of a preoperative localization study for parathyroid tumors. Outcomes assessed were the actual percentage of unilateral exploration when this approach is attempted, and the risk of missing an abnormal gland on the unexplored side of the neck. Initial values for the variables were obtained from textbooks and the literature.

*Results.*—Assumptions were that the frequency of a single adenoma is 80%; hyperplasia, 14%; double adenomas, 4%; triple adenomas, 1%; and carcinomas, 1%; the probability of missing a tumor on the explored side was 5%. The probability of missing a parathyroid tumor on the unexplored side of the neck is determined primarily by the prevalence of multiple adenomas; in half to two thirds of these patients a tumor will be missed. A preoperative localization study that is 80% sensitive should lower the risk of missing a tumor to 2% with unilateral exploration.

*Conclusion.*—Risks and benefits must be weighed in deciding on a unilateral or bilateral approach. If the rate of complications is high, the unilateral approach is favored. Surgeons should be aware that patients more likely to have multiple adenomas (e.g., the elderly) may be at higher risk for missed tumors. A prospective study with randomization to the unilateral or bilateral approach would require 684 patients.

▶ This is another paper that addresses the question of unilateral vs. bilateral neck exploration for primary hyperparathyroidism, this time using a mathematical model. This mathematical model has some problems. For instance, one of the assumptions is that preoperative localization studies are done and that the specificity is 100% (i.e., no false positives). The authors conclude that in patients who undergo unilateral exploration, there is an additional 7% to 8% probability of missing an adenoma, which would have been found if bilateral exploration were performed, and that the risk could be lowered to 2% by a preoperative localization study that is 80% sensitive. As the authors note, between 0% and 10% (average 2.2%) of patients have multiple adenomas. The differences in data may have as much to do with the criteria for determining multiple adenomas vs. hyperplasia by different surgeons and pathologists as with true differences in incidence. Many surgeons do not use localizing studies for the initial operation, because an experienced surgeon is much better at localizing diseased parathyroid glands than currently available radiologic tests are. The authors do not make any firm conclusions as to whether a unilateral or bilateral exploration should be done, but they suggest that a preoperative localization study be performed if the surgeon prefers a unilateral approach because it decreases the risk of missing a tumor.—R.J. Howard, M.D.

### Closed Mediastinal Exploration in Patients With Persistent Hyperparathyroidism

Wells SA Jr, Cooper JD (Washington Univ, St Louis, Mo)
*Ann Surg* 214:555–561, 1991                                    7–12

*Background.*—The management of patients with persistent or recurrent hyperparathyroidism after 1 or more failed neck explorations poses a difficult problem. Two patients with persistent hyperparathyroidism after unsuccessful neck exploration had parathyroid tumors within the thymus gland deep in the anterior mediastinum. In both patients, the tumors were removed during repeat neck exploration through a cervical incision by the closed thymectomy technique.

*Case 1.*—Woman, 18, with hyperparathyroidism, underwent initial neck exploration during which 4 normal parathyroid glands were seen and sampled. No parathyroid tissue was found in the thymus tissue removed from the neck and upper chest. The patient was readmitted with persistent hypercalcemia and underwent a second neck exploration. Because no abnormal parathyroid glands were found in the neck, the entire thymus gland was removed from the mediastinum. An enlarged parathyroid gland was found beneath the anterior surface of the midportion of the thymus gland. The patient's serum calcium concentration remained normal during 7 months of postoperative follow-up.

*Case 2.*—Woman, 38, with hyperparathyroidism, remained hypercalcemic after 2 neck explorations. Computed tomography showed a soft tissue mass in the anterior mediastinum at the level of the aortic arch. Thallium scanning showed increased activity in the mediastinum and left thyroid lobe. During a third neck exploration, the mediastinum was entered through the thoracic inlet and the entire thymus gland was removed. Examination of the thymus gland showed an enlarged parathyroid gland on its anterior surface. The patient's serum calcium values remained normal during 4 months of follow-up.

*Conclusions.*—Closed mediastinal exploration offers the option of extending the primary operation from the neck into the chest when only normal parathyroid tissue is identified at unsuccessful neck exploration. If the missed parathyroid tumor is removed by closed thymectomy, the patient is spared another operation and median sternotomy.

▶ Finding a missed parathyroid adenoma in a patient who has previously undergone neck dissection can be a frustrating problem for the surgeon and the patient as well. It is one place where preoperative radionuclide imaging studies can help to locate the parathyroid gland. The neck should still be examined first in patients who have a missed parathyroid gland. With failure to locate the parathyroid adenoma in the neck, the anterior mediastinum is the next most likely site. In the anterior mediastinum, parathyroid tissue is closely associated with the thymus. The authors demonstrate in 2 patients that it is possible to remove ectopic parathyroid glands located in the anterior mediastinum from the neck without median sternotomy.—R.J. Howard, M.D.

### Parathyroid Carcinoma: Clinical and Pathologic Features in 43 Patients

Wynne AG, van Heerden J, Carney JA, Fitzpatrick LA (Mayo Clinic and Found, Rochester, Minn)

*Medicine* 71:197–205, 1992                                    7–13

*Objective.*—The uncommon endocrine malignancy parathyroid carcinoma is associated with high morbidity and mortality. Parathyroid carcinoma should be considered in the differential diagnosis of hypercalcemic disorders because the prognosis is best with early recognition and operation.

*Patients and Treatment.*—Forty-three patients were treated from 1920 to 1991; there were 22 women and 21 men (mean age, 54 years). Fourteen patients had been reported previously. Two patients had a separate family history. The most common findings at presentation were polydipsia or polyuria, 38%; myalgias or arthralgias, 17%; weight loss, 17%; and nephrolithiasis, 7%. Nearly half had a palpable neck mass. The mean serum level of calcium was 15 mg/dL and phosphorus, 2 mg/dL. All patients tested had elevated parathyroid hormone levels, and most (91%) had hyperparathyroid bone disease. Primary surgical resection was done in all cases; 22 had simple resection of the tumor, 15 had resection with partial or complete thyroidectomy, and 4 had complete excision with debulking of other neck structures. Only 1 patient died within 30 days of surgery.

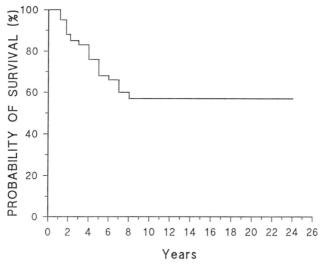

**Fig 7–2.**—Kaplan-Meier survival analysis of 43 patients with parathyroid carcinoma. (Courtesy of Wynne AG, van Heerden J, Carney JA, et al: *Medicine* 71:197–205, 1992.)

*Outcome.*—At a mean follow-up of 7 years, 33% of patients had no evidence of recurrent disease. Of the other 29 patients, 7 never had the serum level of calcium return to normal and 22 had recurrent disease. Almost all patients with recurrence were hypercalcemic, with or without symptoms, on follow-up. Sixty percent of patients eventually went on to have a second operation for recurrent disease, disclosing recurrent or residual neck tumors in most cases. Radiation was used in 5 cases. One patient appeared cured 11 years after tumor invasion of the trachea. Hypercalcemia was controlled effectively by repeated excision of tumor recurrences. The overall 3-year survival rate was 84%, and the 5-year survival rate was 69% (Fig 7–2).

*Discussion.*—The rare diagnosis of parathyroid carcinoma should be considered in patients who have a palpable neck mass, marked elevation in serum calcium and parathyroid hormone levels, and combined renal and bone disease. The best chance of cure is en bloc surgical resection, and effective palliation can be achieved with repeated resections of recurrent tumor. The use of radiation therapy for patients with inoperable, recurrent disease in the neck awaits further study.

▶ Parathyroid carcinoma is so uncommon (1% or less of parathyroid disease) that most surgeons will never encounter such a patient. This series of 43 patients was seen in a 50-year period at the Mayo Clinic. So, even at a large referral institution, there was less than 1 patient per year. Only 7 of the 43 patients had invasion of neck structures. In most patients the diagnosis was made on the finding of mitoses during histologic examination of parathyroid specimens presumed to be parathyroid adenomas. Although in these latter patients the tumor should theoretically have been removed completely, only 33% of the patients had no evidence of recurrent disease on long-term follow-up examination. The authors do not address what surgical steps should be taken at the initial operation if there is evidence of parathyroid carcinoma on histologic examination in an apparent adenoma without local invasion. That is, should one resect the local contiguous structures such as the thyroid gland and adjacent lymph nodes? An aggressive surgical approach is warranted in patients with recurrent disease, because this tumor is resistant to chemotherapy. In fact, 60% of the patients in this series required a second operation. This paper supports the use of aggressive surgical therapy, including multiple operations, in patients who have recurrent tumors that are not amenable to other treatment modalities.—R.J. Howard, M.D.

---

## Hypocalcemia After Thyroidectomy

Demeester-Mirkine N, Hooghe L, Van Geertruyden J, De Maertelaer V (Brugmann Hosp, Brussels, Belgium; Free Univ of Brussels)
*Arch Surg* 127:854–858, 1992                    7–14

---

*Background.*—Transient hypocalcemia after thyroidectomy is a common finding. Although many hypotheses to clarify the mechanisms underlying this phenomenon have been proposed, its causes remain unclear. An attempt was made to clarify the causes and underlying mechanisms of transient postthyroidectomy hypocalcemia.

*Patients and Methods.*—The study population consisted of 101 women and 34 men (mean age, 46 years) undergoing thyroidectomy, and 69 women and 35 men (mean age, 49 years) undergoing a variety of operations of the same magnitude and duration outside the cervical area. Blood samples were obtained on the day before operation and on postoperative days 1 through 4, day 7, and day 10 to measure serum levels of calcium, phosphorus, magnesium, sodium, potassium, chloride, osmolarity, alkaline phosphatase, total protein, albumin, parathyroid hormone, and calcitonin. In addition, 24-hour urine collections were measured for creatinine, calcium, and hydroxyproline excretion.

*Results.*—Total serum calcium levels in thyroidectomized patients and in surgical controls were significantly reduced on the first postoperative day but progressively returned toward preoperative levels during the next 9 days. Serum levels of other electrolytes, osmolarity, proteins, and albumin followed the same pattern of evolution. The evolution of postoperative serum calcium levels in thyroidectomized patients was exactly the same as that in surgical controls and was independent of preoperative functional thyroid status. The extent and duration of hypocalcemia in thyroidectomized patients increased with the extent of surgical thyroid resection. Parathyroid hormone levels on the first postoperative day were slightly reduced in thyroidectomized patients but not in surgical controls. In 3 thyroidectomized patients symptomatic hypocalcemia developed and they required calcium supplementation for 4–6 weeks, but all 3 recovered normal calcium and parathyroid hormone levels within 2–6 weeks after operation. Calcitonin levels were not increased after thyroidectomy. The urinary calcium output did not increase during the first postoperative days.

*Conclusion.*—Postoperative transient moderate hypocalcemia is a multifactorial phenomenon that is not specific to thyroidectomy but is common to all surgical procedures.

▶ This report demonstrates that the serum calcium level falls postoperatively whether the neck has been operated on or whether an operation outside the neck area has been performed. As expected, the more thyroid tissue removed, the greater the degree of hypocalcemia and the decrease in the parathyroid hormone level. With an increasing tendency toward total thyroidectomy for thyroid cancer, permanent hypoparathyroidism becomes a risk, even though a low one. In 3 patients in this series symptomatic hypocalcemia developed, requiring calcium supplementation for up to 6 weeks after thyroidectomy. Being permanently aparathyroid can cause problems that outweigh the potential benefits of total thyroidectomy, even when the patient has neoplastic tissue in both thyroid lobes.—R.J. Howard, M.D.

## Incidentally Discovered Adrenal Tumors: An Institutional Perspective

Herrera MF, Grant CS, van Heerden JA, Sheedy PF II, Ilstrup DM (Mayo Clinic and Found, Rochester, Minn)
*Surgery* 110:1014–1021, 1991                                                    7–15

*Background.*—Questions remain about the evaluation and management of adrenal tumors incidentally discovered on scans. No biochemical or radiologic indicator can reliably differentiate benign from malignant tumors. A large series of patients with incidentally detected tumors was studied to develop guidelines for their evaluation and management.

*Patients.*—During a 5-year period, 61,504 CT examinations were done; 2,066 patients (3.4%) were found to have adrenal masses. Patients with previous or concurrent malignancies, tumors localized after biochemical documentation, and nodules measuring less than 1 cm were excluded, leaving 259 for analysis. An additional 83 patients whose tumors had been found elsewhere were included, for a total of 342 patients (206 women, 136 men; mean age, 62 years). The average tumor diameter was 2.5 cm.

*Findings.*—Half of the patients underwent evaluation of biochemical hyperfunction; 2 of these had a cortisol-producing tumor, and 5 had a pheochromocytoma. Adrenalectomy was done in 55 patients; 4 had a primary and 1 had a metastatic malignancy. The smallest malignant tumor was 5 cm in diameter. No histologic diagnosis was obtained in the remaining 287 patients; 88% were followed clinically for at least 1 year, and 54% underwent a repeat CT scan. No clinical or biochemical adrenal abnormalities were found in this group.

*Conclusions.*—Adrenal tumors are a common incidental finding on CT scan. Biochemical screening is recommended for patients with tumors larger than 1 cm, surgical excision for those with tumors measuring 4 cm or larger, and repeat CT at about 3 months for patients with smaller tumors.

▶ The widespread use of CT scanning has led to the discovery of unsuspected masses in the adrenal gland, the adrenal "incidentaloma." Herrera and his colleagues at the Mayo Clinic report 342 patients with adrenal masses greater than 1 cm who did not have known cancer, and the cancer was not localized after biochemical documentation of disease. In the early days of CT scanning, many surgeons removed all incidentally discovered adrenal masses because of concern that they could be malignant. Few malignancies were actually discovered. This and previous papers have led to the suggestion that masses greater than 4–5 cm in diameter be removed, whereas smaller lesions may be followed as long as there is no biochemical evidence of disease. In this series the smallest malignant tumor was 5 cm in diameter.—R.J. Howard, M.D.

### Survival Rates and Prognostic Factors in Adrenocortical Carcinoma
Icard P, Louvel A, Chapuis Y (Hosp Cochin, Paris)
*World J Surg* 16:753–758, 1992                                        7–16

*Background.*—Adrenocortical carcinoma is a rare malignancy with a poor prognosis. Because of its rarity, the survival rates and prognostic factors for patients undergoing surgical treatment are unknown. The survival rates of 41 consecutively treated patients were assessed and an attempt to identify prognostic factors was made.

*Patients and Treatment.*—The patients, all operated on at a single hospital in a 12-year period, included 7 who had reoperations for local recurrence at an average of 22 months. The 29 women and 12 men had an average age of 42 years, with the men averaging 10 years older than the women. Most of the patients (80%) had secretory tumors. About a third had an abdominal mass. The average time from symptom onset to diagnosis in 25 patients was 10 months. All patients were treated by adrenalectomy and lymphadenectomy. Invasive cancer necessitated extensive resection in 32% of the patients.

*Outcomes.*—There was a 4% rate of operative mortality. There were 24 cancer-related deaths an average of 22 months postoperatively. At an average of 51 months, 37% of the patients were still alive, although 4 had metastases. With curative resection, the 5-year actuarial survival was 45%; with repeat surgery it was 33% (Fig 7–3). The 5-year survival rate was not significantly better in patients with stage I compared with stage II disease, although there was a significant difference between stages II and III (Fig 7–4). Ten patients with metastases had an impressive response to the drug OP'DDD(mitotane). One was alive at 2 years, but all of the rest were dead by 4 months postoperatively. Treatment with mitotane led to no overall prolongation of survival, but 4 patients with metastases had an impressive response and a relatively long survival. Prognosis

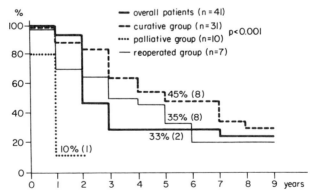

**Fig 7–3.**—Survival rates of patients overall, of patients undergoing curative resection, of patients undergoing palliative resection, and patients undergoing repeat surgery. Numbers in parentheses are patients alive. (Courtesy of Icard P, Louvel A, Chapuis Y: *World J Surg* 16:753–758, 1992.)

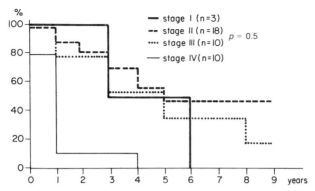

**Fig 7–4.**—Survival rates in each stage of disease. (Courtesy of Icard P, Louvel A, Chapuis Y: *World J Surg* 16:753–758, 1992.)

was not significantly affected by any patient or tumor characteristics.

*Conclusions.*—Adrenocortical carcinoma is most common in women and most often occurs in the 40th year; functional tumors are more common in women. Useful prognostic factors have not been identified. Large controlled trials of adjuvant chemotherapy for this rare malignant tumor are needed.

▶ These authors describe their experience with 41 patients treated for adrenocortical cancer at Hospital Cochin in Paris. These tumors are usually large at the time they become clinically apparent and frequently involve other structures. Eighty percent of the patients had tumors that secreted a hormone causing clinical changes. After an aggressive approach that led to adrenalectomy and regional lymph node dissection in all cases and partial pancreatectomy, nephrectomy, right hepatectomy, intestinal resection, or partial vena cava resection or vena cava thrombectomy in 13 patients and reoperation for recurrent tumor in several others, the 5-year actuarial survival was 45% compared to previously reported survival rates of 15% to 30%. Because these tumors are not very susceptible to chemotherapy or radiation therapy, an aggressive surgical approach is warranted.—R.J. Howard, M.D.

### Pheochromocytoma in Children: 15 Cases

Révillon Y, Daher P, Jan D, Buisson C, Bonnerot V, Martelli H, Nihoul-Fékété C (Hôpital des Enfants Malades, Paris, France )
*J Pediatr Surg* 27:910–911, 1992 7–17

*Background.*—Pheochromocytoma is a rare pediatric diagnosis. A review was made of the case histories of all 15 children treated for pheochromocytoma during the past 28 years.

*Patients and Findings.*—The 9 boys and 6 girls were aged 5–19 years. All 15 had intraperitoneal pheochromocytomas. Six patients had a family history of pheochromocytoma, and 3 of them were brothers and sisters. Symptoms included headache, sweating, visual blurring, polydipsia, and fatigue. Two patients who were brother and sister had café-au-lait spots. Six patients had evidence of hypertrophic and hyperkinetic cardiomyopathy, and 3 had signs of hypertensive encephalopathy. Urinary cathecholamine excretion was markedly increased. The patients underwent a total of 21 operations. Four patients with bilateral pheochromocytomas had bilateral adrenalectomies. Three patients had multiple tumors.

*Results.*—After adrenalectomy, 13 of the 15 patients had a return to normal blood pressure. A second pheochromocytoma was found in the 2 patients in whom the blood pressure remained elevated after operation. Three patients had a recurrence of hypertension 1–5 years later; ، ،estigation identified another pheochromocytoma. Fourteen pheochromocytomas were histologically benign.

*Comments.*—Localization of pheochromocytomas is a major problem, but MRI and angiographic procedures are helpful. Anesthesia is also difficult because the blood pressure must be lowered during operation and hypotension after tumor removal must be avoided. The pheochromocytoma must be resected with great care because manipulation may cause hypertensive episodes. Long-term follow-up is essential inasmuch as recurrences have been reported.

▶ Pheochromocytoma is unusual, and it took 28 years to accumulate these 15 cases from a Paris children's hospital. Six of the 15 patients had familial pheochromocytoma and 1 had multiple endocrine neoplasia type IIB. Pheochromocytomas in children are much more likely to be associated with familial diseases than are the sporadic cases that occur in adults. New diagnostic tests such as MRI have greatly aided in locating pheochromocytomas, especially in children, in whom they can be bilateral, multiple, or outside of the adrenal glands.—R.J. Howard, M.D.

# 8 Metabolism

## Introduction

Surgeons care for patients who sustain catabolic insults such as major operative procedures and life-threatening accidental injuries. When the disease process is prolonged or chronic, several physiologic alterations develop that may be associated with a poor outcome. These include nutritional depletion and its associated weakness, a delay in wound repair, and immunosuppression, often manifested by increased susceptibility to hospital-acquired infections. In the long run, these detriments preclude the immediate return to a productive life and escalate hospital costs enormously.

Recent advances in biotechnology and new information regarding organ nutrition and metabolism will change the way we care for patients in the next decade. Several approaches can be used to attenuate the injury response and/or enhance recovery from catabolic stresses. One current area of intense study focuses on methods of modulating the stress response. Currently employed techniques include the use of anticytokine monoclonal antibodies and cytokine receptor blockade. Two other approaches, which are highlighted in the present section, are the use of growth factors to promote wound healing and anabolism and the use of specialized nutritional support to improve outcome.

Recombinant DNA technology has thrust us into an era that is moving at a pace never before witnessed. We now have the ability to synthesize biological agents in large quantities, clone the specific genes that encode these proteins, transfect cells with genes to accelerate the expression of a certain protein, and cripple certain genes in vivo that may be causally related to a disease process. A good example of this technology is the enormous volume of new information concerning biologically active growth factors. These compounds can be applied topically to wounds or can be given systemically. New knowledge concerning the biochemistry of nonhealing wounds is emerging, including the finding that production of key growth factors by cells that control repair may be impaired. Can we restore normal wound healing with these compounds?

Growth hormone can now be synthesized in large quantities through the use of "smart bacteria." Before this scientific advance was made, human growth hormone had to be extracted from the pituitary gland, a process that was tedious and time consuming, and yielded only tiny amounts of the hormone. Administration of growth hormone to postoperative patients increases strength and skeletal muscle protein synthesis.

Growth hormone promotes a positive nitrogen balance when hypocaloric feedings are given. Growth hormone is now being used by athletes to enhance their performance. The half-life of this compound is short, and the development of antibodies or resistance to it is uncommon. How will the production, distribution, and use of such substances be monitored in the years to come?

We also find ourselves immersed in a complex and complicated era of nutritional pharmacology. Naturally occurring amino acids, which have been ingested orally for years, are being infused into patients in pharmacologic doses and are now considered drugs. Such "industrial-strength" nutritional therapy has important implications in the nutrition industry, a $4 billion market yearly. In our search for a magic bullet, we must remain scientifically sound and as unbiased as possible. Nutritional claims must be based on hard evidence, not on speculation or extrapolation; human nature dictates that we might behave otherwise.

To be meaningful, these new therapies must make a difference. A difference means that the patient, not the rat, clearly benefits. Is recovery enhanced? Does the patient get out of the hospital and return to work quicker? Is survival affected? Does the cost of the new "drug" warrant its use? Who is going to pay for the novel therapy?

This is a terribly exciting time for surgeons because many of the therapeutic advances in the areas of wound healing, nutrition, and metabolism that are taking place apply directly to our patients. Accordingly, in this section, we have focused on recent developments that are likely to influence the care of surgical patients.

**Wiley W. Souba, M.D., Sc.D.**

---

### Factors Influencing Wound Dehiscence

Riou J-PA, Cohen JR, Johnson H Jr (Long Island Jewish Med Ctr, New Hyde Park, NY; Albert Einstein College of Medicine, New York City)
Am J Surg 163:324–330, 1992                                          8–1

---

*Introduction.*—There has been no improvement in the incidence of abdominal wound dehiscence in recent years despite advances in perioperative care. Mortality associated with this complication ranges from 9% to 44%. Records of patients who underwent major intra-abdominal operations were reviewed to determine risk factors for the development of fascial disruption.

*Patients and Methods.*—During a 5-year period, 2,761 major abdominal operations were performed. Thirty-one complete fascial disruptions occurred (1%). Thirty-eight of the patients without dehiscence were randomly selected to serve as controls. The 2 groups were compared for the presence of 22 local and systemic potential risk factors.

Risk Factors Divided Into Significant and Nonsignificant on the Basis of *P* Values Obtained by Multivariate Analysis of Variance

| Significant Factors | Nonsignificant Factors |
|---|---|
| Age over 65 (p < 0.025) | Sex (male) (p = 0.65) |
| Surgery-related factors | Surgery-related factors |
|   Wound infection (p = 0.0001) |   Foreign body in wound |
|   Pulmonary disease (p = 0.007) |   (p = 0.8) |
|   Hemodynamic instability |   Emergency surgery (p = 0.10) |
|   (p = 0.018) |   Type of incision (p = 0.34) |
|   Ostomies in wound (p = 0.04) |   Type of closure (p = 0.44) |
| Systemic factors | Systemic factors |
|   Hypoalbuminemia (p = 0.0001) |   Anemia (p = 0.06) |
|   Systemic infection (p = 0.0001) |   Diabetes (p = 0.39) |
|   Obesity (p = 0.0001) |   Jaundice (p = 0.43) |
|   Uremia (p = 0.0001) | |
|   Hyperalimentation (p = 0.0002) | |
|   Malignancy (p = 0.0002) | |
|   Ascites (p = 0.0004) | |
|   Steroids (p = 0.012) | |
|   Hypertension (p = 0.028) | |

(Courtesy of Riou J-PA, Cohen JR, Johnson H Jr: *Am J Surg* 163:324–330, 1992.)

*Results.*—Multivariate analysis of variance yielded a number of significant risk factors (table) for the development of wound dehiscence. Age older than 65 was a risk factor; male sex was significant by chi-square analysis but not as an independent variable. Surgery-related risk factors included wound infection, pulmonary disease, hemodynamic instability, and ostomies in the incision. Certain systemic factors were also implicated, including obesity, steroid use, malignancy, and hypertension. All patients with more than 8 risk factors had wound dehiscence, and all patients with more than 10 risk factors died. The complication occurred in 30% of patients who had at least 5 significant risk factors.

*Conclusion.*—Wound dehiscence is a dreaded complication of abdominal surgery. Retention sutures placed in high-risk patients (those with 5 or more factors) may help prevent evisceration and dehiscence.

▶ Fortunately, wound dehiscence (fascial disruption) is an uncommon postoperative complication, but it is one that is familiar to all of us who do abdominal surgery on a regular basis. The majority of wound dehiscences are the result of technical errors, which means that they can be prevented by careful attention to suture placement. The diagnosis is a clinical one; in the worst case scenario, evisceration occurs and the patient dies. Generally, once the diagnosis of wound dehiscence is made, a second trip to the operating room for placement of retention sutures is in order. However, we have all managed fascial disruptions (particularly ones that are small or those that occur in very sick patients) in a nonoperative fashion.

The report by Riou and colleagues is worth reviewing because of the large number of patients in the series and because it is from a private institution. Therefore, the vast majority of the patients were very likely to be healthy and reasonably well nourished before the operation. The overall incidence of wound dehiscence was just over 1%. Given this acceptably low incidence of this particular complication, a large sample size is necessary in order to allow clinically relevant conclusions. I learned some things that I found interesting. For example, hypertension is a risk factor but emergency surgery is not. If you have a patient with more than 5 risk factors, it may justify placement of retention sutures at the time the operation is done. The probability of wound dehiscence developing and the patient's likelihood of dying correlate directly with the number of risk factors present.—W.W. Souba, M.D., Sc.D.

---

**Changes in Growth Factor Levels in Human Wound Fluid**
Dvonch VM, Murphey RJ, Matsuoka J, Grotendorst GR (Univ of South Florida, Tampa)
*Surgery* 112:18–23, 1992                                                          8–2

---

*Introduction.*—Platelet-derived growth factor (PDGF) may play a key role in wound healing. It was reported previously that human wound fluid in the immediate postoperative period contains 30-kd of PDGF AA and 12- to 14-kd of monocyte-macrophage–derived growth factor (MDGF). The level of biologically active PDGF AA and MDGF in human wound fluid was assayed in the first 48 hours after surgery.

*Methods.*—Human wound fluid was collected from 6 adolescent patients 6, 12, 20, 28, 36, and 44 hours after undergoing orthopedic surgery. Western blot analysis was performed to measure the amount of PDGF present, and a responsive cell line was used to determine the chemotactic and mitogenic potential of purified wound fluid containing PDGF AA and MDGF. A cell line unresponsive to PDGF AA was used to measure the biological activity of MDGF.

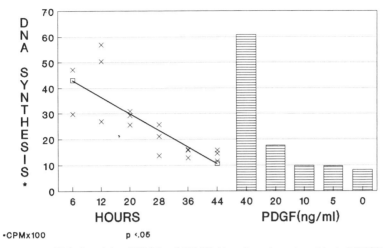

**Fig 8–1.**—Biologic activity of PDGF and MDGF. Note that mitogenic activity in NIH/3T3 cells correlates with mitogenic response. (Courtesy of Dvonch VM, Murphey RJ, Matsuoka J, et al: *Surgery* 112:18–23, 1992.)

*Results.*—The concentrations and biological activity of the 2 factors highest in the immediate postoperative period and had declined to negligible levels by 24 hours. Similarly, the chemotactic activity of MDGF was highest in the immediate postoperative period, declining thereafter (Fig 8–1).

*Conclusions.*—These findings indicate that PDGF and MDGF levels in human wound fluid change over time, bolstering the cascade model of wound healing. The finding that MDGF affects cell lines that are unresponsive to the PDGF AA found in wound fluid suggests that MDGF may also have an important role in wound repair.

---

### *Pseudomonas aeruginosa* Exotoxin A: Its Role in Retardation of Wound Healing

Heggers JP, Haydon S, Ko F, Hayward PG, Carp S, Robson MC (Shriners Burns Inst, Galveston, Tex)

*J Burn Care Rehabil* 13:512–518, 1992                          8–3

---

*Introduction.*—The microorganism *Pseudomonas aeruginosa* (PSAR) results in higher rates of morbidity and mortality than any of the gram-negative organisms associated with infection in burn patients. The most toxic and best studied product of PSAR is exotoxin A. In an animal study, whether exotoxin A from PSAR, rather than the number of bacteria, impedes the wound healing process was investigated.

*Methods.*—Acute granulating wounds were created on 90 Sprague-Dawley rats. The animals were divided into 6 equal groups. Group 1 consisted of uninfected controls and received no topical treatment. Animals in group 2 were treated with exotoxin A 3 times weekly (100 $\mu$g of exotoxin in 100 $\mu$L). Group 3 animals received exotoxin A and anti-exotoxin A (100 $\mu$g/100 $\mu$L for each) 3 times weekly. Group 4 received autoclaved PSAR $10^6$; group 5, $10^6$ viable PSAR inoculated in the wound; and group 6, $10^6$ viable PSAR and anti-exotoxin A. Wound contraction was measured twice a week with computerized digital planimetry, and serial biopsies were performed on all wounds.

*Results.*—When compared with contraction rates in noninfected controls, significantly retarded closure was noted in animals treated with exotoxin A and those given viable PSAR. The animals treated with exotoxin A plus anti-exotoxin and those treated with live PSAR and anti-exotoxin had contraction rates identical to those of controls.

*Conclusion.*—Infection, or the number of organisms present in a wound, is a critical factor in wound healing by contraction. *Pseudomonas aeruginosa* produces innumerable by-products and structures that may contribute to its pathogenicity. This study suggests that exotoxin A is the major mediator for retardation of healing in PSAR wound infections, irrespective of bacterial numbers. Neutralization of the toxin appears to restore the normal healing process.

---

**Transforming Growth Factor-$\beta$ Up-Regulates Elastin Gene Expression in Human Skin Fibroblasts: Evidence for Post-Transcriptional Modulation**
Kähäri V-M, Olsen DR, Rhudy RW, Carrillo P, Chen YQ, Uitto J (Thomas Jefferson Univ, Philadelphia, Pa; Celtrix Labs, Palo Alto, Calif)
*Lab Invest* 66:580–588, 1992                                          8–4

---

*Introduction.*—Relatively little is known of the factors that regulate elastin gene expression. Elevated elastin mRNA levels noted in cultures incubated with transforming growth factor (TGF)-$\beta$1 may result from a combination of enhanced transcriptional activity and reduced turnover of the mRNA. The effects of TGF-$\beta$1 and TGF-$\beta$2 on human elastin mRNA abundance, promoter activity, and mRNA stability were examined in cultured human skin fibroblasts.

*Results.*—There was a dose-dependent increase in elastin mRNA steady-state levels after treatment of cell cultures with varying concentrations of TGF-$\beta$1 or TGF-$\beta$2 for 24 hours. Maximum enhancement was noted with 1 ng/mL. The addition of cycloheximide (10 $\mu$g/mL) did not block upregulation of elastin gene expression by TGF-$\beta$, suggesting that the presence of active protein synthesis is not necessary for this effect. In addition, TGF-$\beta$-elicited enhancement of elastin mRNA levels could be abrogated by tumor necrosis factor-$\alpha$ and partially counteracted by interferon-$\gamma$. Transient transfections of human skin fibroblasts with elastin promoter/chloramphenicol acetyltransferase gene constructs revealed no change in promoter activity in the presence of TGF-$\beta$. But TGF-$\beta$

did appear to stabilize the elastin mRNA transcripts, as determined by Northern hybridizations after inhibition of initiation of the transcription. Thus the elastin mRNA levels were clearly detectable in TGF-β1-treated cultures even up to 48 hours after inhibition of transcription. Those levels were undetectable, however, in the control cells after 24 hours of incubation.

*Conclusion.*—Results indicate that TGF-β can modulate elastin gene expression, but that other cytokines participate in the modulation of elastin synthesis. This effect of TGF-β is mediated, at least in part, post-transcriptionally. The TGF-βs appear to be involved in regulation of elastin deposition during fetal development and tissue repair, as well as in disease conditions.

---

**Platelet-Derived Growth Factor (BB Homodimer), Transforming Growth Factor-β1, and Basic Fibroblast Growth Factor in Dermal Wound Healing: Neovessel and Matrix Formation and Cessation of Repair**

Pierce GF, Tarpley JE, Yanagihara D, Mustoe TA, Fox GM, Thomason A (Amgen, Inc, Thousand Oaks, Calif; Northwestern Univ, Chicago)
*Am J Pathol* 140:1375–1388, 1992                    8–5

*Introduction.*—Soft tissue healing may be hastened by growth factors, specifically recombinant platelet-derived growth factor, BB homodimer (rPDGF-BB), transforming growth factor-β₁ (rTGF-β₁), and basic fibro-

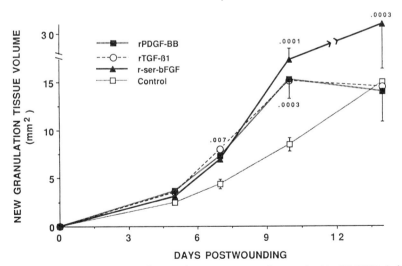

**Fig 8–2.**—Accelerated kinetics of tissue deposition in wounds treated with rPDGF-BB (*solid squares*), rTGF-β₁ (*circles*), or recombinant serine-bFGF (*triangles*) compared with those of untreated controls (*empty squares*). (Courtesy of Pierce GF, Tarpley JE, Yanagihara D, et al: *Am J Pathol* 140:1375–1388, 1992.)

blast growth factor (rbFGF). There are few data on the components of wound matrix induced by these factors or on the molecular mechanisms of accelerated repair and wound maturation, however. The sequence of tissue repair was examined in rabbit ear wounds treated by rPDGF-BB, rTGF-$\beta_1$, and rbFGF.

*Methods.*—Excisional wounds were created in rabbit ears and treated with single applications of optimal concentrations of each growth factor. Specific histochemical and immunohistochemical stains and image analysis techniques were used to assess the composition, quantity, and rate of extracellular matrix deposition within the wounds.

*Results.*—Growth-factor application appeared to accelerate normal healing by 30% (Fig 8-2). Early glycosaminoglycan (GAG) and fibronectin deposition were markedly increased by rPDGF-BB deposition; significantly greater levels of collagen were induced later in the repair process than in untreated wounds. With rTGF-$\beta_1$ treatment, collagen synthesis and maturation were greatly enhanced, with no increase in GAG deposition. A predominantly angiogenic response occurred in rbFGF-treated wounds, including marked increases in endothelia and neovessels and increased wound collagenolytic activity. These wounds did not evolve into collagen-containing scars and continued to accumulate provisional matrix only long after the wound had closed.

*Conclusions.*—Different growth factors appear to affect wound repair in different ways. Whereas rPDGF-BB accelerates deposition of provisional wound matrix, rTGF-$\beta$1 hastens collagen deposition and maturation. The monocellular angiogenic response to rbFGF may result in considerable delays in wound maturation and possible loss of the signal (or signals) to stop the repair process. Thus individual growth factors may selectively regulate components of the repair process and may offer the possibility of targeted therapeutic intervention.

---

**Human Recombinant Transforming Growth Factor-$\beta$1 Modulation of Biochemical and Cellular Events in Healing of Ulcer Wounds**
Chen TL, Bates RL, Xu Y, Ammann AJ, Beck LS (Genentech, Inc, South San Francisco, Calif)
*J Invest Dermatol* 98:428–435, 1992                                                8–6

---

*Background.*—Several animal models have demonstrated the ability of transforming growth factor (TGF) to initiate a series of events leading to enhanced wound healing. Only recently have models allowing quantitative biochemical analysis of alterations induced by recombinant human TGF-$\beta_1$ (rhTGF-$\beta_1$) become available. The effects of rhTGF-$\beta_1$ in a rabbit ear ulcer model were evaluated.

*Methods.*—Full-thickness biopsy ulcers were created in the ears of New Zealand white male rabbits. Wound healing with and without perichondrium was compared in terms of formation of total healing wound

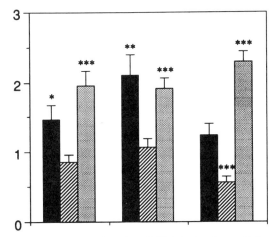

**Fig 8–3.**—Stimulation of collagen synthesis by rgTGF-$\beta_1$ in the ulcers with intact perichondrium. The amount of collagen (*black bar*) and noncollagen protein (*striped bar*) and percentage of collagen synthesis (*gray bar*) are shown. (Courtesy of Chen TL, Bates RL, Xu Y, et al: *J Invest Dermatol* 98:428–435, 1992.)

area over time and the amount of collagen synthesized by the wound tissue on day 5. The total healing wound area was defined as the newly formed connective and granulation tissues within the ulcer. In both models the effect of rhTGF-$\beta_1$ (100 ng by topical application) was assessed. The effect of rhTGF-$\beta_1$ on granulation-tissue-derived fibroblasts was evaluated by measuring DNA and collagen synthesis in response to increasing doses of rhTGF-$\beta_1$.

*Results.*—The total healing wound area reached a plateau at day 7 in ulcers with intact perichondrium, compared with day 14 in the perichondrium-free model. Healing was enhanced with topical application of rhTGF-$\beta_1$; collagen synthesis increased by 100% in ulcers with intact perichondrium and by 40% in perichondrium-free ulcers (Fig 8–3). According to in vitro labeling with [³H]thymidine ([³H]TdR), rhTGF-$\beta_1$ had no effect on DNA synthesis in ulcers with intact perichondrium on day 5. Autoradiography suggested that the main cells labeled were epithelial cells, and that rhTGF-$\beta_1$ treatment enhanced their migration from the wound center to the margin. The percentage of collagen synthesis changed in 2 phases in response to rhTGF-$\beta_1$; a maximal increase of 50% at 20 pM was followed by a decline. There was also a twofold increase in [³H]TdR incorporation, reaching a plateau at 1 nM.

*Conclusions.*—Cellular responses to rhTGF-$\beta_1$ treatment appear to differ in vivo and in vitro. More wound tissue and greater responses to rhTGF-$\beta_1$ stimulation occur in rabbit ear ulcers with intact perichondrium, improving evaluation of biochemical and cellular events. A number of in vivo mechanisms are in operation, possibly involving cell migration and recruitment as a result of numerous interactions between cell and cell and between cell and matrix.

### Independent Modulation of Enterocyte Migration and Proliferation by Growth Factors, Matrix Proteins, and Pharmacologic Agents in an In Vitro Model of Mucosal Healing

Basson MD, Modlin IM, Flynn SD, Jena BP, Madri JA (Yale Univ, New Haven, Conn)
*Surgery* 112:299–308, 1992

8–7

*Objective.*—Healing of the gastrointestinal mucosa occurs by 2 distinct processes: restitution and proliferation. In vivo, however, these 2 effects cannot be distinguished. A study was designed to test the hypothesis that enterocyte mucosal sheet migration is regulated independently from mucosal proliferation and co-regulated by soluble growth factors and the extracellular matrix over which the cells migrate.

*Methods.*—Human Caco-2 enterocytes were cultured on matrix proteins (collagen I, laminin, and fibronectin), with growth factors [epidermal growth factor (EGF) and transforming growth factor-$\beta_1$ (TGF-$\beta_1$)] and with the tyrosine kinase and prostaglandin inhibitors genistein and indomethacin. Monolayer expansion was used as a model of healing, with proliferation assessed by $^3$H-thymidine uptake and restitution by mitomycin-blocked migration.

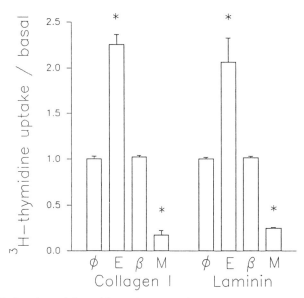

**Fig 8–4.**—Epidermal growth factor (E) stimulates Caco-2 $^3$H-thymidine uptake equivalently on both collagen I and laminin, whereas mitomycin C (M) inhibits Caco-2 $^3$H-thymidine uptake equivalently on both matrix substrates when compared with control conditions ($\phi$) TGF-$\beta_1$ ($\beta$) does not alter Caco-2 $^3$H-thymidine uptake on either substrate. $n = 8$; *$P < 0.05$ compared with basal $^3$H-thymidine uptake over collagen I or laminin, respectively. (Courtesy of Basson MD, Modlin IM, Flynn SD, et al: *Surgery* 112:299–308, 1992.)

*Results.*—Proliferation was unaffected by changing the composition of the matrix. Migration was stimulated 68% more with collagen I, however, than with laminin or fibronectin. At a dose of 30 ng/mL, EGF increased proliferation by 225% on collagen I and by 206% on laminin. It increased migration only on laminin, however. At a dose of 200 pg/mL, TGF-$\beta_1$ stimulated migration over laminin by 210% but inhibited migration of collagen by 89%; it had no effect on $^3$H-thymidine uptake (Fig 8–4). Organization of the $\alpha_2$ integrin subunit was affected by EGF but not by TGF-$\beta_1$ when cultured over laminin. Basal and EGF-stimulated $^3$H-thymidine uptake was inhibited by genistein at a dose of 100 $\mu$mol/L. This treatment also prevented EGF stimulation of replication-blocked migration with no effect on basal replication-blocked migration. At a dose of $10^{-5}$ mol/L, indomethacin had no effect on migration, but it did inhibit basal and EGF-stimulated proliferation by 7%.

*Conclusions.*—Matrix and growth factors seem to affect restitution and proliferation of gut mucosa independently. After surgery or in disease states, mucosal healing may be disturbed by such differential modulation. These findings raise the possibility of targeting specific phases of mucosal healing by pharmacologic agents.

---

**Effect of Transforming Growth Factor Beta and Basic Fibroblast Growth Factor on Steroid-Impaired Healing Intestinal Wounds**
Slavin J, Nash JR, Kingsnorth AN (Univ of Liverpool, Liverpool, England)
*Br J Surg* 79:69–72, 1992                                              8–8

---

*Background.*—Epidermal growth factor, tumor necrosis factor, transforming growth factor-beta (TGF-$\beta$), and platelet-derived growth factor

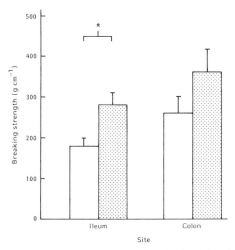

**Fig 8–5.**—Breaking strength of paired treated (*shaded columns*) and control (*white columns*) wounds in steroid-treated animals. Values are mean (SEM). Transforming growth factor-beta: 18 ileum pairs, 6 colon pairs. (Courtesy of Slavin J, Nash JR, Kingsnorth AN: *Br J Surg* 79:69–72, 1992)

applied to skin wounds at the time of wounding accelerate the gain in breaking load of these wounds. Recombinant biotechnology has allowed production of these previously rare peptide growth factors. Steroid impairment of wound healing is well documented. Because intestinal wounds are associated with considerable morbidity and mortality, the effects of steroid therapy and local applications of 2 peptide growth factors were assessed on healing longitudinal enterotomy wounds in pigs.

*Methods.*—One group of 7 pigs was treated with betamethasone twice daily and matched with a group of saline-treated pigs. Statistical comparisons were made of the breaking loads of wounds in the steroid- and saline-treated animals. Another group of 19 pigs was treated with betamethasone before receiving paired wounds in the ileum and colon. One wound was treated with a local application of TGF-$\beta$ or basic fibroblast growth factor (bFGF) at 5 $\mu$g per wound in a collagen suspension, and the second wound was treated with collagen suspension alone.

*Results.*—In the first group of pigs, steroid treatment significantly decreased the breaking load of wounds in the ileum and colon compared with wounds in saline-treated animals. In the pigs with paired wounds, the ileal wounds treated with TGF-$\beta$ were significantly stronger than collagen-treated controls at 7 days (Fig 8–5). A similar but nonsignificant response was seen in colonic wounds treated with TGF-$\beta$. The bFGF-treated ileal wounds had significantly decreased breaking loads and were more cellular compared to the collagen-treated wounds.

*Conclusions.*—Transforming growth factor-$\beta$ is a critical peptide in controlling collagen and matrix deposition. The use of topical wound healing agents in gastrointestinal surgery, particularly in cases of impaired healing, may have therapeutic advantages.

---

### Expression of Epidermal Growth Factor and Epidermal Growth Factor Receptor Genes in Healing Colonic Anastomoses in Rats

Braskén P, Renvall S, Sandberg M (Univ of Turku, Turku, Finland)
*Eur J Surg* 157:607–611, 1991                                                  8–9

---

*Objective.*—Complementary DNA probes were used to determine whether epidermal growth factor (EGF) and EGF receptor genes are activated in healing colonic anastomoses in rats. In previous studies the intraperitoneal application of EGF significantly increased the tensile strength of gastric wounds.

*Methods.*—A single-layer, inverting, submucosal colocolonic anastomosis was constructed in female Sprague-Dawley rats. The anastomosis was removed for examination at days 1, 2, 3, 5, 7, or 14 after operation. Six animals that did not undergo surgery served as controls. In situ hybridization, Northern blotting, and conventional microscopy were used to evaluate the specimens.

*Results.*—All animals convalesced quickly and the abdominal incisions healed without infection. Microscopic healing also progressed normally. Whereas expression of the EGF gene was minimal and not activated by surgery, surgical trauma did increase the expression of the EGF receptor gene (by 2.2 times when compared to day 1). In all specimens, in situ hybridizations localized a strong EGF receptor expression in mucosal cells; a moderate reaction was noted in fibroblasts in the repair tissue in the anastomotic line.

*Conclusion.*—The findings of enhanced EGF receptor gene expression suggest that anastomotic healing is associated with the presence of EGF or an EGF-like substance. This activity increases during the first postoperative week.

---

### Influence of 5-Fluorouracil and Folinic Acid on Colonic Healing: An Experimental Study in the Rat

Graf W, Weiber S, Glimelius B, Jiborn H, Påhlman L, Zederfeldt B (Akademiska Sjukhuset, Uppsala, Sweden; Allmänna Sjukhuset, Malmö, Sweden)
*Br J Surg* 79:825–828, 1992                                            8–10

---

*Introduction.*—The use of 5-fluorouracil (5-FU) as an adjunct to surgery for colorectal cancer has been most effective when administered as an intraperitoneal infusion and in combination with folinic acid. How intraperitoneal 5-FU, with or without folinic acid, affects wound healing in the early postoperative period was assessed in an animal study.

*Methods.*—Two experiments using male Wistar rats were performed. The animals were subjected to colonic resection and randomized to 1 of 4 treatment groups: controls (intraperitoneal NaC; intravenous NaC);

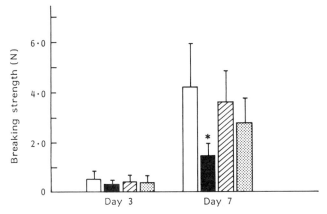

**Fig 8–6.**—Skin breaking strength in experiment 1. *Open bars,* control group; *solid bars,* 5-FU group; *striped bars,* folinic acid group; *stippled bars,* 5-FU-folinic acid group. *$^*P < .01$ 5-FU group vs. control, Duncan's multiple range test. (Courtesy of Graf W, Weiber S, Glimelius B, et al: *Br J Surg* 79:825–828, 1992.)

5-FU group (intraperitoneal 5-FU, intravenous NaC); folinic acid group (intraperitoneal NaC, intravenous folinic acid); 5-FU–folinic acid group (intraperitoneal 5-FU, intravenous folinic acid). Treatment was started immediately after surgery. The 2 experiments differed only in the dose of folinic acid and the time to killing of the animals (3 days or 7 days).

*Results.*—An observer blind to the treatment arm of the study examined the abdomen for anastomotic complications (abscesses or dehiscence). Such complications occurred in 4 of 33 control animals, 12 of 36 given 5-FU, 1 of 32 given folinic acid, and 9 of 36 given 5-FU–folinic acid. Anastomotic and skin breaking strength were similar in the groups on day 3, but were significantly reduced in the group given 5-FU by day 7 (Fig 8–6). Breaking strength was also reduced in animals treated with 5-FU and folinic acid, but to a lesser degree than in those receiving 5-FU alone. In the control animals and those given folinic acid, breaking strengths were similar.

*Conclusion.*—For reasons that are not clear, the intraperitoneal administration of 5-FU impaired colonic healing in this animal model. No further deterioration occurred when folinic acid was added.

▶ Wound repair is a complex process, with different components of healing being regulated selectively by different growth factors. Growth factors are synthesized by a variety of cells in the body. Under certain circumstances, these compounds function to stimulate cell proliferation and control wound healing. Growth factors are present in wound fluids that bathe the operative site after a surgical procedure. Although the exact source of these growth factors is unclear, one might predict that they are synthesized and secreted by injured cells or by inflammatory cells that invade the operative site. It is likely that certain clinical situations are associated with biochemical abnormalities in wound healing. For example, the abnormal wound healing that occurs in keloids and in hypertrophic scars may be associated with a decrease in the elastic fiber content in the extracellular matrix of these lesions. The potential clinical application and use of growth factors is likely to involve targeted therapeutic intervention, which, it is hoped, will lead to improved wound healing and improved outcome.

Infection appears to retard wound repair. As our understanding of the effects of specific bacteria-derived and host-derived products on healing improves, we will be able to produce neutralizing substances to these deleterious compounds. Clinical trials evaluating the use of anticytokine and antiendotoxin antibodies are already in progress.

In vitro models that examine the effects of growth factors on cell proliferation are important because experiments can be done in a very controlled system. In vitro models allow us to study the direct effects of growth factor on biochemical events such as thymidine incorporation and gene expression. Unfortunately, in vitro systems may not reflect the in vivo situation. In vivo studies are critically important, because wound healing involves cell migration and recruitment as well as complex cell-cell interactions, events that are difficult to study in vitro.

With recombinant biotechnology techniques, we have the ability to clone the genes encoding these specific growth factor proteins and synthesize the specific proteins in large quantities. The use of these agents raises a number of provocative questions. Is the concentration and profile of growth factors different in chronic wounds? Do chronic nonhealing wounds produce growth factors at all? Can the antihealing properties of chemotherapeutic agents be abrogated by growth factors? Will growth factors stimulate tumor growth? These compounds may be able to modulate intestinal wound healing as well as the healing of cutaneous and soft tissue wounds. Clinical trials designed solely to evaluate the effects of specific growth factors on healing of the gut mucosa have yet to be done. What would the study group consist of? How would healing be monitored and evaluated? Would the growth factor be applied topically or administered systemically?

Growth factors are likely to plan an important role in the future care of the surgical patient. Before these compounds can be used in the clinical setting, however, it will be important to (1) evaluate their safety and efficacy in patients, (2) identify specific groups of patients who will clearly benefit, and (3) demonstrate conclusively that the use of such peptides will improve outcome and shorten the hospital stay.—W.W. Souba, M.D., Sc.D.

---

## Immediate Postoperative Enteral Feeding Decreases Weight Loss and Improves Wound Healing After Abdominal Surgery in Rats

Zaloga GP, Bortenschlager L, Black KW, Prielipp R (Bowman Gray School of Medicine, Winston-Salem, NC)

*Crit Care Med* 20:115–118, 1992                                                    8–11

---

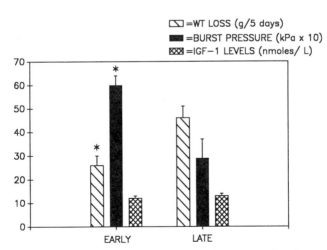

**Fig 8–7.**—Weight (*WT*) loss, abdominal bursting (*BURST*) pressure, and insulin growth factor 1 (*IGF-1*) concentrations in the early (immediate) and late (72 hours) feeding groups. (Courtesy of Zaloga GP, Bortenschlager L, Black KW, et al: *Crit Care Med* 20:115-118, 1992.)

*Background.*—Although nutrients play an important role in wound healing, it is unclear whether giving nutrients in the immediate postoperative period improves wound healing. A prospective, randomized study compared the effects of immediate with delayed postoperative enteral feeding on weight loss and wound healing after abdominal surgery in rats.

*Methods.*—Seventeen male Sprague-Dawley rats underwent midabdominal incisions, placement of a gastroduodenal feeding tube, and closure of the abdominal wound in 2 layers. The rats were then randomly selected to receive immediate enteral feeding with a peptide-based enteral formula or 5% dextrose in water at a rate of 4 mL/hr. Three days later, the latter animals began receiving the peptide formula. A balloon-bursting pressure technique was used to evaluate the strength of the abdominal wound on day 5. Blood insulin growth factor 1 (IGF-1) and the small bowel mucosal protein content also were assessed.

*Findings.*—The early-fed group lost less body weight (26 g versus 46 g) and had greater wound strength (45 mm Hg versus 22 mm Hg) than the late-fed group (Fig 8–7). No significant differences were noted in the circulating IGF-1 or small intestinal mucosal protein concentrations.

*Conclusions.*—This randomized study in rats shows that giving enteral feeding in the immediate postoperative period decreases weight loss and improves wound healing after abdominal surgery. Studies of wound healing in surgical patients are needed before these findings can be generalized to humans.

---

### Enteral Nutrition With Supplemental Arginine, RNA, and Omega-3 Fatty Acids in Patients After Operation: Immunologic, Metabolic, and Clinical Outcome

Daly JM, Lieberman MD, Goldfine J, Shou J, Weintraub F, Rosato EF, Lavin P (Univ of Pennsylvania, Philadelphia; Harvard Med School, Boston, Mass)
*Surgery* 112:56–67, 1992                                                   8–12

---

*Introduction.*—Recent laboratory and clinical studies have shown that individual nutrient substrates improve immunologic function, including the individual nutrients arginine, RNA, and omega-3 fatty acids. Because prospective trials proving the effects of these nutrients on clinical outcome have been lacking, a randomized clinical comparison was made of a supplemental diet containing these nutrients and a standard enteral diet in patients undergoing operation for upper gastrointestinal malignancies.

*Patients.*—The analysis included 77 patients. The mean age in the group given the supplemental diet was 60 years, and that in the group given the standard diet, 65 years. This was the only significant clinical difference between the 2 groups.

Number of Postoperative Complications

| | All patients (n = 85) | | Eligible patients (n = 77) | |
|---|---|---|---|---|
| Complications | Supplemented (n = 41) | Standard (n = 44) | Supplemented (n = 36) | Standard (n = 41) |
| Infectious | 6 | 18 | 5 | 17 |
| Wound healing | 1 | 5 | 0 | 4 |
| Total | 7 | 23 | 5 | 21* |
| Cardiopulmonary | 65 | 60 | 53 | 58 |
| Urinary/Other | 5 | 6 | 4 | 5 |
| Total | 70 | 66 | 57 | 63 |

$P = .02$.
(Courtesy of Daly JM, Lieberman MD, Goldfine J, et al: *Surgery* 112:56–67, 1992.)

*Observations.*—The mean caloric intake was 1,421 kcal/day in the group receiving the supplemental diet and 1,285 kcal/day in the group given the standard diet. In the first 20 patients, the mean nitrogen intake and nitrogen balance were significantly greater in those receiving supplements—16 g/day vs. 9 g/day for nitrogen intake, and −2 vs. −7 g/day for nitrogen balance. In the first 31 patients, in vitro lymphocyte mitogenesis was decreased 1 day after surgery in both groups; the supplemented patients regained normal levels, whereas those given the standard diet did not. Infection and wound complications developed in 11% of the supplemented group and in 37% of the group given the standard (table). On linear logistic models controlling for amount of nitrogen, dietary treatment appeared to be the major factor. The mean hospital stay was 16 days for patients given the supplemental diet and 20 days for those given the standard diet.

*Conclusions.*—Supplementation of the standard enteral diet with arginine, RNA, and omega-3 fatty acids improves the immunologic, metabolic, and clinical outcome in patients undergoing major surgery for upper gastrointestinal malignancies. Aggressive, early postoperative feeding in these patients is possible. More studies are needed to quantify the clinical benefits of supplemental feeding and to optimize nutritional support.

### Fish Oil Fatty Acid Supplementation in Active Ulcerative Colitis: A Double-Blind, Placebo-Controlled, Crossover Study

Aslan A, Triadafilopoulos G (VA Med Ctr, Martinez, Calif; St Mary's Hosp, San Francisco, Calif; Univ of California, Davis)

*Am J Gastroenterol* 87:432–437, 1992

8–13

*Objective.*—Patients with ulcerative colitis have increased levels of leukotriene $B_4$ in their rectal mucosa, and fish oil fatty acids are inhibitors of leukotriene synthesis. The benefits of fish oil fatty acid supplementation in active mild to moderate ulcerative colitis were evaluated.

*Methods.*—Eleven of 18 patients who entered the study completed the 8-month, double-blind, placebo-controlled, crossover trial. All patients had ulcerative colitis involving a minimum of 10 cm to the entire length of the colon as measured continuously from the anus. Patients ingested either fish oil (MAX-EPA) or placebo capsules for 3 months, entered a 2-month washout period, and then took the other capsule for a second 3-month period. Efficacy was assessed by a disease activity index based on patient symptoms and sigmoidoscopic appearance.

*Results.*—The disease activity index showed a significantly greater reduction with MAX-EPA therapy than with placebo (mean decline, 56% vs. 4%). The frequency of bowel movements was not altered significantly in most patients (72%) after MAX-EPA therapy. Therapy with MAX-EPA was associated with a 30% reduction in colonic mucosal leukotriene $B_4$, but placebo administration was accompanied by a similar reduction (26%). Eight patients were able to reduce or eliminate the use of anti-inflammatory drugs during fish oil therapy.

*Conclusion.*—Dietary supplementation with fish oil results in clinical improvement in patients with active mild to moderate ulcerative colitis. Mucosal leukotriene $B_4$ production, however, was not significantly reduced relative to placebo therapy in this series. All patients tolerated fish oil therapy, and none experienced worsening of the disease.

▶ Which surgical patients should receive nutritional support? When is preoperative feeding with total parenteral nutrition (TPN) justified? The recent VA Cooperative Trial (1) demonstrated that only patients who are severely malnourished are candidates for preoperative TPN. The rat study by Zaloga and colleagues (Abstract 8–11) demonstrated that immediate postoperative feedings decrease weight loss and improve wound healing. However, the use of postoperative enteral nutrition in the healthy patient who undergoes abdominal surgery is usually not justifiable. Exceptions include those patients in whom a jejunostomy tube is indicated. The vast majority of healthy patients who undergo abdominal surgery can tolerate a period of 5–7 days of undernutrition in the postoperative period. Thus, although selected patients are good candidates for nutritional support, keep in mind that the majority of patients that we care for do not require specialized nutritional support, and the injudicious use of postoperative enteral nutrition is contraindicated.

It is clear that enteral nutrition is the preferential route of nutrient delivery. One of the best studies demonstrating this is by Kudsk and colleagues (2). Enteral nutrition (compared to TPN) reduced the incidence of major postoperative complications in trauma patients. In this era of nutritional pharmacology, one of the latest hypotheses being tested is whether certain nutrients ought to be provided to the patient in pharmacologic doses. The nutrients that have received the most attention to date are glutamine, arginine, omega-3 fatty acids, and nucleic acids. Clinical studies evaluating these compounds are difficult to do because large numbers of patients are needed and because the diets being compared are usually different in ways other than in the concentration of the specific nutrient being evaluated. For example, arginine may improve wound healing and support immune function. Should we be administering large amounts of arginine to septic patients? Arginine is the exclusive precursor for the biosynthesis of nitric oxide, a bioregulatory molecule that is intimately involved in the pathogenesis of septic shock.

The pathophysiology of ulcerative colitis is still poorly understood, and this makes therapeutic intervention difficult. Aslan et al. (Abstract 8–13) noted a reduction in the disease activity index in patients with ulcerative colitis treated with fish oil. Leukotriene $B_4$ (an inflammatory mediator) levels were diminished, but they decreased in the placebo-treated group as well. The colon uses short-chain fatty acids (e.g. n-butyrate) as a primary energy source. Animal studies have demonstrated that short-chain fatty acids support colonic mucosal metabolism and structure.—W.W. Souba, M.D., Sc.D.

*References*

1. VA Cooperative Trial: N Engl J Med 325:525, 1991.
2. Kudsk, et al: Ann Surg 215:503, 1992.

---

**Effects of Epidermal Growth Factor and Glutamine-Supplemented Parenteral Nutrition on the Small Bowel of Septic Rats**
Ardawi MSM (King Abdulaziz Univ, Jeddah, Saudi Arabia)
*Clin Sci* 82:573–580, 1992                                          8–14

---

*Background.*—Recent studies in experimental animals document the beneficial effects on the intestinal mucosa of glutamine-supplemented parenteral nutrition (PN) after surgery, toxic injury, or radiation treatment. Other reports indicate that epidermal growth factor (EGF), administered with glutamine-supplemented PN, has an additive effect on the intestinal mucosa. The effects of PN, with or without glutamine supplementation, and EGF treatment were assessed in the small bowel of septic rats.

*Methods.*—Parenteral nutrition was started 2 hours after operation for induction of sepsis and catheterization. Septic rats were divided into 4 groups: 24 animals received a conventional hyperalimentation amino acid solution (group 1); 22 received a glutamine-supplemented PN hy-

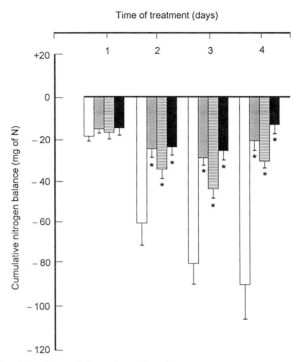

**Fig 8–8.**—Cumulative nitrogen balance during the 4-day PN treatment period. *Open bars,* group 1; *shaded bars,* group II; *striped bars,* group 3; *filled bars,* group 4. \*P < .001 compared with group 1. Values are means with bars indicating 1 SD. (Courtesy of Ardawi MSM: *Clin Sci* 92:573–580, 1992.)

peralimentation amino acid solution (group 2); groups 3 and 4 (22 animals and 24 animals) received the same PN solutions as groups 1 and 2, respectively, but were injected subcutaneously twice daily with .15 μg of EGF/g beginning on the first postoperative day.

*Results.*—The rats infused with glutamine-supplemented PN (with or without EGF) survived sepsis significantly better and had better nitrogen balance (Fig 8–8) than rats given PN alone. The benefits of glutamine-supplemented PN in combination with EGF included increases in jejunal mucosal weight, DNA and protein content, mitotic activity, and villus height and crypt depth, together with greater extraction and metabolism of glutamine by the small bowel.

*Conclusion.*—Survival rates in septic rats were significantly improved by glutamine supplementation, lending support to the hypothesis that glutamine is an essential dietary component for the gut mucosa. Glutamine may have direct cytoprotective effects on the intestinal tract and/or improve gut immune function.

## The Effects of Glutamine-Enriched Total Parenteral Nutrition on Tumor Growth and Host Tissues

Austgen TR, Dudrick PS, Sitren H, Bland KI, Copeland E, Souba WW (Univ of Florida, Gainesville)
*Ann Surg* 215:107–113, 1992                                                8–15

*Introduction.*—Glutamine is the primary amino acid used by rapidly proliferating tissues. When drawn upon by tumors for neoplastic metabolism and growth, glutamine is redistributed from the visceral organs and skeletal muscle. Previous studies have demonstrated that glutamine-enriched total parenteral nutrition (TPN) can help to maintain muscle glutamine concentrations in postoperative patients. The effects of TPN plus glutamine on tumor growth and host tissues were examined in tumor-bearing rats.

*Methods.*—The animals were implanted with methylcholanthrene-induced fibrosarcoma (MCA sarcoma) and studied when the tumors were small (less than 5% of carcass weight) and large (10% of carcass weight). In both small and large tumor experiments, groups of rats were randomized to receive standard glutamine-free TPN (TPN) or TPN plus glutamine.

*Results.*—The provision of 20% of TPN protein as glutamine significantly increased arterial glutamine levels and maintained the skeletal muscle intracellular glutamine concentration. Hindquarter glutamine fractional release increased by nearly threefold in the group given TPN

| | Tumor DNA Flow Cytometrics | | |
|---|---|---|---|
| | $G_1$(%) | S (%) | Aneuploid/Diploid |
| Small tumor | | | |
| TPN – GLN | | | |
| (n = 6) | 54 ± 3 | 29 ± 3 | 0.94 ± 0.14 |
| TPN + GLN | | | |
| (n = 6) | 51 ± 2 | 30 ± 2 | 1.1 ± 0.12 |
| Large tumor | | | |
| TPN – GLN | | | |
| (n = 6) | 62 ± 2 | 22 ± 2 | 1.55 ± 0.043 |
| TPN + GLN | | | |
| (n = 6) | 64 ± 2 | 24 + 2 | 1.86 ± 0.088* |

Note: Values are means ± 1 SEM.
*Abbreviation:* GLN, glutamine.
*P < .05 vs. TPN – GLN.
(Courtesy of Austgen TR, Dudrick PS, Sitren H, et al: *Ann Surg* 215:107-113, 1992.)

plus glutamine. Carcass weight, tumor weight, tumor DNA content, and tumor glutaminase activity were not affected by the addition of glutamine to TPN. The ratio of aneuploid to diploid cells within the tumor mass increased by 20% in animals receiving glutamine, but DNA flow cytometric analysis revealed no difference in percentage of aneuploid tumor cells within the $G_1$, S, or $G_2M$ cell cycles (table).

*Conclusion.*—Glutamine-enriched TPN does not stimulate tumor growth, but it may affect intratumor cell population dynamics. In the patient with cancer, glutamine enrichment might help to maintain nutritional status and prevent cachexia.

---

### Clinical and Metabolic Efficacy of Glutamine-Supplemented Parenteral Nutrition After Bone Marrow Transplantation: A Randomized, Double-Blind, Controlled Study

Ziegler TR, Young LS, Benfell K, Scheltinga M, Hortos K, Bye R, Morrow FD, Jacobs DO, Smith RJ, Antin JH, Wilmore DW (Brigham and Women's Hosp, Boston, Mass; Vrije Universeiteit, Amsterdam, The Netherlands; Mt Clemens Gen Hosp, Mt Clemens, Mich; Tufts Univ, Boston)
*Ann Intern Med* 116:821–828, 1992                                    8–16

*Background.*—Parenteral nutrition attenuates the protein losses associated with bone marrow transplantation. The amino acid formulations of parenteral nutrition usually do not include glutamine because it has a

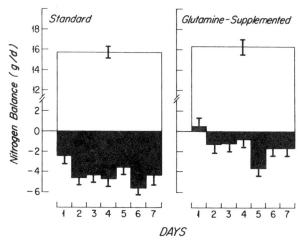

**Fig 8–9.**—Nitrogen balance in the 2 groups of patients receiving isocaloric, isonitrogenous parenteral feedings between days 4 and 11 after transplantation. Nitrogen intake for the week is shown by the *uppermost horizontal line* and balance for each 24-hour period is represented by the *black* or *stippled* areas. The group receiving the standard diet received no glutamine, whereas the group receiving glutamine supplementation received 0.57 g glutamine/kg of body weight per day. Daily nitrogen balance was significantly different between the 2 groups by analysis of variance ($P = 0.001$). (Courtesy of Ziegler TR, Young LS, Benfell K, et al: *Ann Intern Med* 116:821–828, 1992.)

shorter shelf-life than the commonly used amino acids and has been considered a nonessential amino acid. Because some clinical studies have shown improved nitrogen retention with glutamine-enriched parenteral feeding, the effects of glutamine supplementation and standard glutamine-free parenteral feeding on bone marrow transplant recipients were compared.

*Method.*—In a prospective, double-blind, controlled trial, 24 bone marrow transplant recipients received glutamine-supplemented parenteral nutrition and 21 received glutamine-free formulas. Parenteral nutrition was initiated the day after bone marrow transplantation. Nitrogen balance was determined between day 4 and day 11 in 23 patients. The incidence of clinical infection and microbial colonization, time until marrow engraftment, indexes of clinical care, and other data related to hospital morbidity were recorded for all patients.

*Results.*—Although nutrient intake was similar in both groups, nitrogen balance was improved in the glutamine-supplemented patients compared to controls (Fig 8–9). Patients receiving glutamine supplementation also had a significantly lower incidence of positive microbial cultures and clinical infection. The hospital stay of patients receiving glutamine supplementation was 29 days compared to 36 days in the control group.

*Conclusion.*—The positive effects of glutamine supplementation were present despite no differences between the 2 groups in antibiotic requirements, time to marrow engraftment, and the incidence of fever and graft-vs.-host disease.

▶ Several reports from different laboratories indicate that supplemental feeding with the amino acid glutamine is beneficial during certain disease states. Glutamine is abundant in the body, but its stores are quite labile. It may be an essential amino acid during critical illness. The exact mechanism by which glutamine exerts its protective effect is unclear. Although glutamine is an important fuel for the intestinal tract and is required for nucleotide biosynthesis, it is also important for immune function and endothelial function. Provision of large doses of glutamine to postoperative patients improves muscle protein synthesis rates (1). At present, there are few clinical studies that have evaluated, in a carefully designed trial, the impact of glutamine nutrition in critically ill patients. Such studies are likely to emerge in the next several years and presumably will define the route of administration of glutamine as well as the appropriate dose and the specific patients who may benefit from this kind of therapy.

Glutamine is likely to be beneficial to host tissues, but it is also a key fuel for a number of cancers. This raises the question as to whether glutamine should be administered to the patient with malignant disease. Will glutamine feeding stimulate tumor growth? Some researchers believe that tumors extract nutrients from the bloodstream at a maximal rate, and that provision of additional substrate will not influence tumor growth. On the other hand, others have shown that host starvation can decrease tumor growth. Medical oncologists suggest that glutamine stimulation of tumor growth would be beneficial if it improved the efficacy of cell cycle-specific chemotherapeutic agents. These questions are important because patients with cancer often require specialized nutritional support.

The study by Ziegler and colleagues (Abstract 8–16) warrants discussion because it is the best designed trial to date that evaluates the use of glutamine-enriched TPN. The authors chose to study a group of critically ill bone marrow transplant recipients who could not consume adequate amounts of enteral nutrition. Not only was the incidence of infection diminished in the group of patients receiving glutamine, but their hospital stay also was shortened. These investigators have also shown that the bone marrow transplant recipients given glutamine did not "third space." The reduction in hospital stay has been corroborated in a recent separate study by Dr. Paul Schloerb from the Department of Surgery at the University of Kansas. Glutamine is an inexpensive amino acid; the usual supplement provided to patients costs about $3.00 per day. Although glutamine is unstable in solution over the long term, it can be added to the TPN admixture when the pharmacist prepares the final solution. To be a difference, these kinds of dietary manipulations must make a difference. In this capacity, the apparent ability of glutamine to shorten the hospital stay for certain patients is impressive.—W.W. Souba, M.D., Sc.D.

*References*

1. Hammarqvist F, et al: *Ann Surg* 209:455, 1989.
2. Ziegler TR, et al: *Ann Surg* 214:385, 1991.
3. Schloeb R

---

**Excessive Chromium Intake in Children Receiving Total Parenteral Nutrition**

Moukarzel AA, Song MK, Buchman AL, Vargas J, Guss W, McDiarmid S, Reyen L, Ament ME (Univ of California, Los Angeles)
*Lancet* 339:385–388, 1992                                   8–17

*Introduction.*—The essential trace element chromium must be provided in a suitable dose to patients undergoing total parenteral nutrition (TPN), but there is little information about what dose is appropriate. One recommendation for daily chromium intake in children receiving TPN has been .20 μg/kg.

*Study Design.*—Chromium intake, serum chromium level, and renal function were measured in 15 children receiving TPN. The median age was 10 years, and the median duration of TPN therapy was 9.5 years. Age- and sex-matched controls undergoing endoscopy also were studied. The glomerular filtration rate (GFR) was measured by plasma clearance of indium-111-labeled diethylenetriaminepentaacetic acid. Daily chromium intake, serum chromium concentration, and cumulative parenteral chromium intake also were measured. In the second part of the study, chromium supplementation of TPN solutions was discontinued, and the children were reassessed 1 year later.

*Results.*—The patients given TPN had a GFR of 70 mL/min/1.73 m² vs. 110 mL/min/1.73 m² in controls. The average daily chromium intake was .15 μg/kg. The serum chromium concentration, however, was 2.1 μg/L in patients given TPN and .10 μg/L in controls. There was a significant inverse correlation between the GFR and the serum chromium concentration, daily chromium intake, cumulative parenteral chromium intake, and duration of TPN. After discontinuation of chromium supplementation, the patients were still receiving chromium in TPN solutions, fat emulsion, and drinking water for a daily chromium intake of .05 μg/kg. Although the serum chromium concentration decreased to .5 μg/L, it remained significantly higher than in controls. There was no significant change in the GFR and no signs of chromium deficiency.

*Conclusions.*—The current recommended parenteral chromium intake for children is too high; it should be closer to the .05 μg/kg level in breast milk, but this needs further study. The authors have discontinued chromium supplementation of TPN solutions; the concentrations occurring in such solutions appear sufficient to prevent chromium deficiency.

▶ Total parenteral nutrition solutions are generally supplemented with vitamins and minerals. As a general rule, the dose of each trace element has been established based on monitoring circulating micronutrient levels. Inadequate amounts of certain key co-factors are intuitively detrimental to body metabolism. Oftentimes, we think that if some is good, more is better. It is important to keep in mind that excessive amounts of certain nutrients may also be dangerous. In this report by Moukarzel et al., renal function, as measured by the GFR, was inversely correlated with the serum chromium concentration in children receiving TPN. Excessive administration of certain nutrients may be as detrimental as the lack of certain others.—W.W. Souba, M.D., Sc.D.

---

**Recombinant Human Growth Hormone Enhances the Metabolic Efficacy of Parenteral Nutrition: A Double-Blind, Randomized Controlled Study**
Ziegler TR, Rombeau JL, Young LS, Fong Y, Marano M, Lowry SF, Wilmore DW (Brigham and Women's Hosp, Boston, Mass; Hosp of the Univ of Pennsylvania, Philadelphia; New York Hosp-Cornell Med Ctr, New York City)
*J Clin Endocrinol Metab* 74:865–873, 1992                     8–18

---

*Background.*—Prolonged protein breakdown in hospitalized patients results in decreased resistance to infection, poor wound healing, and delayed recovery. Conventional nutritional support may fail to maintain body protein stores, particularly during catabolic states. Whether administration of recombinant human growth hormone (rhGH) increases the effectiveness of total parenteral nutrition (TPN) was investigated.

*Methods.*—Patients recruited for the study had gastrointestinal and/or pancreatic dysfunction and required TPN for at least 3 weeks. All were in stable condition. During a 7-day baseline period, constant maintenance TPN was administered to provide approximately 30 kcal/kg/day and approximately 1.6 g of protein per kg per day. Patients were then randomized, 9 to daily injections of saline and 6 to GH (10 mg/day), for 14 days. Body weight, vital signs, caloric intake, and total intake and output of fluid, nitrogen, potassium, phosphorus, and sodium were obtained daily.

*Results.*—During the baseline week, nutrient balances approached equilibrium in both groups. The administration of GH brought about a significant increase in the nitrogen, potassium, and phosphorus balance. No significant change in those parameters from baseline values occurred in controls. The GH-treated group also had a significantly greater cumulative change in nutrient balances from the baseline week. In addition, GH resulted in a slight rise in the serum level of cholesterol and a fivefold increase in the plasma insulin-like growth factor-I concentration. The only adverse effects of GH were moderate hyperglycemia and mild peripheral edema in a patient also receiving chronic prednisone therapy.

*Conclusion.*—The addition of GH to standard TPN significantly enhances nutrient retention. Thus GH therapy may aid in the recovery of patients requiring specialized metabolic nutritional care.

---

**Growth Hormone Attenuates the Abnormal Distribution of Body Water in Critically Ill Surgical Patients**
Gatzen C, Scheltinga MR, Kimbrough TD, Jacobs DO, Wilmore DW (Brigham and Women's Hosp, Boston, Mass)
*Surgery* 112:181–187, 1992                                                8–19

---

*Background.*—Patients who have sustained severe trauma or burns and those who have undergone major surgery characteristically lose both fat and body cell mass and gain extracellular water. The administration of human growth hormone (GH) increases nitrogen and mineral retention and stimulates protein synthesis. Whether the administration of exogenous GH to critically ill surgical patients might help to preserve the body cell mass was investigated.

*Patients and Methods.*—Of 19 critically ill adults, 10 had complications after major operations, 6 had sustained multiple injuries in traffic accidents, and 3 had large cutaneous thermal burns. All required full nutritional support. Eight patients received standard intensive care unit support and 11 received, in addition, GH (10 mg/kg/day). At the beginning and end of the 2-week study period, body water compartments were measured by the indicator dilution technique.

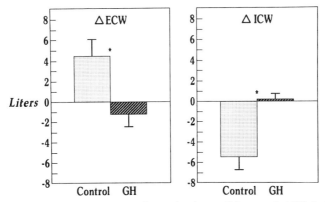

**Fig 8–10.**—Changes in extracellular water (Δ ECW) and intracellular water (Δ ICW) during 2 weeks. Values are means ± 1 SEM. *P < .01 by Mann-Whitney U Test. (Courtesy of Gatzen C, Scheltinga MR, Kimbrough TD, et al: *Surgery* 112:181–187, 1992.)

*Results.*—Body weight and total body water did not change significantly in either group during the 2-week period. A significant difference was observed, however, with respect to extracellular water. Controls gained a mean of 4.4 L, whereas those who received GH either maintained or lost (mean decrease, 1 L) extracellular water. The expansion and disturbance of the extracellular water/total body water ratio in patients receiving standard care was associated with a dramatic reduction of intracellular water, a critical component of the body cell mass.

*Conclusion.*—Critically ill surgical patients treated with GH maintain extracellular and intracellular water (Fig 8–10), indicating preservation of body cell mass. The ratio of extracellular water to total body water became normalized in these patients. Thus GH therapy can be used to reverse the characteristic changes in fluid dynamics that occur during catabolic illness.

## Growth Hormone and Insulin Combine to Improve Whole-Body and Skeletal Muscle Protein Kinetics

Wolf RF, Heslin MJ, Newman E, Pearlstone DB, Gonenne A, Brennan MF (Memorial Sloan-Kettering Cancer Ctr, New York City)
*Surgery* 112:284–292, 1992                                                8–20

*Background.*—Malnutrition remains a problem in some hospitalized patients despite the use of total parenteral nutrition. Previous studies have suggested that insulin may be helpful in decreasing protein loss in skeletal muscle by lowering the rate of whole body protein breakdown. Recombinant human growth hormone (rhGH) also has an anabolic effect with respect to skeletal muscle. The effect of rhGH and insulin administration on whole body and skeletal muscle protein kinetics was investigated.

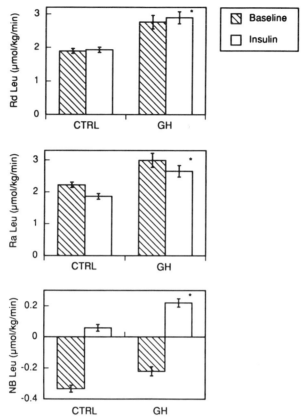

**Fig 8–11.**—Whole body leucine (*Leu*) kinetics: nonoxidative rate of disappearance (*Rd*), rate of appearance (*Ra*), and net balance (*NB*) of leucine. Rd leucine represents protein synthesis; Ra leucine, protein breakdown. *P < .001 vs. control (CTRL)/insulin, paired t test. (Courtesy of Wolf RF, Heslin MJ, Newman E, et al: *Surgery* 112: 284–292, 1992.)

*Methods.*—Twenty-three healthy volunteers took part in the study, 13 serving as controls and 10 receiving rhGH for 3 days before metabolic study. Five subjects treated with rhGH were given a dose of .2 mg/kg/day and 5 received .1 mg/kg/day. All participants then received an infusion of [14]C-labeled leucine and tritiated phenylalanine. Baseline protein kinetics were measured in both control and rhGH-treated groups. A euglycemic insulin infusion (1 mU/kg/min) was then administered concurrently with amino acid, and protein kinetic measurements were repeated at steady state.

*Results.*—There was an increase of whole body and skeletal muscle protein net balance with rhGH and insulin administration alone, and a further increase when the 2 agents were combined. Because substrate availability can influence the response to rhGH and insulin, amino acids were given concurrently during insulin infusion. Insulin levels were higher in the presence of rhGH (Fig 8–11). Although the lower dose of rhGH appeared to conserve more whole body protein, the number of subjects was too small and the treatment period too short to confirm this result.

*Conclusion.*—Loss of body cell mass is associated with poor outcome in surgical patients. Insulin and rhGH, in the setting of amino acid administration, interact to increase the net balance of whole body and skeletal muscle protein.

---

### Growth Hormone Regulates Amino Acid Transport in Human and Rat Liver

Pacitti AJ, Inoue Y, Plumley DA, Copeland EM, Souba WW (Univ of Florida, Gainesville)
*Ann Surg* 216:353–362, 1992                                                  8–21

---

*Objective.*—In surgical patients, human growth hormone (GH) improves nitrogen balance and decreases urea production, probably by increasing protein synthesis in skeletal muscle. The liver has not been studied enough as a site where GH might modulate amino acid uptake and thus divert nitrogen away from ureagenesis. A study was performed in humans and rats to determine whether GH regulates amino acid transport in hepatocytes at the plasma membrane level.

*Methods.*—Twenty healthy surgical patients were given saline solution or GH at a dose of .1 or .2 mg/kg/day for 3 days preoperatively. A 5- to 10-g liver wedge biopsy specimen was obtained at the time of surgery, and hepatocyte plasma membrane vesicles were prepared by Percoll den-

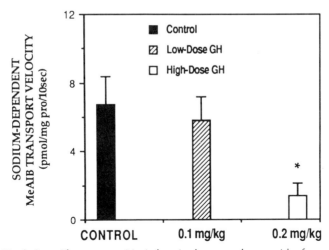

**Fig 8–12.**—Amino acid transport activity in hepatic plasma membrane vesicles from control and GH-treated patients. (Courtesy of Pacitti AJ, Inoue Y, Plumley DA, et al: *Ann Surg* 216:353–362, 1992.)

sity gradient centrifugation. A rapid mixing filtration technique was used to measure vesicle transport of the highly selective system A substrate, [$^3$H]-MeAIB, and the selective system N substrate, [$^3$H]-glutamine. Similarly, rat hepatocyte plasma membrane vesicles were prepared from animals treated with saline or GH—12 hours after chronic GH treatment, 4 hours after acute GH treatment, and 4 hours after chronic GH treatment.

*Findings.*—In the human liver vesicles, low-dose GH decreased system A activity by 13%, whereas high-dose GH caused a 79% decrease (Fig 8–12). There was no effect on system N. In the high-dose GH group, the reduction in MeAIB transport was the result of a 63% decrease in maximal transport velocity ($V_{max}$), with no increase in transport carrier affinity. In preparations from rats receiving chronic GH, system A transport activity was decreased as the result of a 59% reduction in transport $V_{max}$.

*Conclusions.*—In human and rat hepatocytes, chronic GH treatment appears to decrease the activity of system A. This pathway might be one by which GH has the effect of diminishing hepatic ureagenesis and sparing amino acids for peripheral protein synthesis. Studies of the effect of GH treatment on hepatic amino acid transport during catabolic states when amino acid uptake is increased are under way.

▶ Growth hormone is the anabolic agent that has received the most attention in the past several years with regard to its growth-promoting properties. Growth hormone appears to be safe and is associated with few side effects. Insulin and GH may work synergistically to improve protein synthesis in skeletal muscle. Growth hormone most likely exerts its effects through insulin-like growth factor-1.

The paper by Pacitti et al. (Abstract 8–21) demonstrates that GH diminishes amino acid transport across the hepatocyte plasma membrane. This group has gone on to show that GH can also attenuate the endotoxin-induced increase in hepatic amino acid transport. Although this may appear to be beneficial in that amino acids are spared for peripheral tissues, one might wonder what the consequences of this reduced hepatic amino acid availability might be in the long run. Because accelerated hepatic amino acid uptake appears to confer a survival advantage to the host, is a GH induced decrease in hepatic amino acid uptake beneficial? Perhaps GH enhances the efficiency with which the liver uses amino acids so that additional substrate is not as imperative.

This hormone is likely to play an important therapeutic role in patients in the next decade, particularly in combination with specific nutrients and possibly with specific growth factors.—W.W. Souba, M.D., Sc.D.

*Reference*

1. *Arch Surg* 118:167, 1983.

# 9 Gastrointestinal

## Esophagus

INTRODUCTION

For more than 100 years, it has been thought that Zenker's diverticulum develops because of high hypopharyngeal pressure. A recent study indicates that this is indeed the case, and the cause is incomplete relaxation of the upper esophageal sphincter. The cause of the cause, however, remains to be elucidated. Approximately 40% of adult Americans have gastroesophageal reflux and 10% of these have severe disease. A prospective trial comparing medical treatment to Nissen fundoplication indicates that antireflux surgery is significantly more effective than conventional medical therapy in male patients with complications of reflux. When performing antireflux surgery, most surgeons prefer a 360-degree wrap. A recent study suggests, however, that a fundoplication of less than that amount (180 degrees) can normalize acid exposure and increase the length of the high pressure zone, despite esophageal sphincter pressures that are significantly less than those observed with total fundoplication. I will continue to opt for the latter approach, however, particularly in view of a study in which the Belsey repair was compared to the Nissen fundoplication. The Belsey failed significantly more often than did the Nissen, particularly in the face of esophageal stricture.

The serious import of the finding of high-grade dysplasia (HGD) in patients with Barrett's esophagus has been confirmed. Eighteen of 19 patients with HGD underwent esophageal resection, even though none had clinical evidence of carcinoma. Fifty percent were found to have invasive adenocarcinoma histologically. The majority of these were stage 0, in which instance the 5-year survivorship was 100%. The use of flow cytometry in combination with histology in patients with Barrett's esophagus may be useful in identifying that subset of patients at greatest risk for either harboring an invasive malignancy or of having one develop.

Initial experience with thoracoscopic esophagomyotomy a la Heller for achalasia is extremely encouraging. Early results indicate that the technique is safe, effective, durable, and very well tolerated by patients. This approach may well become the standard initial treatment of the disease. A large Western world experience with the Sugiura operation performed in good-risk patients with bleeding esophageal varices has been reported. Although a salutary (i.e., low) incidence of rebleeding, both early and late, was found, the overall survivorship was disappointing, and the fact that esophageal fistulas developed in six patients, with a high mortality rate, is concerning.

Wallace P. Ritchie, Jr., M.D.

## Pharyngeal (Zenker's) Diverticulum Is a Disorder of Upper Esophageal Sphincter Opening

Cook IJ, Gabb M, Panagopoulos V, Jamieson GG, Dodds WJ, Dent J, Shearman DJ (Univ of Adelaide, Adelaide, SA, Australia; Froedtert Mem Lutheran Hosp, Milwaukee, Wis)

*Gastroenterology* 103:1229–1235, 1992                    9–1

*Background.*—In 1878 it was proposed that in posterior pharyngoesophageal diverticulum (Zenker's diverticulum), herniation of the pouch proximal to the cricopharyngeus muscle was caused by high hypopharyngeal pressures, perhaps attributable to defective coordination of the upper esophageal sphincter (UES). Patients with Zenker's diverticulum were investigated to determine whether they have abnormal coordination of pharyngeal and UES motor function and whether increased hypopharyngeal pressures exist during swallowing.

*Methods.*—Fourteen patients with Zenker's diverticula and 9 healthy age-matched controls were examined using simultaneous videoradiography and manometry. Pharyngeal and upper esophageal sphincter pressures were recorded with a perfused side hole/sleeve assembly.

*Results.*—Timing for pharyngeal contraction and sphincter relaxation, opening, and closure did not differ between these 2 groups. Sphincter opening was significantly reduced in the patients as observed in the sagittal and tranverse planes. Manometric sphincter relaxation was normal in

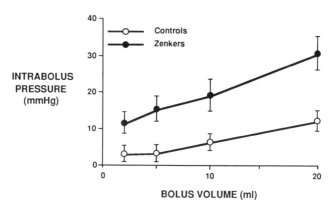

**Fig 9–1.**—Group mean data showing intrabolus pressure for a range of swallowed bolus volumes (mean ± SEM). Overall, pressures were significantly greater in patients than in controls (P = 0.001). (Courtesy of Cook IJ, Gabb M, Panagopoulos V, et al: *Gastroenterology* 103:1229–1235, 1992.)

patients. Intrabolus pressure was significantly greater in patients than in controls (Fig 9–1).

*Conclusions.*—Zenker's diverticulum is a disorder of reduced UES opening. It is not caused by pharyngosphincteric incoordination or lack of sphincter relaxation. Incomplete sphincter opening can lead to dysphagia. Increased hypopharyngeal pressure during swallowing may be important to pathogenesis. Intrabolus pressure measurements are useful as an indirect measure of sphincter compliance in studies of UES pathophysiology.

▶ This elegant study adds significantly to our understanding of the etiology of Zenker's diverticulum. Incomplete upper esophageal sphincter opening, *not* high basal pressure or discoordinate swallowing, is the villain. Why this should occur remains undefined. Nevertheless, the data clearly speak to the necessity of performing adjunctive cricopharyngeal myotomy during operative correction of this condition.—W.P. Ritchie, Jr., M.D.

---

## Comparison of Medical and Surgical Therapy for Complicated Gastroesophageal Reflux Disease in Veterans

Spechler SJ, for the Dept of Veterans Affairs Gastroesophageal Reflux Disease Study Group (Beth Israel Hosp, Boston, Mass)
*N Engl J Med* 326:786–792, 1992                                    9–2

---

*Background.*—About 4 in 10 adult Americans have heartburn, the main symptom of gastroesophageal reflux disease, at least monthly. Medical management involves changes in life-style and, often, combination drug treatment. Those who recommend antireflux surgery believe that an effective operation can spare patients the expense, inconvenience, and risks of long-term medical treatment.

*Study Design.*—Medical treatment with up to 4 medications was compared with the Nissen fundoplication operation in 247 patients with peptic esophageal ulcer, stricture, erosive esophagitis, or Barrett's esophagus. Those assigned to medical treatment were treated either continuously or only when symptoms were present. All but 4 of the patients were men. Follow-up data were available for 176 patients after 1 year and for 106 at 2 years.

*Outcome.*—Activity index scores declined in all of the treatment groups but most markedly in those who were operated on (Fig 9–2). Esophagitis was least evident in the surgically treated patients at follow-up. These patients did significantly better than either group given medical treatment during 2 years of follow-up.

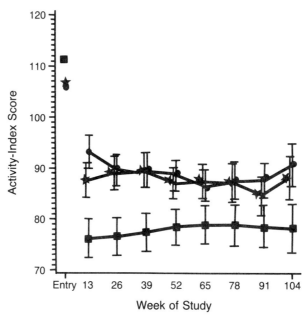

**Fig 9–2.**—Activity index scores for patients with gastroesophageal reflux disease during the 2-year study. Values are means ± 2 SE in the group given continuous medical therapy (*stars*), the group given medical therapy for symptoms only (*circles*), and the group given surgical treatment (*squares*). (Courtesy of Spechler SJ, et al: N Engl J Med 326:786–792, 1992.)

*Conclusion.*—Antireflux surgery was significantly more effective than conventional medical treatment in a chiefly male population of patients with complicated reflux disease.

▶ This important study shows that antireflux procedures performed by skilled and experienced surgeons are significantly more effective than conventional medical therapy (albeit not including omeprazole) in improving the symptoms and endoscopic signs of esophagitis for up to 2 years in male patients with complicated gastroesophageal reflux disease. Whether or not the omission of omeprazole from the nonoperative treatment arm is a fatal flaw, as some medical gastroenterologists have claimed, is problematic in my opinion, because, in our experience at least, patients with disease as advanced as this fare no better with omeprazole therapy than with maximized conventional therapy. The development of laparoscopic antireflux procedures may make the argument moot, however, if they prove as effective at controlling gastroesophageal reflux as they are when performed using the open approach.—W.P. Ritchie, Jr., M.D.

**Lower Esophageal Sphincter Characteristics and Esophageal Acid Exposure Following Partial or 360-Degree Fundoplication: Results of**

## a Prospective, Randomized, Clinical Study

Lundell L, Abrahamsson H, Ruth M, Sandberg N, Olbe LC (Sahlgren's Hosp, Göteborg, Sweden)
*World J Surg* 15:115–121, 1991                9–3

*Background.*—Surgical techniques for preventing gastroesophageal reflux generally result in symptomatic improvement with concomitant objective changes such as healing of esophagitis and prevention of acid reflux. But significant postoperative problems, termed postfundoplication complaints, may occur, including dysphagia, the inability to belch or vomit, postprandial epigastric fullness and pain, and increased flatulence. The results of semifundoplication (180- to 200-degrees, Toupet) were compared to a 360-degree fundic wrap (Rossetti) in terms of gastroesophageal junction function and clinical outcome.

*Method.*—Seventy-one patients were randomized for either partial fundoplication (33) or a 360-degree fundic wrap (38). Each patient underwent endoscopy and clinical assessment before surgery and at 3 and/ or 6 months postoperatively. Pressure data from the gastroesophageal junction was obtained by manometry via a triple-lumen catheter. Pressure in the high pressure zone (HPZ) in the distal esophagus also was measured. The length of the intra-abdominal segment was determined by a "station pull-through" technique. Ambulatory 24-hour pH measurements evaluated acid exposure of the esophageal mucosa.

*Results.*—Both surgical techniques normalized the acid exposure of the esophageal mucosa and increased the length of the HPZ. Patients who received the total fundic wrap had normalization of HPZ pressure, whereas those who underwent the partial fundoplication had significantly lower than normal HPZ pressure (Fig 9–3). There was a higher

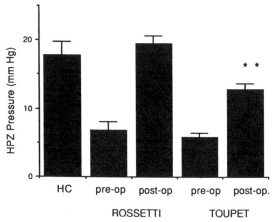

**Fig 9–3.**—The HPZ pressure in healthy controls (HC) and in patients preoperatively and 6 months postoperatively after a Rossetti or Toupet fundoplication (** = P < 0.01). The mean and SEM are given. (Courtesy of Lundell L, Abrahamsson H, Ruth M, et al: *World J Surg* 15:115–121, 1991.)

incidence of dysphagia at 3 months in the group treated by 360-degree fundoplication, but this complication disappeared in the subsequent 3 months.

*Conclusion.*—Both total and partial fundoplication techniques restored the intra-abdominal length of the HPZ and controlled gastroesophageal reflux, but only total fundoplication normalized the HPZ pressure. Clinical assessment showed excellent results with no significant differences between the groups.

▶ All of us have experienced occasional difficulties with postoperative dysphagia in patients undergoing 360-degree fundoplication, even when the wrap is of the "floppy" variety. This report appears to indicate that a partial wrap, which theoretically should produce less dysphagia, can reduce reflux and symptoms about as well as a 360-degree wrap, at least on relatively short-term follow-up. Of interest is the fact that the 360-degree wrap (the Rossetti) increased the HPZ pressure to "normal" levels, but the 180-degree wrap (the Toupet) did not. This suggests that the relative success of the partial wrap may be attributable to its ability to increase HPZ pressure above preoperative levels, but that achievement of "normal" HZP pressure is not necessary for clinical success. A much longer period of follow-up than 6 months is required to adjudicate the validity of that proposition, however.—W.P. Ritchie, Jr., M.D.

---

**Long Term Results After Nissen Fundoplication and Belsey Mark IV Operation in Patients With Reflux Oesophagitis and Stricture**
Vollan G, Stangeland L, Søreide JA, Janssen CW, Svanes K (Univ of Bergen, Bergen, Norway)
*Eur J Surg* 158:357–360, 1992                                              9–4

---

*Objective.*—Because few reports have appeared concerning the long-term outcome of Nissen fundoplication, a review was undertaken to examine the results and failure rate in 105 patients with severe reflux esophagitis who were operated on between 1972 and 1987 and followed for as long as 12 years.

*Patients.*—Forty-three of the 105 patients had a stricture. Eighty-three patients had a Nissen fundoplication operation, whereas 22 had a Belsey Mark IV repair. Most of the patients had been symptomatic for longer than 3 years. The chief indications for surgery were esophagitis with severe symptoms and stricture.

*Results.*—The 1 postoperative death followed a Belsey Mark IV repair. Cumulative recurrence rates were 9% after Nissen fundoplication and 37% after the Belsey repair. About half of the patients with stricture who had the Nissen fundoplication operation required dilatation after surgery. Five of 10 Belsey procedures done for esophageal stricture failed.

Nearly one fifth of the patients having fundoplication had "gas bloating."

*Conclusions.*—Antireflux surgery is a good option for patients having a fibrous stricture secondary to gastroesophageal reflux. A good outcome can be expected even in patients who have required repeated dilatations preoperatively. Most patients who still require dilation after surgery also will have a satisfactory final result.

▶ Although this study is retrospective in nature, it does confirm my bias that a Nissen fundoplication is a safer and more durable operation for patients with reflux esophagitis than is the Belsey Mark IV. This appears to be particularly true in those patients with a dilatable peptic stricture. Under these circumstances, it must clearly be viewed as the procedure of choice provided that significant foreshortening of the esophagus has not occurred.—W.P. Ritchie, Jr., M.D.

### Barrett's Esophagus With High-Grade Dysplasia: An Indication for Esophagectomy?

Pera M, Trastek VF, Carpenter HA, Allen MS, Deschamps C, Pairolero PC (Mayo Clinic and Found, Rochester, Minn)
*Ann Thorac Surg* 54:199–204, 1992                                                      9–5

*Background.*—There is some controversy over the association between high-grade dysplasia and invasive adenocarcinoma in Barrett's disease. Nineteen patients were studied to determine the need for esophageal resection in Barrett's esophagus with high-grade dysplasia.

*Patients.*—The 17 men and 2 women had a median age of 66 years. The most common presenting symptom was heartburn of long duration. None had evidence of invasive adenocarcinoma. In 9 patients, high-grade dysplasia was diagnosed at the time of their initial evaluation for

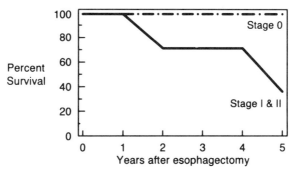

**Fig 9–4.**—Estimated survival of 9 patients with postsurgical stage 0 esophageal carcinoma undergoing esophagectomy for high-grade dysplasia as compared with survival of 9 patients with either postsurgical stage I or stage II disease. Zero time on absicsssa is date of operation. (Courtesy of Pera M, Trastek VF, Carpenter HA, et al: *Ann Thorac Surg* 54:199–204, 1992).

gastrointestinal symptoms. In 10 patients known to have Barrett's esophagus, the diagnosis of high-grade dysplasia was made through surveillance. Eighteen patients underwent esophageal resection; 1 refused the operation.

*Results.*—The most commonly used procedure (12 cases) was an Ivor Lewis esophagogastrectomy. All patients underwent resection of the entire length of Barrett's mucosa. Invasive adenocarcinoma was found in 9 patients, 3 of whom had normal appearing Barrett's mucosa. Postsurgical stage varied with the length of Barrett's esophagus; the median length was 6.5 cm in the 9 patients with stage 0 disease and 12 cm in the 3 patients with stage IIA or IIB disease. At a median follow-up of 34 months, 2 patients who had undergone resection had died of recurrent cancer. The patient who refused surgery was alive and well at 29 months. The 5-year survival rate was 100% for patients with stage 0 disease and 35.7% for those with stage I or II disease (Fig 9–4).

*Conclusion.*—Resection should be performed in patients with Barrett's esophagus and confirmed high-grade dysplasia. The benefits of early intervention in an otherwise fatal disease should outweigh the risks of resection. It is important to remove all areas of Barrett's metaplasia and thoroughly examine lymph nodes histologically. Patients with Barrett's esophagus should undergo biopsy yearly.

▶ This paper is one of many recent reports confirming the fact that about 50% of patients with high-grade dysplasia in the setting of Barrett's esophagus have associated occult invasive adenocarcinoma. Of importance, if resection is done early, the disease-free survival rates are substantially better than those observed in patients first seen with clinically obvious adenocarcinoma. The procedure of choice in my view: transhiatal esophagectomy.—W.P. Ritchie, Jr., M.D.

---

**Flow-Cytometric and Histological Progression to Malignancy in Barrett's Esophagus: Prospective Endoscopic Surveillance of a Cohort**
Reid BJ, Blount PL, Rubin CE, Levine DS, Haggitt RC, Rabinovitch PS (Univ of Washington, Seattle)
*Gastroenterology* 102:1212–1219, 1992                                    9–6

---

*Background.*—Barrett's esophagus is a condition in which the esophageal stratified squamous epithelium is replaced by metaplastic columnar epithelium. This predisposes to the development of esophageal adenocarcinoma. Whether there is a particular at-risk subset of these patients who would benefit from surveillance has not been determined.

*Methods.*—A prospective study was performed on 62 patients with Barrett's esophagus who were free of cancer to determine whether flow-cytometric evidence of aneuploidy and increased G2/tetraploid fractions predispose to neoplastic progression.

*Results.*—Of the 62 patients, 13 had aneuploid or increased G2/tetra-ploid populations on initial flow-cytometric analysis. In 9 of these 13, high-grade dysplasia or adenocarcinoma developed during an average 34 months of follow-up. None of the remaining 49 patients without these abnormalities had progression to high-grade dysplasia or cancer. Those patients in whom dysplasia or cancer developed often had multiple aneuploid cell populations that could be detected by flow cytometry. Patients appeared to progress through a phenotypic sequence that could be recognized histologically.

*Conclusions.*—Neoplastic progression seems to occur in a subset of patients with Barrett's esophagus who have a genomic instability that generates clones with aneuploid or increased G2/tetraploid DNA contents. These subclones may have the ability to eventually become an invasive carcinoma. A combination of histology and flow cytometry can be used to identify the at-risk subset of patients who need more frequent endoscopic surveillance for the early detection of high-grade dysplasia and carcinoma.

▶ This paper is important because it indicates that it is possible, using flow cytometry, to identify a group of patients with Barrett's esophagus at increased risk of esophageal adenocarcinoma before the development of high-grade dysplasia (with all that that implies). An unsettled question is the appropriate management of this group (continuous surveillance versus operation); equally unsettling, however, is the observation that, on follow-up for 18 to 77 months, in 9 of the 13 patients with either aneuploidy or increased numbers of cells in S and G2 phases either high-grade dysplasia developed where none had existed before (4 patients) or frank adenocarcinoma occurred (5 patients). Might not these patients have been better served by transhiatal esophagectomy? A radical suggestion but one worth considering.—W.P. Ritchie, Jr., M.D.

---

**Thoracoscopic Esophagomyotomy: Initial Experience With a New Approach for the Treatment of Achalasia**
Pellegrini C, Wetter LA, Patti M, Leichter R, Mussan G, Mori T, Bernstein G, Way L (Univ of California, San Francisco)
*Ann Surg* 216:291–299, 1992                                   9–7

---

*Background.*—The principal therapy for achalasia for years was extramucosal esophagomyotomy, which required a long hospital stay and much discomfort. Pressure-controlled balloon dilatation replaced it because of the shorter hospital stay and reduced discomfort. This treatment, however, was accompanied by an increased risk of complications and gastroesophageal reflux. An attempt was made to develop thoracoscopic myotomy, to combine the success rate and low rate of complications of myotomy with the low discomfort level of dilatation.

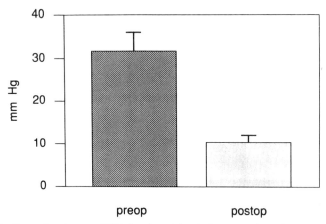

**Fig 9–5.**—Comparison between LES before (n = 14) and after surgery (n = 8) in patients with achalasia. (Courtesy of Pellegrini C, Wetter LA, Patti M, et al: *Ann Surg* 216:291-299, 1992)

*Subjects.*—Seventeen patients with achalasia and dysphagia were studied. Upper gastrointestinal series demonstrated a dilated esophagus and a bird-beak deformity at the cardia in each case. Manometry demonstrated a mean lower esophageal sphincter (LES) pressure of approximately 34 mm Hg, incomplete sphincter relaxation on swallowing, and no primary esophageal peristalsis. Thoracoscopic Heller myotomy was performed in 15 patients and laparoscopic Heller myotomy in 2.

*Outcome.*—After operation, the mean LES pressure was approximately 10 mm Hg (Fig 9–5). Fifteen patients could swallow on the second postoperative day. The average hospital stay was 3 days, and there were no major complications. In 3 of the patients treated early in the series, the myotomy was not carried far enough into the stomach and a second myotomy was necessary to alleviate dysphagia. Therefore, endoscopic examination during the procedure was important to determine the length of the myotomy. Early exposure of the mucosa was also an important step. Final dysphagia elimination was excellent in 12 patients, good in 2, fair in 2, and poor in 1.

*Conclusions.*—Heller myotomy can be performed safely with minimally invasive techniques to relieve dysphagia with minimal postoperative pain, hospital stay, and time before return to normal activity. It appears to be the preferred procedure in patients with achalasia.

▶ This report details the initial experience of the UCSF group with 17 patients subjected to either thoracoscopic (15 patients) or laparoscopic (2) esophagomyotomy for achalasia. In 2 additional patients the "mini-access" approach had to be abandoned for an open one. On follow-up to 13 months, 14 of the 17 patients had good or excellent results with respect to relief of dysphagia. As is universally true with any evolving technique, there is a learning curve: The 3 failures occurred in the first 3 patients, in all of whom myotomy was inadequate. An important technical point: The esophagoscope was used to define the esophagus during dissection, to detect any mucosal injuries, and to help determine the extent of the myotomy. Eight of the 17 patients had follow-up manometry, with significant reductions in the LES pressure seen in all. Unfortunately, only 4 of the 17 had follow-up 24-hour pH monitoring; 2 of these demonstrated abnormal esophageal acid exposure. This raises the same question that is frequently voiced relative to the open approach: Is an antireflux procedure necessary? Many would say "yes"; Pellegrini and his colleagues have not as yet tested enough of their 17 patients to say "no" with any real confidence. Regardless, it seems clear to me that the bell may be tolling for both surgeons and gastroenterologists who treat achalasia in the "conventional" way.—W.P. Ritchie, Jr., M.D.

---

**Elective Treatment of Bleeding Varices With the Sugiura Operation Over 10 Years**

Orozco H, Mercado MA, Takahashi T, Hernández-Ortiz J, Capellán JF, Garcia-Tsao G (Instituto Nacional de la Nutricion Salvador Zubiran, Mexico City, Mexico)

*Am J Surg* 163:585–589, 1992                                                    9–8

---

*Introduction.*—The Sugiura operation for bleeding esophageal varices consists of esophagogastric devascularization, esophageal transection to interrupt submucosal varices, vagotomy, pyloroplasty, and splenectomy. It has proven effective, with low rates of rebleeding and postoperative encephalopathy. A 10-year experience with this procedure as an alternative to selection shunts was evaluated.

*Patients.*—The Sugiura operation was done on an elective basis in 100 patients (57 males, 43 females) in whom it was not possible to place a shunt. The mean age was 44 years. In 69%, portal hypertension resulted from cirrhosis and severe portal fibrosis. Sixty-three patients were in Child's class A, 32 were in class B, and 5 were in class C. Fifteen patients had both stages in 1 operation, 51 had both stages with a delay between, and 34 had only 1 stage.

*Outcomes.*—One patient undergoing a single operation died, for a mortality rate of 6%. Eight patients in Child's class A died; this group underwent a total of 111 operations. Their operative mortality rate was 12%, and in terms of number of procedures, it was 7%. There was a 4% incidence of rebleeding in the early postoperative stage and a 6% incidence in the long term. The 1-year survival rate was 75%; 5-year survival, 70%; and 10-year survival, 69%. There were 6 secondary esophageal fistulas.

*Conclusions.*—The Sugiura operation is an excellent alternative to selective shunting to prevent recurrent variceal bleeding. It maintains portal flow and is associated with a low rate of encephalopathy. This operation should be chosen based on the patient's characteristics and the surgeon's experience.

▶ This series is probably the largest in the Western world evaluating the Sugiura procedure (esophagogastric disconnection) in patients with portal hypertension. The results are reasonably salutary: 12% operative mortality, minimal rebleeding both in the postoperative period and on relatively long-term follow-up, and a low incidence of "severe" encephalopathy. It's important to note, however, that the vast majority of patients were in Child's class A, and that all procedures were performed on an elective basis. Esophago-pleural fistulas developed in 6 patients and resulted in a sobering 50% mortality rate. Finally, of course, the Sugiura procedure is not the definitive treatment for esophageal varices, bringing to mind the old adage that the biggest mistake one can make after operating on cirrhotic patients is to operate on them again. In any case, one wonders about the place of the Sugiura procedure in today's world, particularly when TIPS procedures are becoming increasingly available.—W.P. Ritchie, Jr., M.D.

## Stomach

Introduction

The widely held view that life expectancy is reduced after peptic ulcer surgery has been confirmed. However, that reduction occurs almost exclusively in male patients, most of whom have been operated on for gastric ulcers. Excess mortality is not a function of operation per se, but is related to heavy smoking. This is hardly surprising, given the strong correlation between smoking and the development of gastric ulcer in the first place. A carefully done prospective trial clearly indicates that a pyloroplasty is an indispensable adjunct to operations in which the stomach is used as an esophageal substitute following resections for cancer.

Traditional bariatric procedures have not met with great success in the "superobese." However, the use of a longer than normal limb (150 cm) of jejunum to construct a Roux Y gastric bypass appears to be associated with improved weight loss in this group without excessive attendant protein deficiency, hepatic dysfunction, or diarrhea. Endoscopic approaches to the control of bleeding peptic ulcer continue to be popular and are certainly applicable in community hospital settings. This is particularly true of those techniques that involve direct injection of epinephrine or sclerosant into the ulcer bed. What is really needed, in my opinion, is a comparison of the long-term outcomes of these approaches to those of a definitive surgical procedure. The hypothesis that primary duodenogastric reflux can occur and be pathologic continues to be investigated. Specifically, the effects of the "duodenal" switch operation have recently been studied in dogs. The results indicate that stomal ulcers are few and gastric emptying is normal. Whether or not this procedure deserves widespread clinical application remains controversial.

Wallace P. Ritchie, Jr., M.D.

### Long-Term Prognosis After Partial Gastrectomy for Benign Conditions: Survival and Smoking-Related Death of 2633 Amsterdam Postgastrectomy Patients Followed up Since Surgery Between 1931 and 1960

Tersmette AC, Offerhaus GJA, Giardiello FM, Brand R, Tersmette KWF, Tytgat GNJ, Vandenbroucke JP (Univ Hosp, Leiden, The Netherlands; Academic Med Ctr, Amsterdam, The Netherlands; Johns Hopkins Univ, Baltimore, Md)

*Gastroenterology* 101:148–153, 1991                                    9–9

*Introduction.*—Some studies have suggested a reduced life expectancy after peptic ulcer surgery, for reasons that are not clear.

*Methods.*—The results of a 50-year follow-up study of patients in Amsterdam who underwent gastrectomy for ulcer disease between 1931 and 1960 were reviewed. By the end of the study in 1987, 1,761 patients died.

*Results.*—The survival of postgastrectomy patients was significantly reduced by 12 years after operation (Fig 9–6). The effect was chiefly the result of reduced survival among men, mostly those with gastric ulcers. Men with duodenal ulcers had significantly reduced survival only after 40 years of follow-up. Women's survival did not differ significantly from

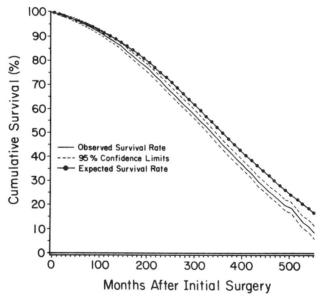

**Fig 9–6.**—Cumulative survival in an Amsterdam cohort of 2,633 postgastrectomy patients operated on in 1931–1960 for benign disease in comparison with survival in the general Dutch population adjusted for sex, age, and calendar time. (Courtesy of Tersmette AC, Offerhaus GJA, Giardello FM, et al: *Gastroenterology* 101:148–153, 1991).

that of the general population. Most of the excess mortality from cancer was caused by lung carcinoma.

*Conclusion.*—Smoking appears to have an important role in the excess mortality seen after remote ulcer surgery. The same may be the case for patients treated with drugs to reduce gastric acid secretion.

▶ Any report involving more than 2,600 postgastrectomy patients followed for 30 to 60 years certainly deserves our attention. Smoking is clearly a major risk factor for the development of peptic ulcer, particularly in the stomach. This study suggests that continued smoking after gastrectomy, particularly by men who have undergone surgery for gastric ulcer, is the single most important factor contributing to excess mortality and a shortened life expectancy. Of interest, excess mortality attributable to tobacco use has also been observed on much shorter follow-up in patients taking $H_2$ receptor antagonists. The authors conclude, quite correctly in my view, that smoking cessation may provide the greatest improvement in the long-term prognosis of patients with peptic ulcers, regardless of treatment. Easier said than done, unfortunately.—W.P. Ritchie, Jr., M.D.

---

**Pyloroplasty Versus No Drainage in Gastric Replacement of the Esophagus**
Fok M, Cheng SWK, Wong J (Queen Mary Hosp, Hong Kong)
*Am J Surg* 162:447–452, 1991                                        9–10

---

*Introduction.*—It is not clear whether pyloroplasty is required when the stomach is used to reconstruct the esophagus after resection of cancer. In a prospective, randomized study, 200 patients were enrolled and followed for up to 6 years after surgery for esophageal cancer. Half of the patients underwent pyloroplasty.

*Results.*—Resection was considered to be curative in 47% of those having pyloroplasty and in 40% of the others. The median survival was about 10 months in both groups. An adequate length of stomach was consistently achieved in the group that had pyloroplasty, and no leakage occurred at the site of pyloroplasty. Thirteen patients without drainage had symptoms of gastric outlet obstruction, and 4 had consequent pulmonary complications. Two of these patients died of aspiration. Postoperative morbidity was significantly less frequent in the group having pyloroplasty. Gastric emptying times in patients without drainage were nearly 4 times those in patients who had pyloroplasty (Fig 9–7). Pyloroplasty allowed more patients to tolerate normal amounts of solid foods.

*Conclusion.*—Pyloroplasty is justified when the stomach is used to replace the esophagus after esophagectomy. The procedure is safe and effective; normal gastric emptying cannot be assured unless drainage is provided.

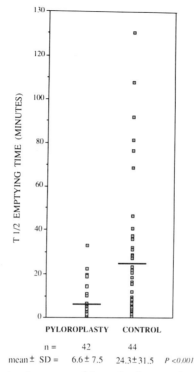

**Fig 9–7.**—Gastric emptying times measured 6 months after operation showing significantly longer adjusted half-life ($T_{1/2}$) in patients without pyloroplasty. (Courtesy of Fok M, Cheng SWK, Wong J: *Am J Surg* 162:447–452, 1991).

▶ This study has all of the virtues we have come to expect from the reports of John Wong and his colleagues in Hong Kong: a carefully designed, appropriately stratified, and astutely performed prospective, randomized trial asking an important question. The answer is clear and should settle the issue at hand permanently: The performance of a pyloroplasty, in this case the 2-layer Heineke-Mikulicz variety, is mandatory for patients in whom the whole stomach is used for reconstruction after esophagectomy. The results are almost certainly applicable to the Ivor Lewis esophagogastrectomy as well. Parenthetically, it is doubtful that any other clinic in the world could amass a total of 200 patients to study the issue in only 6 years. The rigorous academic approach adopted by this group to solve real clinical problems is truly exemplary.—W.P. Ritchie, Jr., M.D.

### Long-Limb Gastric Bypass in the Superobese: A Prospective Randomized Study

Brolin RE, Kenler HA, Gorman JH, Cody RP (UMDNJ-Robert Wood Johnson Med School, New Brunswick, NJ)
*Ann Surg* 215:387–395, 1992                                         9–11

*Introduction.*—Surgical treatment of obesity has been reserved for patients 100 lb or 100% above their ideal weight. Conventional gastric restrictive operations, however, have been less effective in the "superobese"—those at least 200 lb above their ideal weight. Whether a modification of the conventional Roux-en-Y gastric bypass (RYGB) results in greater weight loss in superobese patients was determined.

*Methods.*—Two modifications of RYGB were compared prospectively in 45 patients. Both procedures resulted in greater diversion of bile and pancreatic secretions away from the functional gastrointestinal tract. The length of the defunctionalized jejunum was 75 cm in the RYGB-1 group (22 patients) and 150 cm in the RYGB-2 group (23 patients). Patients were evaluated postoperatively for weight loss, calorie intake, improvement of medical problems, and complications.

*Results.*—Weight loss stabilized in all but 1 patient within 24 months after surgery (Fig 9–8). This patient had a high level of physical activity and lost 50 more lb during the third postoperative year. At 24 months and 36 months, the mean weight loss was significantly greater in the RYGB-2 group. Both groups had a significantly reduced mean daily calo-

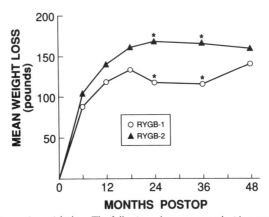

**Fig 9–8.**—Postoperative weight loss. The following values correspond with mean ± SD weight loss shown in the graph. *Significant difference between groups (P ≤ .02 by unpaired Student's t test). (Courtesy of Brolin RE, Kenler HA, Gorman JH, et al: *Ann Surg* 215:387–395, 1992).

|        | 6 mo | 12 mo | 18 mo | 24 mo | 36 mo | 48 mo |
|--------|------|-------|-------|-------|-------|-------|
| RYGB-1 | 88 ± 23 | 118 ± 35 | 133 ± 40 | 117 ± 38* | 115 ± 49* | 140 ± 63 |
| RTGB-2 | 104 ± 37 | 140 ± 41 | 161 ± 51 | 168 ± 52* | 165 ± 50* | 159 ± 70 |

*Significant difference between groups (P ≤ 0.02 by unpaired Student's t test.)

rie intake after operation. All but 3 patients had obesity-related medical illnesses before surgery; these were either resolved or improved with surgery in all but 4 patients. There were no perioperative deaths, and the only late death occurred 6 years after operation in a patient with congestive heart failure who was a heavy drinker.

*Conclusion.*—Weight loss was increased, without protein deficiency, hepatic dysfunction, or diarrhea, in these superobese patients who underwent long-limb modification of RYGB. In both groups, weight loss maintenance was related to the postoperative calorie intake. Patients who lost at least 50% of their excess weight had improvement of both coexisting medical problems and general life-style.

▶ A major challenge to the bariatric surgeon is the appropriate surgical treatment for the superobese, i.e., those patients whose weight is more than 225% of ideal. In up to 30% of these unfortunate individuals, conventional gastric restrictive procedures fail, even when combined with Roux-Y. The present carefully performed study evaluated the use of a longer than usual Roux Y limb during gastric bypass in superobese individuals. The procedure itself represents a compromise between conventional Roux-Y bypass and the biliopancreatic bypass procedure described by Scopinaro (1). The latter produced excellent weight loss but at the expense of a high rate of severe metabolic complications. The outcome of the current effort: an apparently more effective operation for the superobese, resulting in substantial weight loss but without excessively untoward side effects. One note of caution: The average follow-up reported here is only 4 years. Some believe that a minimum of 5 years is necessary to evaluate adequately the results of bariatric surgery.—W.P. Ritchie, Jr., M.D.

*Reference*

1. Scopinaro N, et al: *Am J Clin Nutr* 33:506, 1980.

---

**Controlled Trial of Endoscopic Injection Treatment for Bleeding From Peptic Ulcers With Visible Vessels**
Oxner RBG, Simmonds NJ, Gertner DJ, Nightingale JMD, Burnham WR (Old-church Hosp, Essex, England)
*Lancet* 339:966–968, 1992                                            9–12

---

*Introduction.*—Trials conducted in major research centers show endoscopy and the injection of epinephrine or sclerosant to be successful treatment for bleeding peptic ulcers. Endoscopic treatment of upper gastrointestinal bleeding has not yet become routine in general hospitals. The effectiveness of endoscopic injection treatment for bleeding peptic ulcers was evaluated in the general hospital setting.

*Methods.*—Endoscopy was performed on all patients with suspected upper gastrointestinal bleeding. Ninety-three of 98 patients found to

Clinical Outcome in Control and Injected Patients

|  | Injection treatment (n = 48) | Conservative treatment (n = 45) |
|---|---|---|
| Rebleeding | 8 (16·7%) | 21 (46·7%)* |
| Mean (range) blood units transfused | 5 (0–22) | 7·5 (0–27) |
| Mean (range) hospital stay (days) | 9·5 (2–35) | 10 (0–37) |
| Surgery | 4 (8·3%) | 8 (17·8%) |
| Deaths | 4 (8·3%) | 9 (20·0%) |

*$P = .011$ ($\chi^2$ with 1 degree of freedom).
(Courtesy of Oxner RBG, Simmonds NJ, Gertner DJ, et al: *Lancet* 339:966–968, 1992.)

have an ulcer with a visible vessel were randomized at the time of endoscopy to injection (48) or no treatment (45). Treatment consisted of 1–2 mL of epinephrine 1:10,000 injected at 4 to 6 sites around the ulcer. Epinephrine and 5% ethanolamine oleate, 1–2 mL, were then injected directly into the vessel. All patients with serious rebleeding were to undergo reendoscopy and open injection.

*Results.*—The 2 groups were comparable in age, initial hemoglobin concentration, shock, and ulcer site, but the overall clinical outcome was better in the group receiving injections (table). These patients had an incidence of rebleeding significantly lower than that in controls (16.7% vs. 46.7%). Treatment was also associated with a lower rate of mortality (8.3% vs. 20%), less need for surgery (8.3% vs. 17.8%), and reduced transfusion requirements (5 vs. 7.5 units). No patient in either group died of bleeding alone.

*Conclusion.*—In this small group of patients with upper gastrointestinal bleeding and at high risk of further bleeding, injection treatment reduced rebleeding and transfusion requirements. When performed by endoscopists experienced in injection treatment, this inexpensive and effective method can be used in most general hospitals.

▶ This study shows that injection of epinephrine or sclerosant into those peptic ulcers with a high risk of continued bleeding or rebleeding in the hospital (i.e., those with a visible vessel) is more effective in controlling hemorrhage than is no treatment—not surprising. Unfortunately, it doesn't tell us anything about the patients in whom this approach does not work, which is precisely the kind of information we as surgeons need to know. It is my distinct impression that sick patients with bleeding peptic ulcers are made to jump over numerous nonoperative hurdles in an attempt to "avoid surgery." As a result, they arrive in the operating room even sicker, with greater transfusion requirements and higher operative mortality rates. Is this an advance?—W.P. Ritchie, Jr., M.D.

## Effect of Duodenal Switch Procedure on Gastric Acid Production, Intragastric pH, Gastric Emptying, and Gastrointestinal Hormones

Welch NT, Yasui A, Kim CB, Barlow AP, Hinder RA, DeMeester TR, Polishuk PV, Clark GWB, Adrian TE (Creighton Univ, Omaha, Neb; Univ of Southern California, Los Angeles)

*Am J Surg* 163:37–45, 1992                                        9–13

*Background.*—Excessive duodenal gastric reflux can be a significant problem, requiring Roux-en-Y gastrojejunostomy. This procedure diverts all gastric juice from the duodenum and requires both vagotomy and antrectomy to prevent stomal ulcers. Suprapapillary Roux-en-Y duodenojejunostomy, or the duodenal switch, maintains gastric continuity with the proximal 3–7 cm of duodenum. This should be enough to block excessive reflux, while avoiding vagotomy and antrectomy, yet preventing ulcers. This hypothesis was examined in dogs.

*Methods.*—Twelve dogs with Pavlov pouches were randomized to receive either a duodenal switch or Roux-en-Y procedure on an intact stomach. Gastric acid secretion, gastrointestinal hormones, and gastric emptying were compared. Intragastric pH was monitored at 5 different levels in the dogs. These results were compared to those in 12 human patients who underwent the duodenal switch.

*Results.*—After the Roux-en-Y procedure, stomal ulcers developed in 2 of the 6 dogs; the rest demonstrated stomal hyperemia, despite ranitidine treatments to inhibit acid secretion between tests. In the group undergoing duodenal switch, none of the dogs had ulcers. Gastric emptying, plasma gastrin levels, cholecystokinin, secretin, gastric inhibitory polypeptide, peptide YY, and neurotensin levels were similar after the 2 procedures. Intragastric pH monitoring in both dogs and humans demonstrated that the duodenal switch did not cause any significant changes in intragastric pH.

*Conclusions.*—The duodenal switch operation prevents stomal ulcers without requiring vagotomy or gastric resection. It does not affect gastric pH or slow gastric emptying. Therefore, the duodenal switch is a good surgical alternative for patients who have not had gastric resection previously and for patients with severe duodenogastric reflux that does not respond to medical therapy.

▶ The innovative and prolific group at Creighton University has contributed much over the years to our understanding of the pathophysiology and treatment of gastroesophageal reflux disease. Of late, however, their focus has shifted toward investigating the possibility that primary and pathologic duodenogastric reflux exists and is susceptible to correction using the "duodenal switch" operation. That operation is designed to preserve the pylorus and the proximal 3–7 cm of duodenum in continuity with the stomach while diverting pancreaticobiliary secretions distally. The present study is primarily an experimental one and demonstrates, not surprisingly, that drainage of an innervated whole stomach preparation using the classic Roux procedure can produce stomal ulcers with great regularity, whereas the "switch" does not. This is undoubtedly because the proximal duodenum has a striking ability to neutralize HC.

I confess to a sense of deja vu when considering the hypothesis under consideration and its operative correction. Twenty years ago there was considerable enthusiasm for the possibility that, after operations for peptic ulcer, excessive enterogastric reflux would lead to a unique postgastrectomy syndrome, so-called alkaline reflux gastritis. Two decades later, the hypothesis remains totally unproven, and some of the therapies that we use to try to correct the problem are as bad as the putative disease itself. What is needed, I believe, is to fulfill Koch's postulates with respect to the possibility that de novo excessive enterogastric reflux is a problem in those who are otherwise classified as the "nervous pukers" of the world. That is, symptoms should always occur in the presence of excessive reflux, never occur in its absence, and be eliminated (and permanently) by eliminating reflux. It is to be hoped that this will be the direction taken in future studies of this problem.—W.P. Ritchie, Jr., M.D.

## Biliary Tract

INTRODUCTION

The explosive growth of laparoscopic surgery in general, and of laparoscopic procedures on the biliary tract in particular, has produced several studies of interest. First, it is now clear that laparoscopic techniques are well taught within the traditional curriculum of a surgery residency program—good news, indeed. It is also clear that extirpation of the gallbladder is best accomplished laparoscopically in the morbidly obese. Concern about laparoscopic bile duct injuries continues, however. Risk factors appear to include chronic scarring in the region of the triangle of Calot, acute inflammation and/or cholecystitis, bleeding that obscures the field of dissection, and obesity. Whether or not routine cholangiography will reduce the incidence of this major complication is not certain.

Endoscopically directed decompression of the common bile duct using nasobiliary drainage is superior to emergent operative decompression in patients with severe acute cholangitis. Biliary ascariasis is a major problem worldwide. Methods of diagnosis, indications for operation, and techniques for clearing the biliary tree of ascarids are similar to those used for choledocholithiasis. Postoperative bile duct strictures continue to be a frustrating problem. For most afflicted patients, reconstruction with a Roux-en-Y anastomosis appears to be the treatment of choice; percutaneous transhepatic biliary dilatation is of limited value under these circumstances. Using cholecystectomy as a model, a new method of reporting negative outcomes has been proposed that, if widely adopted, could facilitate comparison of surgical results between different centers or comparison of results of surgical versus nonsurgical approaches in a variety of conditions.

Wallace P. Ritchie, Jr., M.D.

### Incorporation of Laparoscopy Into a Surgical Endoscopy Training Program

Schirmer BD, Edge SB, Dix J, Miller AD (Univ of Virginia, Charlottesville)
*Am J Surg* 163:46–52, 1992                                              9–14

*Background.*—With rapid gains in the popularity of endoscopy, it is necessary to include this procedure in training programs for surgical residents. Many surgeons who did not practice flexible gastrointestinal endoscopy are now performing laparoscopic procedures. The effect of incorporating laparoscopy into the gastrointestinal endoscopy training of general surgery residents was assessed.

*Observations.*—All endoscopic procedures performed at a single medical center, both in inpatient and outpatient settings, were analyzed. An attending surgeon was present for all procedures. The number of flexible gastrointestinal endoscopic procedures increased from 268 in 1988 to 339 in 1989 to 532 in 1990. When the total number of procedures (both flexible and laparoscopic) was considered, the increase was 117% from 1989 to 1990. In 59% of therapeutic laparoscopies, a resident stood in the "surgeon's" position. A resident served as either surgeon or "first assistant" in 86% of all therapeutic laparoscopies and in 94% of all diagnostic laparoscopies. For diagnostic procedures, complication rates were .3% in 1989 and .2% in 1990. For therapeutic procedures, the complication rate was 4%, regardless of whether a resident served as the surgeon.

*Conclusions.*—Laparoscopy can be safely introduced into a surgical residency program. This is especially true for programs with an established program in endoscopy. In the described program, residents average about 80 cases in a 2-month surgical endoscopy rotation. Residents learn the skills necessary for laparoscopy by serving in the role of assistant, rather than in a formal animal surgery course.

▶ The rush to join the minimal access surgical bandwagon has led to such a proliferation of informal, loosely structured, and frequently very brief (although costly) training venues that hospital credentialing and privileging committees everywhere must be tearing their collective hairs out. The long-term solution, of course, is to incorporate such procedures into the traditional general surgical training program. This paper proves the feasibility of such an approach. Residents can safely be taught laparoscopic cholecystectomy, at least, with minimal or no previous animal training if the attending surgeon is sufficiently experienced (and patient!). In the interim, Credentials Committees would do well to heed the sage guidelines of SAGES (the Society of American Gastrointestinal Endoscopic Surgeons) (1).—W.P. Ritchie, Jr., M.D.

*Reference*

1. The Society of American Gastrointestinal Endoscopic Surgeons: *Surg Endoscopy* 7:67, 1993.

---

### Endoscopic Biliary Drainage for Severe Acute Cholangitis
Lai ECS, Mok FPT, Tan ESY, Lo C-m, Fan S-t, You K-t, Wong J (Queen Mary Hosp, Hong Kong)
*N Engl J Med* 326:1582–1586, 1992                                    9–15

*Background.*—Substantial morbidity and mortality are associated with emergency surgery in patients with severe acute cholangitis caused by choledocholithiasis. Recent research suggests that emergency endoscopic drainage may improve the outcome of such patients. A prospective study was done to determine the role of this procedure as initial treatment.

*Methods.*—In a 43-month period, 82 patients with severe acute cholangitis from choledocholithiasis were assigned randomly to either surgical decompression of the biliary tract or endoscopic biliary drainage followed by definitive treatment. Linear discriminant analysis was used to study prognostic determinants.

*Results.*—Complications associated with biliary tract decompression and definitive treatment developed in 34% of those treated with endoscopic biliary drainage and in 66% of those treated surgically. The time needed for normalization of temperature and stabilization of blood pressure was similar in the 2 groups. More surgically treated patients needed ventilatory support. The hospital death rate was significantly lower for those undergoing endoscopy (10%) than for those having surgery (32%). Other independent determinants of mortality in both groups were the presence of concomitant medical problems, a low platelet count, a high serum urea nitrogen concentration, and a low serum albumin concentration before biliary decompression.

*Conclusions.*—Endoscopy can be valuable in reducing mortality associated with severe acute cholangitis. Endoscopic biliary drainage seems to be a safe, effective method for initially controlling severe acute cholangitis caused by choledocholithiasis.

▶ This paper clearly demonstrates that, in patients with severe acute cholangitis secondary to choledocholithiasis, nasobiliary drainage of the common bile duct is far preferable in terms of outcome than is operative decompression of the duct using a T tube. The availability of a skilled endoscopist is, of course, of paramount importance (and those who participated in this study were certainly skilled: all patients randomized to receive nasobiliary drainage were successfully cannulated, 4 without the need of a concomitant papillotomy; the average time required to place the nasobiliary catheter was in the neighborhood of 30 minutes). The beauty of this approach is that, once sepsis has been controlled, all of the many options extant to treat choledocholithiasis are still available, and there are many more patients alive to take advantage of them.—W.P. Ritchie, Jr., M.D.

**Biliary Ascariasis: Surgical Aspects**
Wani NA, Chrungoo RK (Sher-i-Kashmir Inst of Med Sciences, Srinagar-Kashmir, India)
*World J Surg* 16:976–979, 1992                                                9–16

*Background.*—Ascariasis is one of the most common helminthic diseases in human beings. It involves hundreds of millions of persons in countries where standards of public health and personal hygiene are low. Adult worms normally live in the intestinal lumen without causing significant symptoms, but they do cause acute abdominal distress when they invade ectopic sites, most commonly the hepatobiliary tree. Surgical experience with biliary ascariasis in Kashmir where *Ascaris* infestation is highly endemic was reviewed.

*Patients.*—During a 5-year period, 204 patients were treated for biliary ascariasis. Among the 204 patients were 109 children and young adults aged 10–20 years (53.4%); 11 (5.4%) were younger than age 10 years. Upper abdominal pain was the presenting symptom in 166 patients (81.4%), and 10 of them had a history of previous biliary surgery. Whereas 86 of the patients with upper abdominal pain had typical biliary colic suggestive of intraluminal biliary obstruction, 61 had clinical evidence of cholecystitis, and 4 had symptoms suggestive of pancreatitis. Twenty-two patients had obstructive jaundice and 5 had ascardial biliary peritonitis. Abdominal ultrasonography was performed in 183 patients (89.7%), endoscopic retrograde cholangiopancreatography in 28 (13.7%), T tube cholangiography in 16 (7.8%), and laparotomy for peritonitis in 5 (2.45%). Patients were initially treated conservatively and were followed by serial ultrasound until the worms moved from the bile ducts into the gut, usually within 4–5 weeks.

*Results.*—Forty patients who had no response to conservative treatment and had persistent pain underwent surgical exploration of the common bile duct; 36 of them had cholecystectomy. Indications for surgical exploration included ultrasound evidence of *Ascaris* in 11 patients, ultrasound evidence of dead worms in the biliary system in 6, deepening jaundice in 4, biliary stones in 11, peritonitis in 5, and a nonfunctioning gallbladder seen on oral cholecystography in 3. Microscopic examination revealed *Ascaris* ova in the center as a nidus of the stone of 1 patient. Two patients admitted with biliary peritonitis died of septicemia in the postoperative period.

*Recommendations.*—Hepatobiliary ultrasound is the imaging method preferred in the diagnosis of biliary ascariasis. Endoscopic retrograde cholangiopancreatography is also helpful. In areas where *Ascaris* infestation is endemic, mass deworming campaigns should be undertaken at the public health level.

▶ Global travel and transmigration have made the planet a small place. It would behoove the Western surgeon to be aware of this entity because ascariasis is a very common disease: more than 25% of the world's population may be infested. Of interest, biliary ascarids can be diagnosed and managed much like retained or recurrent common bile duct stones—ultrasound and possibly endoscopic retrograde cholangiopancreatography extraction—with operation reserved for patient deterioration or failed extraction.—W.P. Ritchie, Jr., M.D.

---

**Laparoscopy: The Preferred Method of Cholecystectomy in the Morbidly Obese**

Miles RH, Carballo RE, Prinz RA, McMahon M, Pulawski G, Olen RN, Dahlinghaus DL (Loyola Univ, Maywood, Ill; Resurrection Hosp, Chicago)
Surgery 112:818–823, 1992                                              9–17

---

*Introduction.*—Laparoscopic cholecytectomy (LC) has become the preferred treatment for symptomatic cholelithiasis. Morbid obesity, however, has been considered a contraindication to LC. To investigate whether LC can be performed in morbidly obese patients, 201 patients who had undergone LC were reviewed.

*Methods.*—The outcome of 21 morbidly obese patients (weighing at least 100 lb over ideal body weight) was compared to that of nonobese patients and to 11 morbidly obese patients who underwent standard open cholecystectomy. All groups were comparable with regard to age, sex, and symptoms. Operative time, resumption of normal diet, postoperative hospitalization, complications, conversion to open procedure, and ability to perform cholangiography were assessed.

*Results.*—There were no significant differences between the obese and nonobese patients who underwent LC in any of the above parameters.

---

Outcome in Operative Groups

|  | *Operative time (min)* | *Time to general diet (days)* | *Time to discharge (days)* |
|---|---|---|---|
| Nonobese LC | 151.7 ± 4.0 | 1.2 ± 0.1 | 2.0 ± 0.1 |
| Obese LC | 160.7 ± 9.9 | 1.1 ± 0.1 | 1.8 ± 0.2 |
| Obese standard | 117.6 ± 11.6* | 3.1 ± 0.2† | 4.6 ± 0.4† |

Note: All data are mean ± SEM.
*P < 0.05 by analysis of variance and Student-Newman-Keuls test.
†P < 0.01 by analysis of variance and Student-Newman-Keuls test.
(Courtesy of Miles RH, Carballo RE, Prinz RA, et al: *Surgery* 112:818–823, 1992.)

Operative time was shorter in obese patients who underwent open cholecystectomy. Time to achieve a normal diet and the length of postoperative hospitalization, however, were both significantly longer in that group (table), and there were more complications among these patients.

*Conclusions.*—The use of LC is safe and effective in the morbidly obese and should be preferred for symptomatic cholelithiasis in this group of patients.

▶ Those experienced in the technique of laparoscopic cholecystectomy will not be surprised in the least by the results of this study. In the obese, laparoscopic cholecystectomy is easier for both surgeon and patient than is open cholecystectomy. The key is longer trochars and angled scopes. One caveat, however: Obese men may be more difficult to operate on than obese women because they are more likely to be fat on both the inside and the outside.—W.P. Ritchie, Jr., M.D.

---

**Laparoscopic Bile Duct Injuries: Risk Factors, Recognition, and Repair**
Rossi RL, Schirmer WJ, Braasch JW, Sanders LB, Munson JL (Lahey Clinic Med Ctr, Burlington, Mass)
*Arch Surg* 127:596–602, 1992                                                9–18

---

*Introduction.*—Early studies suggest that laparoscopic cholecystectomies result in more injuries to the bile duct than the traditional open procedure. To determine specific risk factors for such injuries and evaluate methods of repair, the records of 11 patients were examined.

*Methods.*—Eight women and 3 men were treated for injuries to the bile duct sustained during laparoscopic cholecystectomy; the median age was 35 years. Five were clinically obese. Operative notes were reviewed, as were hospital records and roentgenographic films.

*Findings.*—The operative notes described some difficulty with operative dissection in 10 cases. Problems included chronic scarring or fibrosis in the region of Calot's triangle, acute inflammation and/or cholecystitis, bleeding that obscured the field of dissection, and obesity. In 7 patients injuries to the bile duct were not recognized during the original laparoscopic procedure but were suspected postoperatively when symptoms suggested a complication. Anorexia, ileus, pain, ascites, and jaundice were among the presenting symptoms. Ductal injury was diagnosed in these patients by endoscopic retrograde cholangiopancreatography. All required hepaticojejunostomies. During initial exploration for repair, the most typical finding (8 cases) was high transection of the common hepatic duct. Two patients had multiple lateral rents in the common duct, and 1 had a clip placed across the common hepatic duct. The average total hospital stay for these patients was 28.6 days.

*Conclusion.*—During open cholecystectomy, distortion of the common duct is minimized (Fig 9–9). In contrast, traction produces angula-

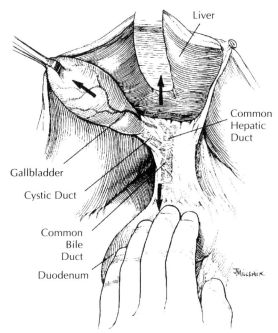

Liver

Common
Hepatic
Duct

Gallblatter

Cystic Duct

Common
Bile
Duct

Duodenum

**Fig 9–9.**—During open cholecystectomy, the common duct is placed under axial traction, minimizing angulation during lateral retraction of the gallbladder. (Copyright 1991, Lahey Clinic. Courtesy of Rossi RL, Schirmer WJ, Braasch JW, et al: *Arch Surg* 127:596–602, 1992.)

tion of the common duct during laparoscopic cholecystectomy (Fig 9–10). This anatomical distortion must be appreciated to avoid injuries during the latter procedure. Early conversion to an open procedure and the use of cholangiography are recommended whenever a question arises about anatomy. With heightened surgical judgment, the risk of ductal injury can be reduced.

▶ This case study of 11 laparoscopic common bile duct injuries referred to a major center for definitive repair makes the important point that the technique of open cholecystectomy differs from that of laparoscopic cholecystectomy in one important respect. During the former, axial traction is placed on the common duct, minimizing its angulation during lateral traction of the gallbladder. Conversely, during the latter, the traction placed on the gallbladder produces angulation of the common duct, which may lead the unwary surgeon into wrongly identifying it as the cystic duct. Eleven common duct injuries in a short period of time seems impressive; however, because we have no idea what the denominator figure is, we should be cautious about drawing hard and fast conclusions. Nevertheless, some things stand out. Only 1 patient had a laparoscopic cholangiogram (and that was misinterpreted). Eight of the 11 had scarring or inflammation around Calot's triangle, which

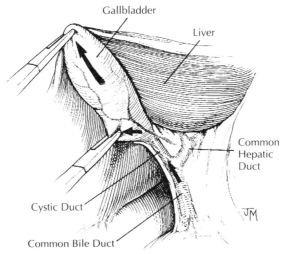

Gallbladder

Liver

Common
Hepatic
Duct

Cystic Duct

Common Bile Duct

**Fig 9–10.**—During laparoscopic cholecystectomy, traction is applied only to the gallbladder. Traction in a cephalad and lateral fashion produces angulation of the common duct. (Copyright 1991, Lahey Clinic. Courtesy of Rossi RL, Schirmer WJ, Braasch JW, et al: *Arch Surg* 127:596-602, 1992.)

may have magnified the angulation problem alluded to. Finally, most injuries were not recognized at the original operation.

The lesson is that surgeons should be very cautious in the setting of dense adhesions or severe inflammation. Cholangiography may avoid common bile duct transection, but this remains to be determined conclusively. All of us should remember that a "lost surgeon" is more common than a biliary anomaly, and that conversion to an open cholecystectomy is no sin.—W.P. Ritchie, Jr., M.D.

---

**Mechanisms of Major Biliary Injury During Laparoscopic Cholecystectomy**
Davidoff AM, Pappas TN, Murray EA, Hilleren DJ, Johnson RD, Baker ME, Newman GE, Cotton PB, Meyers WC (Duke Univ, Durham, NC; Mem Mission Med Ctr, Asheville, NC)
*Ann Surg* 215:196-202, 1992                                                   9–19

---

*Introduction.*—Laparoscopic cholecystectomy is the preferred means of surgically removing the gallbladder, but bile duct injuries are of concern. Undetected injuries to the common or hepatic duct have been infrequent but produce serious effects.

*Observations.*—Data were reviewed on 12 patients treated for bile duct injuries incurred during laparoscopic cholecystectomy in an 11-month period. Of the initial procedures, 7 were considered to have been uncomplicated, and 5 were difficult because of inflammatory reaction around the gallbladder or in the portal region. Significant intraoperative

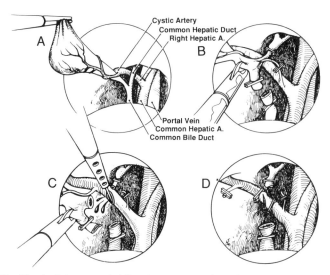

**Fig 9–11.**—The classic laparoscopic biliary injury. **A,** normal portal anatomy. **B,** misidentification of the common duct for the cystic duct, with subsequent ligation and division. **C,** misidentification of the small arterial supply to the common duct for the cystic artery, with subsequent ligation and division. Note also injury of the right hepatic artery that invariably occurred during proximal division of the common hepatic duct. **D,** ligation of the right hepatic artery and complete obstruction of the biliary system. (Courtesy of Davidoff AM, Pappas TN, Murray EA, et al: *Ann Surg* 215:196-202, 1992.)

bleeding was reported by 5 surgeons. Cholangiography established the diagnosis in all patients. In 8 patients, biliary obstruction resulted from ligation of the biliary system, which was complete in 4 patients (Fig 9–11). In 4 patients, there was subhepatic leakage and bile but no ductal obstruction. All 3 strictures involved the common hepatic duct system. In 8 patients, the injuries occurred when the common duct was mistaken for the cystic duct. Excessive cautery or laser application in the area of the common duct, producing a stricture resulted in 3 complications. In 1 patient, the distal common duct was clip ligated and the cystic duct divided proximally.

*Results.*—In 10 patients, a Roux-en-Y hepaticojejunostomy was necessary to obtain adequate bile drainage. Direct common duct repair was successful in 1 patient and 1 patient had endoscopic dilatation.

*Conclusion.*—Classically, these injuries occur when the common duct is incorrectly identified as the cystic duct, part of the common and hepatic ducts are resected, and the right hepatic artery is injured. Most patients do well after hepaticojejunostomy.

▶ This paper complements the previous report in that it, too, suggests that the classic faux pas leading to injury during laparoscopic cholecystectomy appears to be misidentification of the common duct as the cystic duct, probably because of angulation. This, in turn, can lead to resection of a portion of the common and hepatic ducts and to an associated right hepatic arterial

injury by the mechanisms illustrated in Figure 9–11. In an accompanying editorial, Way makes the important point that most duct injuries that occur during laparoscopic cholecystectomy can be avoided by more thorough proctor-
ing of neophyte laparoscopic surgeons, associated with a low threshold for
converting to open cholecystectomy when the dissection becomes bloody or
is otherwise difficult.—W.P. Ritchie, Jr., M.D.

---

### Management of Bile Duct Strictures: An Evolving Strategy

Millis JM, Tompkins RK, Zinner MJ, Longmire WP Jr, Roslyn JJ (Univ of California, Los Angeles)
*Arch Surg* 127:1077–1084, 1992                                    9–20

---

*Objective.*—Postoperative bile duct strictures can be a frustrating
problem. Although endoscopic and radiologic techniques have provided
alternative methods of relieving biliary obstruction, outcome may be better for patients who have definitive surgical repair of benign postoperative strictures. The role of interventional radiologic, endoscopic, and surgical techniques in the management of benign biliary strictures was
evaluated.

*Patients.*—Of a total 194 consecutive patients, 138, comprising group
1, were treated from 1955 through 1979; 56, comprising group 2, were
treated from 1980 through 1989, after the technology used for nonoperative treatment of benign biliary strictures became available. In the latter
group, 47 patients were treated primarily by surgery and 9 initially had
nonoperative balloon dilation. There were 136 women and 58 men
(mean age, 54 years). Jaundice was the most common presenting symptom, followed by cholangitis and pain. The most common reconstructive
procedure was Roux-en-Y biliary-enteric anastomosis. Transhepatic
stents were placed in 49% of group 1, 94% of group 2 patients who
were surgically treated, and all of the group 2 patients who were treated
nonoperatively. All patients were followed for at least 2 years, and 92%
were followed for longer than 3 years.

*Outcomes.*—Strictures recurred in 21% of group 1 and 23% of group
2. Reoperation rates, however, were 21% and 6%, respectively. Twenty
patients in group 2 underwent percutaneous transhepatic biliary dilation;
the success rate was 93% in patients with anastomotic strictures and 50%
in those with primary strictures.

*Conclusions.*—For most patients with bile duct injuries, reconstructive
surgery with Roux-en-Y anastomosis remains the preferred treatment.
Although percutaneous transhepatic biliary dilation is of limited use in
patients with primary strictures, it should be considered as initial treatment for those with anastomotic strictures. In most cases, patients with

bile duct strictures benefit from early referral to centers with experience in dealing with these problems.

▶ This is a timely report given the growing impression that, at least early in a surgeon's experience, common bile duct injury is more common during laparoscopic cholecystectomy than during an open procedure. The authors make the important point that bile duct injuries leading to stricture are usually found proximal to the cystic duct and respond poorly to balloon dilatation. Strictures are best repaired by an experienced team the first time around, using a stented reconstruction to a Roux-en-Y limb of jejunum. Interestingly, anastomotic strictures can be ballooned more successfully than those observed in the nonreconstructed duct (are the latter longer?). One unresolved issue: the length of time the stent should be left in place.—W.P. Ritchie, Jr., M.D.

**Proposed Classification of Complications of Surgery With Examples of Utility in Cholecystectomy**
Clavien P-A, Sanabria JR, Strasberg SM (Mount Sinai Hosp, Toronto, Ont, Canada)
*Surgery* 111:518–526, 1992                                               9–21

*Background.*—The number and severity of complications reported with results of surgery may be used to improve a standard surgical procedure, to select management options, and to compare results. Interpretation of the surgical literature is difficult, however, because the reporting of negative outcomes is not uniform. An attempt was made to define and classify negative outcomes by differentiating complications, sequelae, and failures, and by classifying complications into 4 grades.

*Method.*—In all, 650 elective cholecystectomies were reviewed with the proposed 4-grade classification of complications. The risk factors for the development of complications of cholecystectomy were determined in terms of odds ratio. The classification was also used to analyze the value of a modified Acute Physiology and Chronic Health Evaluation (APACHE II) system as a preoperative prognostic score.

*Classification.*—By definition, complications and sequelae result from procedures, adding new problems to the underlying disease. Complications are unexpected events not intrinsic to the procedure, whereas sequelae are inherent to the procedure. Failures are events in which the purpose of the procedure is not fulfilled. Grade I complications are alterations from the ideal postoperative course, are non–life-threatening, and cause no lasting disability, e.g., gastric distention treated by nasogastric suction and pancreatitis not requiring specific therapy. Grade II complications are potentially life-threatening but without residual disability. Grade IIa comprises complications requiring only the use of drug therapy, total parenteral nutrition, or blood transfusion, e.g., wound infections requiring antibiotics and evidence of continued bleeding after surgery managed by transfusion alone. Grade IIb complications are those requiring therapeutic imaging procedures, therapeutic endoscopy, or reoperation, and all other life-threatening complications not fitting grade IIa or III criteria, e.g., gastrointestinal hemorrhage requiring therapeutic endoscopy, postoperative bowel obstruction requiring reoperation, and pancreatitis requiring therapeutic endoscopy, drainage, or surgery. Grade III complications cause residual and lasting disability and include the presence of persistent and objective signs of life-threatening diseases or organ resection, e.g., myocardial infarction, impending infarction, and unstable angina. Grade IV complications result in death.

*Conclusion.*—The classification of complications was useful in analyzing risk factors and in predicting complications in a modified APACHE II score. Advantages of the 4-grade classification of complications include increased uniformity in reporting results, the ability to compare surgical results between centers or in a single center or to compare results of surgical versus nonsurgical measures, the ability to perform adequate meta-analysis, and the ability to objectively identify preoperative risk factors and prognostic scores.

▶ This paper has been selected for inclusion because it represents a thoughtful attempt to bring relative order out of what is frequently chaos in the reporting of surgical experience. It deserves reading in its entirety because the methodology outlined might well increase our ability to compare similar data from several studies or centers in a more meaningful way than at present. Furthermore, it could be applied in a statistically valid fashion to meta-analyses and to prospective studies of common surgical problems with low complication rates (e.g., bile duct injury during laparoscopic cholecystectomy) as well as to uncommon surgical problems with higher complication rates (e.g., liver failure after major hepatic resection).—W.P. Ritchie, Jr., M.D.

## Pancreas

INTRODUCTION

It is becoming increasingly clear that biliary sludge can be an important cause of so-called idiopathic pancreatitis. Sludge may also be a precursor of the development of frank cholelithiasis in some patients. Hereditary pancreatitis is a rare variant of this disease but appears to behave in a manner similar to pancreatitis from other causes (although patients are afflicted much earlier). In addition, traditional surgical approaches are associated with reasonably good long-term results in most affected patients.

When to use percutaneous or endoscopic drainage techniques for pancreatic pseudocysts remains an unsettled question. An algorithm based on endoscopic retrograde cholangiopancreatography has been proposed, the essence of which is this: In the absence of either pseudocyst communication with the pancreatic duct or pancreatic ductal obstruction, percutaneous drainage should be attempted. On the other hand, in the presence of either of these findings, surgical drainage is required. The natural history of pseudocysts, i.e., whether or not they resolve spontaneously, appears to be related more to the underlying etiology of the pancreatitis than to either pseudocyst size or to acute or chronic presentation. Specifically, pseudocysts associated with postoperative or biliary tract pancreatitis are extremely unlikely to resolve without active intervention.

Serous cystadenomas of the pancreas may be difficult to distinguish from inflammatory pseudocysts or mucinous cystadenomas. In general, however, their clinical course is benign, and nonoperative therapy with continued observation is a very acceptable approach under certain circumstances.

Wallace P. Ritchie, Jr., M.D.

---

**Biliary Sludge as a Cause of Acute Pancreatitis**
Lee SP, Nicholls JF, Park HZ Univ of Washington, Seattle; (Univ of Auckland, Auckland, New Zealand)
*N Engl J Med* 326:589–593, 1992                                    9–22

*Objective.*—No cause of acute pancreatitis is found in 20% to 40% of cases, which are termed idiopathic. An attempt was made to learn how often biliary sludge (a suspension of cholesterol monohydrate crystals or calcium bilirubinate granules) is present in patients with this disease.

*Method.*—Eighty-six patients seen from 1980 to 1988 with acute pancreatitis were followed prospectively. The disease was considered to be idiopathic in 31 patients (36%). The mean follow-up period was 4 years.

*Findings.*—Twenty-three patients with acute idiopathic pancreatitis (74%) had biliary sludge demonstrated by ultrasonography or microscopic study of bile. Two of these patients had dilated bile ducts. Nine of the remaining 29 patients had predominantly cholesterol crystals. Ultrasonography was more likely to detect calcium bilirubinate granules than to detect cholesterol crystals. Patients who underwent cholecystectomy or papillotomy had fewer recurrences of acute pancreatitis during follow-up than did untreated patients.

*Conclusions.*—Biliary sludge apparently is a more frequent cause of acute idiopathic pancreatitis than has been recognized. A majority of patients with idiopathic pancreatitis had biliary sludge. Ultrasound study frequently failed to detect sludge composed of cholesterol monohydrate crystals. The presence of sludge should be ruled out before idiopathic pancreatitis is specified.

▶ The clinical significance of gallbladder sludge—thickened gallbladder mucoprotein with tiny entrapped cholesterol crystals—is becoming increasingly clear. In this study, for example, 74% of patients thought to have acute idiopathic pancreatitis had biliary sludge, observed either by ultrasonography or on microscopic examination of bile. In this group, patients treated by cholecystectomy or papillotomy had fewer recurrences of acute pancreatitis during a 7-year follow-up than did untreated patients, differences that were statistically significant. Thus at least 1 of Koch's postulates has been fulfilled with respect to the hypothesis that idiopathic pancreatitis may, in fact, be related to biliary sludge in many instances. In an important complementary study, Lee and his colleagues followed a group of 96 patients with biliary sludge for a mean of 38 months (1). In the vast majority, the sludge disappeared and reappeared, at least ultrasonographically, during this period. However, gallstones developed in 14 patients, 6 of whom were symptomatic and required cholecystectomy. An additional 6 patients with gallbladder sludge but without stones underwent cholecystectomy for pancreatitis with resolution of their symptoms in every case. All of this leads one to the conclusion that the finding of gallbladder sludge associated with biliary tract symptoms, including pancreatitis, is hardly a benign condition.—W.P. Ritchie, Jr., M.D.

*Reference*

1.  Lee SP, et al: *Gastroenterology* 94:170, 1988.

---

**The Surgical Spectrum of Hereditary Pancreatitis in Adults**
Miller AR, Nagorney DM, Sarr MG (Mayo Clinic and Found, Rochester, Minn)
*Ann Surg* 215:39–43, 1992                                                              9–23

*Background.*—Hereditary, or familial, pancreatitis is inherited as a non–sex–linked autosomal dominant trait with incomplete penetration. It is a rare form of chronic progressive pancreatic inflammation and parenchymal destruction associated with a variable clinical course. Operative intervention for other types of chronic pancreatitis is generally accepted, but the indications for surgical therapy in hereditary pancreatitis have not been clearly defined. The immediate and long-term results of operative therapy in adults with hereditary pancreatitis were reviewed.

*Method.*—A retrospective medical record review identified 22 patients treated surgically for hereditary pancreatitis between 1950 and 1989. The disease was defined as acute recurrent or chronic pancreatic inflammation in patients with 2 or more relatives who had documented pancreatitis. Records were analyzed by patient age at onset of disease symptoms, age at operative intervention, spectrum of clinical presentation, preoperative management, and diagnostic evaluation. Operative therapy was categorized by surgical procedure, pathologic review, perioperative morbidity, and long-term clinical results. Follow-up information was obtained by telephone, personal interview, or written correspondence.

*Results.*—The mean age at onset of symptoms was 15 years, with surgery at a mean age of 31 years. Pain was the primary indication for sur-

Operative Procedure According to Status of the Pancreatic Duct

| | Persistent Pain Relief | |
| --- | --- | --- |
| | Ductal Dilatation (15 patients) | Small Duct (7 patients) |
| Pancreaticojejunostomy | 7/10* | |
| Distal pancreatectomy and proximal pancreaticojejunostomy | 1/1 | 2/2† |
| Distal pancreatectomy | 2/2 | 0/1† |
| Other | | |
|   Pseudocyst drainage | 0/1‡ | |
|   Cholecystectomy | | |
|     Alone | — | 1/2 |
|   With sphincteroplasty | — | 1/2 |
| Pancreatic drainage abscess | 1/1 | |

\* Two patients subsequently required resection.
† The patient without relief of symptoms went on to completion (total) pancreatectomy without success.
‡ Pseudocyst recurred requiring pancreatic resection.
(Courtesy of Miller AR, Nagorney DM, Sarr MG: *Ann Surg* 215:39–43, 1992.)

gery, but nausea, vomiting, weight loss, and diarrhea were common symptoms. About two thirds of the 22 patients (68%) had ductal dilatation, 73% had pancreatic parenchymal calcifications, 36% had pseudocysts, and 18% had splenic vein thrombosis. The operative strategy used in patients with hereditary pancreatitis was dictated by the anatomy of the pancreatic duct (table). The morbidity rate was 14% and included intra-abdominal abscess, wound infection, and urinary tract infection. There were no perioperative deaths. Five of 9 patients with a recurrence of symptoms underwent reoperation. On follow-up of all patients for a median of 85 months, 82% were clinically improved or asymptomatic. Symptoms persisted in 4 patients, and 2 patients died of pancreatic carcinoma.

*Conclusion.*—Surgical results in a highly selected group of 22 patients with hereditary pancreatitis were safe and efficacious. Patient selection and surgical results in the management of hereditary pancreatitis can be based on the same criteria used for nonhereditary chronic pancreatitis.

▶ Familial pancreatitis is a rare disease—at this major referral center, no more than 1 patient per year is operated on with this diagnosis. The pathophysiology and molecular genetics are unknown. However, symptoms start early, and most patients have pancreatic ductal dilatation by the time they come to the attention of surgeons. The operative procedure in this group should be based on traditional considerations, i.e., the anatomy of the pancreatic duct. Interestingly, 2 patients ultimately died of pancreatic carcinoma. One had seen both parents die of the same disease. Perhaps (as the authors speculate) total pancreatectomy should be entertained in those patients with hereditary pancreatitis who have a clear family history of pancreatic malignancy.—W.P. Ritchie, Jr., M.D.

---

**An Endoscopic Retrograde Cholangiopancreatography (ERCP)-Based Algorithm for the Management of Pancreatic Pseudocysts**
Ahearne PM, Baillie JM, Cotton PB, Baker ME, Meyers WC, Pappas TN (Duke Univ, Durham, NC)
*Am J Surg* 163:111–116, 1992                                                   9–24

---

*Introduction.*—Percutaneous and endoscopic drainage have become alternatives to surgery in some patients with pancreatic pseudocysts. Surgical drainage, however, is associated with fewer recurrences. To identify those cases in which percutaneous drainage will result in a high recurrence rate, the use of an endoscopic retrograde cholangiopancreatography (ERCP)-based algorithm was proposed.

*Methods.*—Surgical treatment is required for pancreatic pseudocysts associated with main pancreatic duct obstruction or pseudocyst communication. Nonelective cases are directed to immediate percutaneous drainage or percutaneous biopsy. An ERCP is performed in elective cases and further treatment is based on findings of pseudocyst communication or pancreatic duct obstruction. Percutaneous drainage is not performed in the presence of either finding (Fig 9–12). The algorithm was evaluated in a series of 102 patients, 73 with symptomatic pseudocysts requiring treatment.

*Results.*—The 73 patients underwent 88 interventional procedures, 69 performed on an elective basis and 19 on a nonelective basis. Forty of 49 elective treatments performed after ERCP had radiographs adequate for

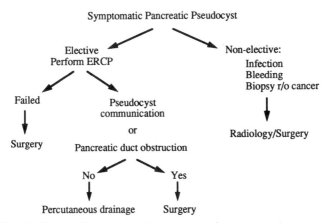

**Fig 9–12.**—Algorithm used in a retrospective assignment of treatment in the management of 40 cases of pancreatic pseudocysts. (Courtesy of Ahearne PM, Baillie JM, Cotton PB, et al: *Am J Surg* 163:111–116, 1992.)

review. Twenty patients had a pancreatic duct obstruction and 16 had pseudocyst communication; in 2 patients ERCPs showed both. In 26 cases, treatment retrospectively followed the algorithm; 14 patients had a treatment course that differed from the algorithm. Adverse outcomes occurred in 12% of the former and 43% of the latter cases, supporting the validity of the algorithm.

*Conclusion.*—Small, asymptomatic pseudocysts can be observed. Treatment is required, however, in pseudocysts larger than 5–6 cm and older than 6 weeks, as well as for all symptomatic cysts. Treatment can then be allocated according to ERCP findings.

▶ The problem with evaluating clinical algorithms retrospectively is that they are frequently evolved (in this case by a very good group of pancreatologists) from the same group of patients on whom they are then tested. This absolutely guarantees that the algorithm will work! Nevertheless, it makes good sense in the present instance. In the elective setting, ERCP should be done in patients with symptomatic pseudocysts. If it can be shown that the cyst communicates with the main ductal system, or that the main pancreatic duct is obstructed (or if ERCP is unsuccessful), operative internal drainage is indicated. Without the above, however, percutaneous drainage may well succeed. I await (but don't necessarily expect to see) a prospective evaluation of this very reasonable therapeutic plan.—W.P. Ritchie, Jr., M.D.

### Influence of the Etiology of Pancreatitis on the Natural History of Pancreatic Pseudocysts

Nguyen B-LT, Thompson JS, Edney JA, Bragg LE, Rikkers LF (Univ of Nebraska, Omaha)
*Am J Surg* 162:527–531, 1991                                                9–25

*Objective.*—Pancreatic pseudocysts, a common complication of pancreatitis, can resolve spontaneously or require surgical drainage to prevent the development of complications. Whether the etiology of the underlying pancreatic disease affects the natural history of a pancreatic pseudocyst was examined in 90 patients with pancreatic pseudocysts.

*Patients.*—Acute pancreatitis in 57 patients (63%) was caused by alcohol in 15, postoperative pancreatitis in 14, biliary pancreatitis in 12, and other causes in 16. Chronic pancreatitis in 33 patients (37%) was caused by the use of alcohol in 27 patients and other causes in 6.

*Outcome.*—Overall, 64% of patients had surgery: 18% of pseudocysts resolved spontaneously, including 11% that resolved within 8 weeks; and 8% of patients had complications. Multiple pseudocysts occurred significantly more often in patients with acute alcoholic pancreatitis than in all other groups combined. Although pseudocysts associated with acute pancreatitis were significantly larger than those associated with chronic pancreatitis, the rates of spontaneous resolution, need for operation,

# Moving?

I'd like to receive my *Year Book of Surgery* without interruption.
Please not the following change of address, effective:

Name: _____

**New Address:** _____

_____

City: _____ State: _____ Zip: _____

**Old Address:** _____

_____

City: _____ State: _____ Zip: _____

# Reservation Card

Yes, I would like my own copy of *Year Book of Surgery*. Please begin my subscription with the current edition according to the terms described below.* I understand that I will have 30 days to examine each annual edition. If satisfied, I will pay just $63.95 plus sales tax, postage and handling (price subject to change without notice).

Name: _____

Address: _____

City: _____ State: _____ Zip: _____

Method of Payment
○ Visa   ○ Mastercard   ○ AmEx   ○ Bill me   ○ Check (in US dollars, payable to Mosby, Inc.)

Card number: _____ Exp date: _____

Signature: _____

LS-0908

# *Your *Year Book* Service Guarantee:

When you subscribe to the *Year Book*, we'll send you an advance notice of future volumes about two months before they publish. This automatic notice system is designed to take up as little of your time as possible. If you do not want the *Year Book*, the advance notice makes it quick and easy for you to let us know your decision, and you will always have at least 20 days to decide. If we don't hear from you, we'll send you the new volume as soon as it's available. And, of course, the *Year Book* is yours to examine free of charge for 30 days (postage, handling and applicable sales tax are added to each shipment.).

# BUSINESS REPLY MAIL

FIRST CLASS MAIL   PERMIT No. 762   CHICAGO, IL

**POSTAGE WILL BE PAID BY ADDRESSEE**

Chris Hughes
Mosby-Year Book, Inc.
200 N. LaSalle Street
Suite 2600
Chicago, IL  60601-9981

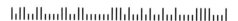

# BUSINESS REPLY MAIL

FIRST CLASS MAIL   PERMIT No. 762   CHICAGO, IL

**POSTAGE WILL BE PAID BY ADDRESSEE**

Chris Hughes
Mosby-Year Book, Inc.
200 N. LaSalle Street
Suite 2600
Chicago, IL  60601-9981

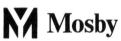

**M** Mosby

*Dedicated to publishing excellence*

Outcome of Pseudocysts According to Cause of Pancreatitis

| | Spontaneous Resolution after 8 wks | Operation after 1 yr (%) | Unre- solved | Recur- rence |
|---|---|---|---|---|
| Acute pancreatitis | | | | |
| Alcoholic (n = 15) | 3 | 9 (60) | 3 | 3 |
| Postoperative (n = 14) | 0 | 12 (86) | 2 | 1 |
| Biliary (n = 12) | 0 | 8 (67) | 4 | 0 |
| Others (n = 16)* | 2 | 8 (50) | 6 | 1 |
| Total (n = 57) | 5 | 37 (65) | 15 | 5 |
| Chronic pancreatitis | | | | |
| Alcoholic (n = 27) | 3 | 19 (70) | 5 | 3 |
| Miscellaneous (n = 6)† | 2 | 2 (33) | 2 | 0 |
| Total (n = 33) | 5 | 21 (64) | 7 | 3 |

° Others: idiopathic, traumatic, tumor, pancreas divisum.
† Miscellaneous: cystic fibrosis, familial, idiopathic.
(Courtesy of Nguyen B-LT, Thompson JS, Edney JA, et al: *Am J Surg* 162:527–531, 1991.)

and recurrence were similar with either acute or chronic presentation (table). Similarly, the outcome of pseudocysts was similar regardless of size (larger then 6 cm or smaller than 6 cm). Pseudocysts less than 6 cm in size that required operative management were significantly more common in chronic pancreatitis. None of the pseudocysts associated with postoperative or biliary pancreatitis resolved spontaneously. Mortality was significantly higher among patients with postoperative pancreatitis than in all other groups. The rate of recurrence was similar in all groups, although recurrences tended to be more frequent in patients with alcoholic pancreatitis.

*Conclusion.*—The etiology of the underlying pancreatitis is a more important determinant of pseudocyst outcome than pseudocyst size or presentation.

▶ This retrospective study of 90 patients with pancreatic pseudocysts seen over a 10-year period challenges what has become conventional wisdom by suggesting that their outcome is determined more by the etiology of the pancreatitis than by either the acuity/chronicity of presentation or by pseudocyst size. Specifically, pseudocysts secondary to gallstone pancreatitis did not resolve even after 8 weeks of observation. The same was true for pseudocysts secondary to postoperative pancreatitis, which also carried a very high morbidity and mortality. The other observations are quite similar to those generally expressed in the literature: Pseudocysts associated with acute pancreatitis of any etiology are larger than those associated with chronic pancreatitis; small pseudocysts needing operation are usually those that occur in the setting of chronic pancreatitis; and multiple pseudocysts are most uncommon in the alcoholic patient with acute pancreatitis.

It is disappointing to note that the investigators did not make significant use of endoscopic retrograde cholangiopancreatography either in establishing the diagnosis or in planning management. Also, percutaneous and endoscopic drainage techniques were rarely used. As every pancreatic surgeon knows, both procedures are in hot competition with surgical drainage as definitive treatment. Unfortunately, the efficacy claimed for them by their proponents is more often based on anecdote than on rigorous experiential review.—W.P. Ritchie, Jr., M.D.

---

**The Spectrum of Serous Cystadenoma of the Pancreas: Clinical, Pathologic, and Surgical Aspects**
Pyke CM, van Heerden JA, Colby TV, Sarr MG, Weaver AL (Mayo Clinic and Found, Rochester, Minn)
*Ann Surg* 215:132–139, 1992                                                   9–26

---

*Background.*—Serous cystadenoma of the pancreas, a rare and normally benign lesion, has usually been managed conservatively. Some physicians now advocate a more aggressive surgical approach because of the difficulty in distinguishing this tumor from mucinous cystadenocarcinoma.

*Methods.*—Clinical records of 40 patients treated between 1936 and 1991 were reviewed and follow-up obtained by death certificate or patient contact. The group included 26 women and 14 men (mean age, 63

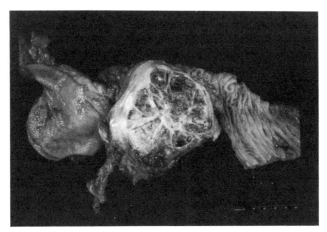

**Fig 9–13.**—Gross features of serous cystadenoma. In this specimen from a Whipple procedure, the microcystic adenoma of the head of the pancreas has been cut across to show the presence of gross cysts as well as stellate central scarring. The opened duodenum lies adjacent to the tumor. (Courtesy of Pyke CM, van Heerden JA, Colby TV, et al: *Ann Surg* 215:132–139, 1992.)

years). The median follow-up was about 2 years, with a maximum of 22 years.

*Findings.*—About a third of the patients were asymptomatic at diagnosis, with the lesion found during examination for another problem. Most (69%), however, reported an abdominal pain or mass, nausea and vomiting, and weight loss—symptoms thought to result from the local pressure effects of the cystic neoplasm. Symptomatic and asymptomatic lesions did not differ significantly in mean size (7.5 cm vs. 6 cm). Preoperative CT, used since 1974, could not make an unequivocal diagnosis. Only 10 of 27 patients undergoing celiotomy for a known or presumed pancreatic mass had a preoperative diagnosis of serous cystadenoma. Four of the 36 patients who underwent resection died, and 15 had significant postoperative complications. Twenty-three patients are still alive.

*Conclusion.*—The serous cystadenoma is usually composed of numerous cystic areas, some small or microscopic and others larger (Fig 9–13). Additional CT findings may include calcification, a central scar, the absence of metastases, and hypervascularity. The decision to undertake resection should be based on the confidence of preoperative diagnosis, clinical presentation and symptoms, safety of resection, and potential consequences of conservative therapy. The possibility of associated conditions should also be considered in patients with serous cystadenoma of the pancreas.

▶ This paper suggests that symptomatic serous cystadenomas of the pancreas are best treated by resection (if the procedure can be accomplished safely). On the other hand, incidentally discovered lesions should be evaluated with ultrasound, CT, aspiration for pathologic and biochemical studies, and, on occasion, arteriography. If the diagnosis of serous cystadenoma is fairly certain once all of this has been accomplished, patients should be observed and periodically reevaluated because the risk of life-threatening complications (e.g., malignant transformation, hemorrhage) may be far lower than the operative mortality of resection (10% in this series). The astute reader will recognize, of course, that none of the aforementioned discussion applies to the mucinous cystadenoma, which has clear malignant potential.—W.P. Ritchie, Jr., M.D.

## Small Intestine

INTRODUCTION

A diagnostic-therapeutic algorithm has been proposed for those extremely difficult patients who have chronic gastrointestinal bleeding of obscure origin. The algorithm includes preoperative enterscopy, surgical exploration with additional intraoperative enteroscopy, and occasional intraoperative scintigraphy. A positive bleeding site was found in each of 71 patients evaluated in this way; 56 had no further bleeding.

Although stricturoplasty has become a common method of dealing with small bowel strictures secondary to Crohn's disease, an occasional leak does develop. A recent report suggests that a side-to-side bypass proximal and distal to the stricture may offer some advantages over the conventional approach in this regard.

Although the numbers of autopsies on patients with surgical diseases of the digestive tract have decreased dramatically, the information gained from them clearly has not. Autopsies in 77 patients with a primary diagnosis of nonmalignant disease of the gastrointestinal tract indicated one or more discrepancies with the clinical impressions formed during life in almost half and an incorrect treatment regimen leading to a negative outcome (death) in almost 10%.

Wallace P. Ritchie, Jr., M.D.

## Surgical Approach to Occult Gastrointestinal Bleeding
Szold A, Katz LB, Lewis BS (Mount Sinai Med Ctr, New York City)
*Am J Surg* 163:90–93, 1992                                    9–27

*Background.*—Approximately 95% of bleeding gastrointestinal lesions may be discovered by endoscopy, but routine diagnostic work-up may fail to reveal the source of bleeding in the remaining 5% of patients. Angiography, small bowel enteroscopy, surgical exploration, and intraoperative scintigraphy have been used in patients with obscure gastrointestinal bleeding. A diagnostic-therapeutic "algorithm" was developed for treating patients with obscure gastrointestinal bleeding.

*Method.*—Thirty-eight male and 33 female patients underwent extensive diagnostic work-ups, including barium contrast studies, endoscopy, angiography, multiple bleeding scans, Meckel scans, and surgical explorations for obscure gastrointestinal bleeding. According to the diagnostic-therapeutic sequence, all patients underwent endoscopy, and 68 of the 71 patients underwent enteroscopy and surgery. Enteroscopy was aborted in the remaining 3 patients when "watermelon stomach" was diagnosed.

*Findings.*—In 30 patients in whom the bleeding site was not apparent at exploration, intraoperative enteroscopy was performed. Intraoperative scintigraphy was used in 2 patients who were actively bleeding when intraoperative enteroscopy failed to localize the bleeding site. Bleeding originated in small bowel arteriovenous malformations in 28 patients, leiomyoma in 8, primary small bowel malignancies in 11, and from other causes in 24. On follow-up averaging 20 months, 56 patients had no further bleeding after resection of the affected bowel, 9 patients with multiple small bowel arteriovenous malformations had, rebleeding but are alive, 6 patients died of recurrent bleeding, and 6 patients died of metastatic cancer.

*Conclusion.*—A diagnostic-therapeutic algorithm, including enteroscopy, surgical exploration with additional intraoperative enteroscopy, and occasional intraoperative scintigraphy, had a 100% yield in 71 patients evaluated. Preoperative enteroscopy excludes patients with unresectable disease and can localize the bleeding lesion in many patients. Application of the diagnostic-therapeutic algorithm resulted in a low complication rate with only minimal bowel injury.

▶ This clearly must be one of the largest series extant dealing with those extremely difficult patients with occult gastrointestinal hemorrhage in whom the source is not readily identifiable on routine (and frequently repetitious) diagnostic work-up. The proposed algorithm (preoperative enteroscopy, operative exploration with more enteroscopy, and occasional intraoperative scintigraphy) must be a good one, because a bleeding lesion was identified in every instance. Forty percent were found to be arteriovenous malformations, and 33% were previously undetected small bowel tumors. The proof of the pudding is in the eating: 79% of patients were free of bleeding at an average follow-up of 20 months.—W.P. Ritchie, Jr., M.D.

---

**Stapled Strictureplasty for Crohn's Disease**
Keighley MRB (Queen Elizabeth Hosp, Birmingham, England)
*Dis Colon Rectum* 34:945–947, 1991                                              9–28

---

*Background.*—Strictureplasty is commonly done in patients with recurrent Crohn's disease of the small bowel, especially if there is only limited residual disease and the recurrence is well localized. In 7 of 56 patients undergoing this operation, however, an early postoperative leak developed. An alternative method of strictureplasty was examined using an enterotomy some distance from the disease site and accomplishing enteroplasty by side-to-side stapling.

*Technique.*—A small enterotomy is made 7 cm proximal and distal to the area of the recurrence. Stay sutures are used to approximate the bowel loop above and below the stricture. The Ethicon Autosuture device is inserted through the 2 enterotomies. A side-to-side bypass, or strictureplasty, is then created by construction of a staple line to the apex of the intestinal loop. A transverse continuous, inverting, extramucosal prolene suture is used to close the enterotomy to make sure that the bowel lumen is not compromised. There were no complications in 22 patients undergoing this procedure.

*Discussion.*—This technique of stapled strictureplasty offers some advantages over conventional sutured strictureplasty. Enterotomy is done away from the site of the recurrence, enteroplasty is wider, and tissue reaction can be minimized by use of nonabsorbable suture material. The absence of leakage may be another advantage.

▶ This technique is basically a side-to-side anastomosis designed to bypass a stenotic segment of small bowel that is too long for stricturoplasty. The anastomosis comes right up to the stricture, minimizing the bypass length. The use of staples may be superfluous, but the fact that no leaks occurred in 26 patients in whom suture lines were created in potentially diseased bowel is impressive. One interesting question: Does the bypassed segment recover any form or function? It might, once distal obstruction is relieved.—W.P. Ritchie, Jr., M.D.

### The Results of Autopsy of Patients With Surgical Diseases of the Digestive Tract

Barendregt WB, de Boer HHM, Kubat K (Univ Hosp Nijmegen, The Netherlands)
*Surg Gynecol Obstet* 175:227–232, 1992                                    9–29

*Background.*—Autopsy aids awareness of the inaccuracy of clinical diagnosis and can help to detect errors of management that may be preventable.

*Methods.*—An analysis of autopsy results was performed to identify missed diagnoses and incorrect therapy in 77 patients who died with surgical disease of the digestive tract. None had malignant disease. Premortem and postmortem findings were compared, and treatment and diagnostic procedures were evaluated in light of autopsy findings.

*Findings.*—All diagnoses were correct in 51% of the patients, but there was at least 1 discrepancy in 49% of the patients. Failed or inadequate diagnostic methods were significantly associated with treatment

Table 1.—Instances of Incorrect Treatment With Clear Adverse Effect

|  | No. of pts. |
|---|---|
| Failure to operate in duodenal stump leakage | 1 |
| Failure to operate in bleeding gastric ulcer | 1 |
| Failure to debride infected pancreatic haematoma | 1 |
| Failure to reoperate leaking intestinal anastomosis | 1 |
| Failure to reoperate intra-abdominal bleeding | 1 |
| Failure to drain hepatic abscesses and purulent peritonitis | 1 |
| Failure to debride pancreatic necrosis | 1 |

(Courtesy of Barendregt WB, de Boer HHM, Kubat K: *Surg Gynecol Obstet* 175:227–232, 1992.)

Table 2.—Instances of Incorrect Treatment With Possible Adverse Effect

|  | No. of pts. |
|---|---|
| Failure to débride pancreatic necrosis | 1 |
| Failure to drain rest abscesses and fecal peritonitis. | 1 |
| Inadequate early shock treatment, hypovolemic and septic | 1 |
| Failure to give antibiotics in bronchopneumonia. | 1 |
| Failure to administer adequate coronary care | 1 |

(Courtesy of Barendregt WB, de Boer HHM, Kubat K: *Surg Gynecol Obstet* 175:227-232, 1992.)

failure. Postmortem examination revealed an error in treatment in 12 patients with a clear adverse effect on the disease course in 7 patients (Table 1). In the remaining 5 patients, the harmful effect was possible but unclear (Table 2). The most common error was failure to reoperate on patients with an intra-abdominal complication. In 6 of 9 patients who died suddenly or unexpectedly, the direct cause of death had not been correctly estimated clinically. Septic shock and myocardial infarction were the most important causes of unexpected death.

*Conclusion.*—In an autopsy analysis of 77 patients who died because of surgical disease of the digestive tract, primary diagnoses had been correct in 95%, but complications were diagnosed correctly in only 57%. Incorrect treatment, given to 12 patients, had a clear negative impact on the clinical course in 7 of them. Sudden, unexpected death and failed or inadequate diagnostic procedures had a significant negative influence on clinical accuracy.

▶ Because surgeons have available to them such a large array of sophisticated diagnostic imaging modalities, it is widely assumed that postmortem examination can add little information of value in cases with the ultimate untoward outcome. This study clearly refutes that notion. Twelve of 77 surgical patients were treated inappropriately during life, and that treatment resulted in the demise of 7. A particularly disturbing note is that 5 of the 7 had intra-abdominal sepsis from potentially correctable causes. The message is simple: Autopsies are extremely instructive learning exercises for surgeons, and many more of them should be done.—W.P. Ritchie, Jr., M.D.

## Colon and Rectum

INTRODUCTION

Mucosal proctectomy with ileal pouch-anal anastomosis has become the surgical treatment of choice for patients with ulcerative colitis and familial polyposis. Controversy remains, however, about the necessity of performing a protective loop ileostomy under these circumstances. One recent randomized trial of carefully selected patients suggests that it may be safe to omit this step. In general, however, most experienced surgeons continue to advocate the performance of a diverting ileostomy to obviate the development of pelvic sepsis.

The use of metaclopramide to reduce postoperative ileus in patients undergoing colorectal operations has been evaluated and, once again, has been found wanting. A policy of routine, as opposed to selective re-implantation of a patent inferior mesenteric artery appears to decrease the incidence of ischemic colitis in patients undergoing aortic recon-structive surgery.

Mini-access surgery using the laparoscope is inexorably working its way south. A prospective, randomized trial of laparoscopic versus open appendectomy demonstrated the clear superiority of the former tech-nique. An ingenious application of the methodology involves laparo-scopic fixation of the sigmoid colon in patients who have experienced sigmoid volvulus.

**Wallace P. Ritchie, Jr., M.D.**

---

### Randomized Trial of Loop Ileostomy in Restorative Proctocolectomy

Grobler SP, Hosie KB, Keighley MRB (Queen Elizabeth Med Ctr, Birmingham, England)

*Br J Surg* 79:903–906, 1992
9–30

---

*Introduction.*—Restorative proctocolectomy with construction of an ileoanal anastomosis is performed routinely with temporary diversion via an ileostomy. Restorative proctocolectomy without protective ileostomy, however, may not increase the risk of anastomotic complications. The risks and benefits of performing restorative proctocolectomy with and without a protective ileostomy were compared in a randomized, con-trolled clinical trial.

*Patients and Methods.*—During a 3-year period, 59 patients under-went standard totally stapled abdominal restorative proctocolectomy. Only patients who were not being treated with systemic corticosteroids and in whom intraoperative testing revealed that all staple lines were in-tact and without tension were included in the study. Thus 45 patients met the entry criteria. After construction of the ileoanal anastomosis, 23 patients were allocated to receive a loop ileostomy and 22 were allo-cated to receive no ileostomy. Follow-up examinations, including pouch endoscopy, were performed at 1, 3, and 6 months after operation and every 6 months thereafter. The median follow-up period was 20 months.

*Results.*—There were no deaths. Two ileoanal anastomotic leaks oc-curred, 1 in a patient with an ileostomy and 1 in a patient without. Five patients with an ileostomy (22%) and 1 patient without (5%) had ileoa-nal stenosis. One patient without an ileostomy required early reopera-tion and pelvic packing for pelvic hemorrhage. Major wound sepsis occurred in 2 patients with ileostomies and in 1 without. Twelve of 23 patients with ileostomies (52%) had 1 or more ileostomy-associated complications. The median total hospital stay was 23 days for patients with ileostomies and 13 days for those without. Both groups had similar functional outcomes.

*Conclusion.*—Restorative proctocolectomy without a defunctioning ileostomy is a safe alternative to temporary diversion.

▶ This is an excellent prospective study from an experienced surgical group. It should be read carefully by all surgeons engaged in performing restorative proctocolectomy. The essence of the message is this: Although it appears to be safe, and even preferable, not to perform a routine ileostomy under these circumstances, the patients chosen for this procedure must be very carefully selected (uncomplicated operation, no preoperative steroids, tension-free anastomosis, and water-tight suture lines). Further, both surgeon and patient should be prepared for prompt reoperation and total diversion should a leak occur.—W.P. Ritchie, Jr., M.D.

---

**Ileal Pouch–Anal Anastomosis: Patterns of Failure**
Gemlo BT, Wong WD, Rothenberger DA, Goldberg SM (Univ of Minnesota, Minneapolis)
*Arch Surg* 127:784–787, 1992                                    9–31

---

*Background.*—The ileal pouch–anal anastomosis for ulcerative colitis or polyposis has been well accepted and has yielded satisfactory functional results. Nevertheless, the risk of failure is a significant source of anxiety for both patients and physicians, partly because of the difficulty of reconstruction after pouch failure.

*Patients.*—Data were reviewed on 253 patients having 253 ileoanal reservoirs constructed between 1980 and 1990. About 75% of the patients were available for review. Pouch failure developed in 25 patients (10%).

*Findings.*—Crohn's disease became evident in 13 patients after surgery, and in 6 of them, this condition resulted in pouch loss from perianal sepsis or a pouch fistula. Pouchitis developed in 78 patients and accounted for 4 failures. Pouchitis did not, as Crohn's disease did, increase the risk of pouch failure. Thirteen patients had significant pelvic sepsis not associated with Crohn's disease, and 5 of them lost their pouches. Seven pouch failures were ascribed to poor functional results. One failure each was caused by pouch infarction, hemorrhage, and pouch obstruction by a desmoid tumor.

*Discussion.*—The true pouch failure rate in this series was 10%. The learning curve for ileal pouch–anal anastomosis is both personal and institutional. Poor functional results are the most common cause of ileal pouch failure. It is hoped that improvements in the technique of pouch construction and in ileoanal anastomosis will better preserve anal sphincter function.

▶ This is a large series from a very experienced group analyzing the patterns of failure after ileal pouch–anal anastomoses. Of 253 patients undergoing the procedure (90% had a "S" pouch), 196 (77%) were available for review. Twenty-five patients (10% of the total) lost their pouches (more than half within 2 years) because of poor function, i.e., incontinence (7 patients), unrecognized Crohn's disease (6), pelvic sepsis (5), pouchitis (4), and a miscellany of other reasons (3). Interestingly, in contrast to unrecognized Crohn's disease, the development of pouchitis per se did not significantly increase the risk of pouch failure. On the other hand, the high risk of such failure associated with the development of pelvic sepsis has led the Minnesota group to be very liberal in the use of pelvic drains and has prompted them to perform a diverting ileostomy in virtually every case.—W.P. Ritchie, Jr., M.D.

---

### Does Metoclopramide Reduce the Length of Ileus After Colorectal Surgery: A Prospective Randomized Trial

Cheape JD, Wexner SD, James K, Jagelman DG (Cleveland Clinic Florida, Ft Lauderdale)
*Dis Colon Rectum* 34:437–441, 1991                                    9–32

---

*Background.*—Metoclopramide stimulates gastric motility, but its effects on the postoperative return of bowel function have not been well defined. A randomized, prospective, controlled trial of patients who had undergone elective colorectal surgery was undertaken to examine the effects of this drug on postoperative ileus.

*Methods.*—Group 1 consisted of 40 patients who received metoclopramide intravenously every 8 hours from the end of surgery until the beginning of a solid food diet. Group 2 consisted of 53 patients who did not receive the drug.

*Results.*—There were no significant differences between groups 1 and 2 in mean length of time before liquid intake, mean length of time before solid intake, or prolonged ileus.

*Conclusions.*—Administration of metoclopramide does not significantly change the course of postoperative ileus in patients undergoing elective colorectal surgery. The routine use of this drug cannot be advocated.

▶ The authors are to be commended for attempting to answer an interesting, perhaps even important, clinical question using acceptable statistical methodologies. They may have bitten off more than they could chew, however, for several instructive reasons. In the first instance, the end points of the study—the ingestion of liquid or regular diets based on the passage of flatus and stool—were almost of necessity subjective and vague (as all other students of ileus have found, to their distress). Also, the patients studied were not necessarily homogeneous: They had 16 different diagnoses and underwent 11 different operative procedures, ranging in magnitude from formation of a colostomy to creation of an ileoanal reservoir. Finally, despite the statistical power of the study detailed in the paper, it is still possible that a type 2 error might have occurred. None of this is meant to disparage the efforts of the authors, which were commendable. On the other hand, the report does point to some of the major difficulties that may be encountered, even in well-designed, prospective trials.—W.P. Ritchie, Jr., M.D.

---

### Routine Reimplantation of Patent Inferior Mesenteric Arteries Limits Colon Infarction After Aortic Reconstruction

Seeger JM, Coe DA, Kaelin LD, Flynn TC (Univ of Florida, Gainesville; VA Med Ctr, Gainesville)

*J Vasc Surg* 15:635–641, 1992                                                              9–33

---

*Background.*—Ischemic colitis leading to colonic infarction after reconstructive surgery on the aorta is associated with a high mortality rate. Reimplanting all patent inferior mesenteric arteries should lessen mortality, but the method is justified only if it is both effective and safe.

*Methods.*—A review was made of 337 aortic reconstructive procedures performed between 1982 and 1989. In 151 operations done in the last 3 years of this period, patent inferior mesenteric vessels were reimplanted when possible. Previously, these vessels were ligated selectively on the basis of bowel appearance, colonic mesenteric Doppler signals, and stump pressures in the inferior mesenteric arteries.

*Results.*—No patient in the later part of the review period had colonic infarction. Five earlier patients (2.7%) did have colonic infarction and perforation, and 4 died. The operative mortality rate was 14.5% early in the series and 4% when the mesenteric arteries were reimplanted if possible. Transfusion requirements did not differ significantly in the 2 periods.

*Conclusion.*—Routine reimplantation of patent inferior mesenteric arteries appears to lower the risk of colonic infarction after reconstruction of the aorta.

▶ Although this paper suffers from the debits of being retrospective, especially those related to the use of historical controls, it does make a very good case (the best yet, in my view) for routine as opposed to selective reimplantation of a patent inferior mesenteric artery in the patient undergoing aortic reconstruction.—W.P. Ritchie, Jr., M.D.

## A Prospective Randomized Trial of Laparoscopic Versus Open Appendectomy

Attwood SEA, Hill ADK, Murphy PG, Thornton J, Stephens RB (St James's Hosp, Dublin, Ireland)

*Surgery* 112:497–501, 1992

9–34

*Introduction.*—Laparoscopic appendectomy is reportedly safe and effective. Open and laparoscopic appendectomies were compared to determine whether the laparoscopic approach offers advantages to the patient.

*Methods.*—Patients with suspected acute appendicitis were randomized, 30 to laparoscopy and 32 to open appendectomy. Postoperative recovery, complications, and return to normal activities were assessed.

*Results.*—The patients having laparoscopy were discharged significantly earlier and had fewer complications. Follow-up indicated less pain, shorter stay in bed at home, and faster return to normal activity after laparoscopy than after open appendectomy (table).

*Conclusions.*—Laparoscopic appendectomy is superior to open appendectomy with regard to patient comfort, complication rate, and early and late recovery. Therefore, laparoscopy is recommended as the preferred treatment in patients with acute appendicitis.

▶ This paper indicates that appendectomy performed laparoscopically is not only a safe procedure but also appears to permit the patient to return to normal activity much more rapidly than does open appendectomy. We and many others have also found that laparoscopic exploration of the abdomen is in and of itself a useful maneuver, particularly in those female patients in whom the diagnosis is unclear and when hospital observation to "rule out appendicitis" for 24–48 hours has been standard in the past. In general, if such patients show no clinical improvement within 6–8 hours, they are sub-

Recovery of Patients After Discharge From Hospital After Laparoscopic and Open Appendectomy

| Days | Laparoscopic appendectomy (n = 26) | | Open appendectomy (n = 28) | | |
|---|---|---|---|---|---|
| | Median | Range | Median | Range | p Value* |
| In bed at home | 0 | 0-14 | 2 | 0-28 | 0.017 |
| Pain | 0 | 0-14 | 13 | 0-91 | 0.014 |
| To work | 10 | 1-25 | 16 | 2-84 | 0.001 |
| To sport | 14 | 1-75 | 21 | 2-90 | 0.07 NS |
| To full fitness | 21 | 5-120 | 38 | 5-150 | 0.02 |

*Abbreviation:* NS, not significant.
* Wilcoxon rank sum test, significant if *p* < 0.05.
(Courtesy of Attwood SEA, Hill ADK, Murphy PG, et al: *Surgery* 112:497–501, 1992.)

jected to laparoscopy. It has been our practice to remove the appendix irrespective of whether or not it is inflamed, admittedly an unsettled issue.—W.P. Ritchie, Jr., M.D.

## Laparoscopic Fixation of Sigmoid Volvulus

Miller R, Roe AM, Eltringham WK, Espiner HJ (Bristol Royal Infirmary, Bristol, England)

*Br J Surg* 79:435, 1992          9–35

*Case Report.*—Man, 75, was admitted with a 4-day history of abdominal colic, distention, and constipation. Plain radiography revealed a sigmoid volvulus. He underwent decompression with a rigid sigmoidoscope, which was repeated when the distention recurred. After removal of the flatus tube following the second procedure, symptoms and signs of obstruction recurred and laparoscopic fixation of the colon was performed. Under general anesthesia, the colon was sutured to the inner layer of the rectus sheath at a point under the tenth rib. A second point of fixation on the sigmoid loop was established in the left upper quadrant. The third point of fixation was established in the left iliac fossa (Fig 9–14). At the 14-month follow-up, the patient was asymptomatic with no further episodes of volvulus.

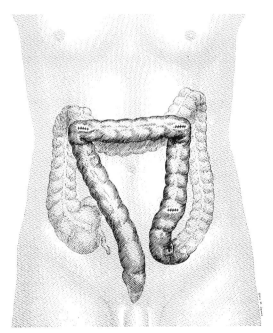

**Fig 9–14.**—Position of the colon after laparoscopic fixation. (Courtesy of Miller R, Roe AM, Eltringham WK, et al: *Br J Surg* 79:435, 1992.)

*Conclusion.*—If endoscopic measures fail to decompress a sigmoid volvulus or if there are frequent recurrences, fixation of the sigmoid volvulus is the preferred treatment. Suture fixation with a laparoscopic approach avoids the morbidity associated with the large abdominal wound required for laparotomy, but it may be associated with a higher risk of recurrence compared to resection. Laparoscopic fixation was particularly useful in this elderly patient with poor lung function.

▶ Surgeons are nothing if not inventive. This looks like a potentially safe, simple, and effective method of dealing with a difficult problem in patients who are usually not exceptionally fit for open colon resection.—W.P. Ritchie, Jr., M.D.

## Liver and Spleen

INTRODUCTION

The results achieved in 70 patients with idiopathic thrombocytopenic purpura subjected to splenectomy in a 6-year period confirm the safety and efficacy of this approach. Interestingly, the response to preoperative IgG therapy was a better predictor of splenectomy outcome than was the response to corticosteroid therapy.

Wallace P. Ritchie, Jr., M.D.

**Surgical Treatment of Immune Thrombocytopenic Purpura**
Chirletti P, Cardi M, Barillari P, Vitale A, Sammartino P, Bolognese A, Caiazzo R, Ricci M, Muttillo IA, Stipa V (Università degli Studi di Roma "La Sapienza," Rome, Italy)
*World J Surg* 16:1001–1005, 1992                                    9–36

*Background.*—Immune thrombocytopenic purpura (ITP) is an idiopathic autoimmune disease characterized by a reduced circulating platelet count because of platelet destruction in the spleen. Corticosteroids represent the standard initial treatment for ITP, but response is often only transient. Splenectomy may be a valid alternative to immunosuppressive steroid therapy.

*Patients and Methods.*—During a 6-year period, 70 patients with ITP aged 6–56 years underwent splenectomy. Fifteen patients were younger than 12 years of age. All patients had been treated with steroids for at least 3 months. Initially, 33 patients had transient complete response and 27 had a partial response to steroids. Indications for operation were a platelet count lower than 80,000/mm$^3$, a history of abnormal bleeding, easy bruisability, purpura, ecchymosis or petechiae of at least 3 months' duration, inability to taper high steroid doses or no response to steroid therapy, and the presence of serum antiplatelet antibodies. Eight patients who were at standard risk for intraoperative bleeding were given tranexamic acid 2 hours before operation and 62 high-risk patients were given high doses of IgG 2 days before operation. All patients had a positive antiplatelet antibody titer.

*Results.*—Forty-three patients (69%) had a complete response to pre-operative IgG infusion and required no further treatment before operation. Accessory spleens were identified on the preoperative ultrasonography scans of 5 patients and found at operation in 11 patients (16%). There was no perioperative mortality. Fourteen patients had minor post-operative complications. After a mean postoperative follow-up of 21 months, 63 patients (90%) responded completely and 7 patients had no response. All 7 nonresponders to splenectomy also had not responded to preoperative IgG therapy. On radionuclide imaging studies with [111]In-labeled platelets, accessory spleens were detected in the gastrocolic omentum of 2 nonresponders. Both patients had complete resolution of ITP after undergoing accessory splenectomy.

*Conclusion.*—Splenectomy is a safe and effective treatment for ITP. The response to preoperative IgG therapy is predictive of splenectomy outcome.

▶ With standard preoperative evaluation, patients with ITP can expect to experience a complete response to splenectomy (platelet counts greater than 150 K/mm$^3$) in 80% to 90% of instances. This series is no exception: Only 5 of 70 patients (7%) were permanent nonresponders. Of interest, 4 of the 5 demonstrated an increase in platelet count during preoperative steroid treatment, a response thought by many (apparently erroneously) to predict a good surgical result. The authors found that nonresponsiveness to IgG was a much better predictor of a poor surgical outcome than was nonresponse to steroids. Two patients required reoperation to remove accessory spleens. We have been impressed by the ability of preoperative scintigraphy to alert us to this possibility before splenectomy, especially in patients with very low platelet counts.—W.P. Ritchie, Jr., M.D.

# 10 Oncology

## Introduction

This was a particularly productive year in the literature with regard to oncology and basic research. Rather than be all inclusive, I have tried to select studies that will have an impact on the management of patients with cancer, both immediately and in the future. This is true not only of the subjects dealing with various disease categories but also in the basic science literature where studies have been selected because of their large numbers and overall impact or because of their prospective nature. Retrospective and anecdotal studies, no matter how prestigious the author or how valid the subject matter, have largely been omitted.

With regard to breast cancer, the year began with the success of the *Lancet* articles (Abstracts 10-1 and 10-2). These two publications have in large part strengthened the resolve of medical oncologists to treat patients over the age of 50 with tamoxifen and to a large degree those under the age of 50 with chemotherapy. New trials have already been designed to answer some of the questions that have been raised from these overviews, such as the length of time of tamoxifen administration and the use of sequential chemotherapy and tamoxifen, as well as the selection of patients who are node negative for systemic treatment. Because breast cancer is so ubiquitous to the practice of most general surgeons as well as surgical oncologists, I have further broken down this category into subtopics such as pathologic features. In this area, several articles discuss new molecular biological techniques that are associated with prognosis. In the future, one would expect an ever-increasing number of papers addressing angiogenesis, marker genes, and marker proteins that will influence not only prognosis but also the selection of patients for inclusion in adjuvant therapy trials.

There has been a significant increase in the number of manuscripts involving the new stereotactic biopsy approach. Whereas this new technology increases the armamentarium of procedures for the early diagnosis of breast disease, its true place in the management of patients with mammographic and/or palpable abnormalities is as yet undefined. Articles have also been included that concern the outcome of conservative surgery and radiation therapy as well as address the questions as to whether or not to perform axillary dissection, and if performed, how many nodes should be removed and what technique should be used.

Colorectal cancer remains one of the most common malignancies in the United States. The importance of patterns and screening has been emphasized in several articles dealing with the utility of stool guaiac or more invasive means for detection and screening of large patient populations. The manuscript by Sariego et al. (Abstract 10–22) reporting a 25-year experience documents the rightward shift in incidence of colorectal cancer, as well as the significance of earlier diagnosis, most likely because of colonoscopy. Similarly, I have included two articles (10–30 and 10–31) reporting the monoclonal antibody detection of occult colorectal tumors. This reflects a recent fad, but these studies not only document the utility of this technique but also point out some of its limitations.

With respect to colorectal treatment, I have included several manuscripts dealing with topics that we all must manage in our daily practice: the proper management of polyps with invasive carcinoma as well as large unresectable tumors treated with preoperative radiation. There are some very nice studies from well-respected institutions that may help to affect the day-to-day care of our patients.

In the section on tumor biology/basic science, I have attempted to choose articles that examine various aspects of basic science mechanistically. Many topics that deal with some of the more common entities in basic tumor biology are discussed, such as stimulation of effector cells, side effects of interleukin-2 therapy, and either gene markers or other cytokines in their potential antitumor roles. The articles selected amplify the wide range of basic science problems that, when answered, will have a positive impact on the future management of our patients with malignancy.

With respect to gastric cancer, there have been several large series from Korea and Japan that report not only on the surgical technique of gastric resection but also on the immuno/adjuvant treatment of this difficult malignancy. Gastric cancer in the Pacific Basin does not appear to be similar to its presentation in the United States. However, much can be learned from the surgical techniques and the combination of treatments. The latter is also pointed out in the Brennan article (Abstract 10–55), which addresses multidrug regimen chemotherapy in patients with gastric cancer. The role of endoscopic ultrasound and dynamic CT is also evaluated in the staging and management of patients with gastric cancer.

Several excellent articles by the Memorial group regarding the indications for amputation as well as limb-sparing procedures in adult soft tissue sarcomas are included in the section on sarcomas (Abstracts 10–59 and 10–60). Additionally, manuscripts on such common topics as prognosis, long-term salvageability following recurrence, and ability to diagnose with core needles can also be found in this section.

With respect to melanoma, several large series that examined patient characteristics and prognostic features were reported. Most alarming was the study from the American College of Surgeons (Abstract 10–64), which documented that even in that series a large number of patients did not have adequate pathologic staging consisting of Clark's level and

Breslow thickness. Only through uniform staging will treatments be standardized and therefore be able to be compared.

This has been an excellent year for reporting several large and significant trials that deal with various malignancies, as well as for making meaningful strides in basic biological mechanisms that eventually will have an effect on clinical therapies. The coming year will be accompanied by a heightened level of expectation for additional excellent reviews in the YEAR BOOK OF SURGERY.

Timothy J. Eberlein, M.D.

# Breast

INTRODUCTION

As would be expected, the incidence of breast cancer in the United States has stimulated the production of a large number of articles on various aspects of this disease. In this volume, the studies have been categorized by such topics as pathologic features or novel treatment practices. The year began with the meta-analysis published in 2 parts in the *Lancet*. For nonstatisticians, these manuscripts may be somewhat daunting; however, they are helpful in formuating treatment policies around the world and are recommended for reading in their entirety.

Timothy J. Eberlein, M.D.

OVERVIEW

**Systemic Treatment of Early Breast Cancer by Hormonal, Cytotoxic, or Immune Therapy: 133 Randomised Trials Involving 31,000 Recurrences and 24,000 Deaths Among 75,000 Women**
Early Breast Cancer Trialists' Collaborative Group (Radcliffe Infirmary, Oxford, England)
*Lancet* 339:1–15, 1992                                                  10–1

*Objective.*—A worldwide collaborative effort was undertaken to analyze recurrences and deaths in randomized trials, begun before 1985, that dealt with systemic adjuvant treatment for early breast cancer. Data were available for 75,000 women, about 90% of those ever randomized into trials. About one third of these women had died and another 10% had had recurrences. There were about 30,000 women in trials of tamoxifen and 3,000 in trials of ovarian ablation.

*Tamoxifen.*—Tamoxifen use lowered recurrences by 25% and deaths by 17%. In addition, it reduced the risk of contralateral breast cancer by 39%. Tamoxifen was of value in women older than age 70 years. Recurrences were chiefly lowered in the first 4 years of follow-up.

*Ovarian Ablation.*—Women younger than age 50 years who were managed by ovarian ablation had a 26% reduction in recurrences and a 25% decline in mortality. Ablation at older ages was ineffective.

*Polychemotherapy.*—In 11,000 women participating in trials of polychemotherapy, recurrences were reduced by 28% and mortality declined by 16%. As with tamoxifen, recurrences were avoided chiefly in the first years of follow-up, but mortality remained lowered after this time. Polychemotherapy was significantly more effective than single-agent chemotherapy. Treatment for 6 months was at least as effective as long-term treatment. In women aged 50–69 years, chemotherapy plus tamoxifen was more effective than chemotherapy alone. With combined chemoendocrine therapy in middle-aged women, the absolute improvement in 10-year survival was about twice as great for node-positive as for node-negative patients.

---

### Systemic Treatment of Early Breast Cancer by Hormonal, Cytotoxic, or Immune Therapy: 133 Randomised Trials Involving 31,000 Recurrences and 24,000 Deaths Among 75,000 Women

Early Breast Cancer Trialists' Collaborative Group
*Lancet* 339:71–85, 1992                                                   10–2

---

*Introduction.*—A review was made of the results of cytotoxic and immunotherapy in a worldwide collaborative study that included data on some 75,000 women overall.

*Results of Chemotherapy.*—The findings of 47 trials involving 18,000 women provided evidence that some form of chemotherapy can affect both recurrence and survival. Prolonged polychemotherapy was associated with the greatest therapeutic effect. Shorter regimens (mean, 6 months) were not significantly more beneficial, however, than longer regimens (mean, 16 months). Gains in recurrence-free survival occurred primarily during the first 5 years. The effects of polychemotherapy on survival, however, were far more definite at 10 years than at 5 years.

*Results of Immunotherapy.*—A total of 6,300 women in 24 trials received bacille Calmette Guerin (BCG) vaccine, levamisole, or other agents. Neither recurrence-free survival nor overall survival was significantly improved with the use of immunotherapy. There appeared to be an adverse effect with BCG.

*Conclusion.*—The definite effects of the older regimens of cyclophosphamide, methotrexater, and 5-fluorouracil and tamoxifen suggest that adjuvant treatment may now offer greater improvement in 10-year mortality. Patients with estrogen-receptor (ER)-positive tumors benefited most from tamoxifen, yet those with ER-poor tumors, especially women older than age 50 years, also had favorable results. In addition, tamoxifen, which substantially reduces blood cholesterol levels, was associated with a marginally significant reduction in vascular mortality. Although the reported data make no recommendations as to the treatment that should be used, physicians who treat early breast cancer should review the trial's results.

▶ These 2 papers (Abstracts 10–1 and 10–2) that appeared in *Lancet* in the beginning of 1992 present an analysis of 133 randomized trials involving 75,000 women before 1985. Although this study is a monumental achievement in statistical analysis, it suffers somewhat from the fact that multiple different trials from around the world are compared. For example, there is a preponderance of trials involving early breast cancers and breast cancers with good prognoses (i.e., participants from Japan), however, because of the statistical power when grouped in large numbers, the conclusions of the smaller trials are rendered significant.

In general, although adjuvant treatments are relatively brief, (a median of only 2 years for tamoxifen, median of 1 year for polychemotherapy), there appears to be additional divergence in mortality after the first 5 years occurring many years after the treatments had ended. This is highly significant and surprising to most collaborators and reviewers.

The reader should be further cautioned from overanalyzing or performing subset analyses that were not originally anticipated in the design of the trials. With these caveats, several points require emphasis.

*Tamoxifen*—The most widely tested regimen consisted of 20 mg/day for 2 years. This dose seemed to be sufficient, but, longer-term tamoxifen may well be more effective. Currently, trials are underway testing tamoxifen for 5 or more years. As would be expected, patients with ER-positive tumors benefited most, especially if they were older than 70 years. However, women with ER-negative tumors, especially those older than 50, also appeared to have benefited from tamoxifen treatment. There was a marginally significant reduction in vascular mortality.

*Chemotherapy*—In general, polychemotherapy regimens were much more effective than single agents. A minimum of 6 months of treatment was found to be significant. There were no outstanding differences between the various forms of polychemotherapy. Thus chemotherapy with cyclophosphamide, methatrexate, and 5-fluorouracil remains a standard of treatment. Chemotherapy concurrent with tamoxifen was less effective, but chemotherapy with tamoxifen in women older than age 50 was more effective than chemotherapy alone. There appeared to be a significant reduction in risk regardless of whether patients had positive nodes or negative nodes.

*Ovarian Ablation*—Women younger than age 50 seem to benefit by ovarian ablation, with or without chemotherapy. Ablation after the age of 50 appeared ineffective.

*Immunotherapy*—Immunotherapy appeared to have no benefit for women with breast cancer.

Analyses of these trials have helped to formulate the following treatment policies:

Women older than age 50 with ER-positive tumors and positive nodes should receive adjuvant tamoxifen; women with ER-negative tumors may receive tamoxifen or be enrolled in chemotherapy trials; and for women with negative nodes, therapy recommendations must be individualized.

For node-positive patients younger than age 50, multidrug regimen chemotherapy should be used. Higher-dose chemotherapy is appropriate in patients with multiple positive nodes, and bone marrow transplantation should be considered for patients with 10 or more positive nodes. In node-negative women, therapy recommendations need to be individualized. Pathologic criteria such as lymphatic vessel invasion and ER-negative status are highly significant in directing patients toward participation in chemotherapy trials.—T.J. Eberlein, M.D.

PATHOLOGIC FEATURES

**Association of Overexpression of Tumor Suppressor Protein p53 With Rapid Cell Proliferation and Poor Prognosis in Node-Negative Breast Cancer Patients**
Isola J, Visakorpi T, Holli K, Kallioniemi O-P (Univ of Tampere, Tampere, Finland; Univ Hosp of Tampere)
*J Natl Cancer Inst* 84:1109–1114, 1992                                          10–3

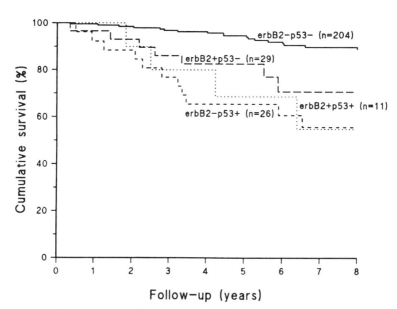

**Fig 10–1.**—Long-term survival of 270 patients with axillary node-negative breast cancer according to overexpression of the p53 and c-*erb* B-2 proteins. Difference in survival between patients with no overexpression of p53 or c-*erb* B-2 and patients with overexpression of either one or both of the proteins was highly significant (P < .0001, Mantel-Cox test). (Courtesy of Isola J, Visakorpi T, Holli K, et al: *J Natl Cancer Inst* 84:1109-1114, 1992.)

Independent Predictors of Survival in Invasive Axillary-Node Negative Breast Cancer According to a Multivariate Cox Regression Analysis

| Prognostic parameter | RR | CI | *P* value |
|---|---|---|---|
| Without inclusion of S phase | | | |
| p53 overexpression, yes or no | 2.7 | 1.5-5.1 | .0002 |
| Tumor size, 2-5 cm or <2 cm | 2.3 | 1.1-4.6 | .016 |
| c-erbB-2 overexpression, yes or no | 1.9 | 0.9-3.8 | .09 |
| After inclusion of S phase | | | |
| S-phase fraction, ≥8% or <8% | 3.8 | 2.0-7.1 | <.0001 |
| Tumor size, 2-5 cm or <2 cm | 2.5 | 1.2-5.1 | .007 |

*Abbreviations:* RR, relative risk of death; CI, 95% confidence interval.
*Note:* Results of the Cox analysis are shown without inclusion of the S-phase in the model (no. = 270) and after inclusion of S-phase (no. = 213). Other factors tested in the Cox model were histologic grade, estrogen receptor content, progesterone receptor content, DNA index, age, and menopausal status.
(Courtesy of Isola J, Visakorpi T, Holli K, et al: *J Natl Cancer Inst* 84:1109–1114, 1992.)

*Background.*—Some breast cancer patients with negative axillary nodes apparently benefit from adjuvant therapy, but reliable markers are needed to identify these patients. The p53 gene codes for a DNA-binding phosphoprotein that inhibits the progression of cells through the cell cycle. Mutations of this gene often lead to overexpression of the gene protein and are commonly found in a wide range of human cancers, including breast cancer.

*Objective.*—The prognostic import of overexpression of p53 protein was examined in 289 patients with axillary node-negative breast cancers less than 5 cm in size, the great majority of whom had undergone mastectomy. Immunostaining of more than 20% of tumor cells signified overexpression of p53 protein.

*Findings.*—Overexpression of p53 protein was found in 34% of high-grade tumors and 3% of low-grade tumors. Correlation with tumor size was not impressive, but overexpression was more frequent in tumors negative for hormone receptors. Tumors with p53 protein overexpression had a higher mean S-phase fraction than others. Patients with overexpression of either p53 or *c-erb* B-2 protein had a significantly poorer prognosis than patients whose tumors lacked oncoprotein abnormalities (Fig 10-1, table).

*Implications.*—Overexpression of p53 protein indicates a relatively high malignant potential in patients with axillary node-negative breast cancer. Correlation of the overexpression of both the p53 and *c-erb* B-2 proteins with an increased S-phase fraction suggests that they confer a proliferative advantage on cancer cells.

▶ This is a randomly selected study of preserved tumor samples in an epidemiologically defined population-based cohort of breast cancer patients from the Finnish Cancer Registry. All of the patients had negative nodes, and all of their tumors were less than 5 cm in size. Because this study was performed on preserved tumor samples, there exists a high degree of variability. Thus, although p53 expression (and c-*erb* B-2 protein overexpression) were associated with poor prognosis in this study, the reader should be cautioned that variability of expression may represent intratumor heterogeneity, cell cycle phase-dependent variability in protein expression, or inherent difficulties in the assay technique. Thus expression of these proteins may be helpful in selecting patients for adjuvant therapies but most likely will not definitively tell the whole story.—T.J. Eberlein, M.D.

---

### Overexpression of HER-2/neu and Its Relationship With Other Prognostic Factors Change During the Progression of In Situ to Invasive Breast Cancer

Allred DC, Clark GM, Molina R, Tandon AK, Schnitt SJ, Gilchrist KW, Osborne CK, Tormey DC, McGuire WL (Univ of Texas, San Antonio; Hosp Clinico Provincial, Barcelona, Spain; Beth Israel Hosp, Boston, Mass; Univ of Wisconsin, Madison)

*Hum Pathol* 23:974–979, 1992                                          10–4

---

*Background.*—The transforming gene *neu*, found in the DNA of chemically induced rat neuroblastoma, is partly homologous with the epidermal growth factor receptor gene. The human equivalent of *neu* was cloned from a cDNA library and termed HER-2. Recent studies have suggested that HER-2/*neu* is amplified or overexpressed, or both, in as many as 30% of invasive breast cancers.

*Methods and Cases.*—Immunohistochemical study of permanent sections served to assess the role of HER-2/*neu* in the development of breast cancer. Expression of the gene was measured in 30 hyperplastic, 15 dysplastic, and 708 malignant neoplastic lesions of the breast duct epithelium. The malignant series included 649 infiltrating ductal carcinomas, all node negative, and 59 pure ductal carcinomas in situ.

*Results.*—None of the hyperplastic or dysplastic lesions overexpressed HER-2/*neu*. More than half of the pure ductal carcinomas in situ (56%) and 77% of comedo variants expressed the gene, as did 15% of infiltrating ductal carcinomas. In the latter group overexpression was most frequent when an element of ductal carcinoma in situ was prominent.

*Interpretation.*—It appears that HER-2/*neu* is more important in the initiation of ductal breast cancers than in their progression. Many invasive cancers probably arise de novo through mechanisms that do not involve the gene.

▶ This study examined 753 specimens using permanent section immunohistochemistry. These authors found that none of the benign epithelial lesions showed evidence of HER-2/*neu* overexpression. There was, however, a high rate of overexpression in the pure ductal carcinoma in situ, (DCIS). In fact, these authors present several instances in which patients had negative expression of HER-2/*neu* in atypical ductal hyperplasia samples, but positive expression in areas of ductal carcinoma, indicating that HER-2/*neu* overexpression may be associated with the first histologic manifestation of malignant transformation. The fact that 56% of the ductal carcinomas expressed HER-2/*neu*, yet only 22% of the infiltrating tumors associated with DCIS expressed HER-2/*neu*, begs for an explanation. This may come by arguing against the assumption that histologically distinct patterns of breast cancer remain stable during tumor progression, or may challenge the popular notion that comedo DCIS is the most likely subtype of in situ disease to progress to invasion. Like previous authors, these authors found overexpression of HER-2/*neu* correlated with other poor prognostic factors (1, 2).—T.J. Eberlein, M.D.

*References*

1. Slamon DJ, et al: *Science* 255:177, 1987.
2. Zeillinger R, et al: *Oncogene* 4:109, 1989.

---

**Estrogen Receptor Immunohistochemistry in Carcinoma *In Situ* of the Breast**
Bur ME, Zimarowski MJ, Schnitt SJ, Baker S, Lew R (Univ of Massachusetts, Worcester; Beth Israel Hosp, Boston, Mass)
*Cancer* 69:1174–1181, 1992                                                10–5

---

*Background.*—A great deal of research has addressed the estrogen receptor (ER) content of invasive breast cancer and its clinical significance. There are fewer data, however, on the ER expression of carcinoma in situ (CIS) of the breast and its correlates.

*Methods.*—One hundred paraffin-embedded specimens of breast carcinomas were studied using a monoclonal antibody to ER and an indirect immunoperoxidase technique. The percentages of positive and strongly positive nuclei among the various histologic types of CIS and between CIS and invasive carcinoma were compared, and the relationships among histologic features, patient age, and ER status were studied. Estrogen receptor findings in pure CIS and CIS with adjacent invasive carcinoma were also compared.

*Findings.*—Overall, 80% of CIS specimens were ER positive. Fifty-seven percent of comedo CIS were ER positive, compared with 91% of noncomedo and 100% of lobular CIS specimens. The best independent predictor of ER negativity was a predominance of large cells; invasion was the next best predictor. There was a 98% correlation between ER in CIS and ER in invasive carcinoma. When CIS was not associated with invasive carcinoma, it was usually weak or negative for ER. Estrogen receptor status did not predict tumor extent. The percentage of nuclear staining of CIS was no different in women younger and older than 50 years of age, although the older women had a higher proportion of strongly positive cells.

*Conclusions.*—This study demonstrates a correlation between the ER expression of CIS of the breast and the pathologic features of differentiation. Estrogen receptor expression of these tumors is similar to that of invasive carcinoma. Immunohistochemistry appears better suited than biochemical analysis for evaluating ER expression of CIS.

▶ It is difficult to obtain ER status in patients with ductal CIS who undergo biopsy. Because of otherwise grossly normal tissue, this study documents that using the immunohistochemical method for determining ER is much better than attempting biochemical analysis. Sensitivity and specificity were excellent for both frozen and paraffin-embedded sections. The finding that CIS associated with invasive carcinoma was more frequently ER positive was somewhat unexpected. Multivariate analyses showed that invasion remained a predictor of ER status and CIS second only to large cell type. Thus there appears to be a relationship between cytologic/histologic differentiation and ER expression as well as ER expression in CIS and coexistent invasive carcinoma of the breast.

This article not only demonstrates the practical methodology for obtaining ER, but also looks at the biological relationship between ER expression and subtypes of human breast cancer.—T.J. Eberlein, M.D.

---

### Stefins and Lysosomal Cathepsins B, L and D in Human Breast Carcinoma

Lah TT, Kokalj-Kunovar M, Štrukelj B, Pungerčar J, Barlič-Maganja D, Drobnič-Košorok M, Kastelic L, Babnik J, Golouh R, Turk V (J Stefan Inst, Ljubljana, Yugoslavia; Inst of Oncology, Ljubljana)
*Int J Cancer* 50:36–44, 1992                                    10–6

---

*Background.*—In a previous study, most human sarcomas showed a reduced potential for cathepsin (Cat) B inhibition, probably because of the impaired potential of stefin A to bind to cysteine proteinase (CP). Proteolytic inactivation by other proteinases (e.g., Cat D) is another possible explanation for the imbalance between CP and its inhibitors (CPIs) in disease states. Cathepsin D, Cat L, and Cat B were correlated with total CPI activity to explore the associations between various cathepsins and endogenous CPIs.

*Methods and Findings.*—Fifty matched pairs of breast carcinomas and normal breast tissues were compared. Activity of CPs was increased by an average of 18.5 times in the breast carcinomas and that of Cat B and Cat L by 52.5 times. About two thirds of the carcinomas showed reduced CPI activity, whereas the rest had similar or higher CPI activity. Those with reduced CPI activity had a significantly higher relative increase in specific activity of Cat B and Cat L. Although these patients were more likely to have grade III tumors and negative estrogen and progesterone receptor levels, metastatic regional lymph node involvement was similar. After 2 years of follow-up a significant inverse correlation was observed between disease-free survival and increased Cat L activity. There were no significant differences between patients with high vs. low CPI activity. The mean Cat D activity was 5.8 times higher in tumor than in controls on measurement of 20 matched pairs. The absence of correlations between corresponding activities was evidence against the hypothesis that elevated Cat D activity increased CP activity and/or lowered tumor CPI activity as a result of posttranslational proteolytic modifications. Most of the breast carcinoma specimens had a reduced stefin A protein and mRNA content on immunoassay and Northern blot analysis.

*Conclusions.*—The activity of Cat D, Cat B, and Cat L is elevated in breast carcinoma samples. Many tumors show reduced CPI activity in association with increased Cat B and Cat L values. Stefin A is correlated with CPI activity, suggesting that it makes a significant contribution to total inhibition potential. Most tumor samples show lower levels of stefin A transcripts on Northern blot analysis; this inhibitor may be useful in the diagnosis or prognosis of breast carcinoma.

▶ This study details 50 matched pairs of breast carcinomas in normal breast tissue looking at proteolysis. In general, lysosomal enzymes, Cat D, Cat B, and Cat L, were elevated in all tumor samples. The relatively small numbers in this study, however, prevent possible correlation to differentiation, progression, stage of the tumor, or clinical status of the patient. The authors have shown that cysteine-dependent proteolysis may play an important role in the progression of breast cancer. It is probably not directly related, however, to metastatic spread. This work requires further study of a larger patient population before more definitive conclusions can be derived.—T.J. Eberlein, M.D.

---

**The Continuing Dilemma of Lobular Carcinoma In Situ**
Walt AJ, Simon M, Swanson GM (Wayne State Univ, Detroit, Mich; Michigan State Univ, East Lansing)
*Arch Surg* 127:904–909, 1992                                     10–7

---

*Introduction.*—Lobular carcinoma in situ (LCIS) of the breast was thought to be rare, but its frequency has increased over time. The natural course of LCIS remains poorly understood, and the optimal surgical treatment has not been defined. The natural course and outcome of LCIS, were examined.

*Patients.*—The study population consisted of 250 women (mean age, 50.7 years) in whom LCIS was diagnosed from 1973 through 1986. The women were followed up through late 1989 for the development of second primary breast carcinomas. In this analysis, mastectomy included

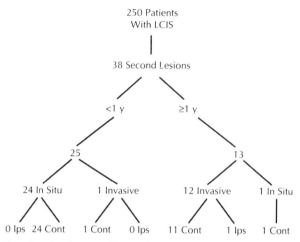

250 Patients
With LCIS

38 Second Lesions

<1 y          ≥1 y

25                    13

24 In Situ    1 Invasive        12 Invasive    1 In Situ

0 Ips  24 Cont    1 Cont    0 Ips        11 Cont    1 Ips    1 Cont

**Fig 10–2.**—Flow chart showing second lesions developing in patients with LCIS. *Cont,* contralateral; *Ips,* ipsilateral. (Courtesy of Walt AJ, Simon M, Swanson GM: *Arch Surg* 127:904–909, 1992.)

subcutaneous, total, modified radical, and radical mastectomies, and "less than mastectomy" included segmental or partial mastectomy, lumpectomy, quadrantectomy, wedge resection, nipple resection, and excisional biopsy. Of 250 patients, 212 (74%) underwnet mastectomy and 65 (26%) had less than mastectomy. The average follow-up period was 93 months.

*Results.*—In 38 patients new lesions developed, 1 in the ipsilateral breast and 37 in the contralateral breast (Fig 10–2). Twenty-five second lesions developed within the first year after surgical treatment for LCIS. Of the 38 new lesions, 25 were in situ cancers and 13 were invasive. Seventeen patients died, 2 of breast cancer and 13 of non–breast–related causes. The mortality from breast cancer was .8% for known deaths caused by breast cancer and 1.6% if 2 unknown deaths are assumed to have been breast cancer deaths. The frequency of mastectomy was 78% for the period 1973–1983 and 52% for the period 1984–1986, reflecting the growing move away from mastectomy.

*Recommendations.*—In the absence of a strong family history, previous invasive cancer, florid LCIS, or a patient's inability to cope with uncertainty, patients with LCIS may be managed by excision of the involved area and annual follow-up evaluations that should include physical examination and mammography.

▶ This article addresses many issues surrounding LCIS. The first is the treatment of LCIS with mastectomy in the 1970s. This trend, however, has been significantly reversed.

Of the 25 lesions detected less than 1 year after the initial diagnosis, 23 were LCIS, only 1 lesion was a ductal carcinoma in situ, and 1 was an invasive cancer. After 1 year from initial diagnosis, 12 of 13 tumors were invasive.

The recommended treatment remains unchanged; LCIS should be treated as a marker for potential malignancy. Thus patients with LCIS should be treated with excision and follow-up. Mastectomy should be reserved for individual patients with a strong family history or inability to cope with this diagnosis.—T.J. Eberlein, M.D.

DIAGNOSIS

▼ The next 2 reviews describe a new stereotactic technique for diagnosing breast cancer.—T.J. Eberlein, M.D.

---

### Nonpalpable Breast Lesions: Stereotactic Automated Large-Core Biopsies

Parker SH, Lovin JD, Jobe WE, Burke BJ, Hopper KD, Yakes WF (Radiology Imaging Associates, Englewood Col; Fitzsimons Army Med Ctr, Aurora, Col; Pennsylvania State Univ, Hershey)
*Radiology* 180:403–407, 1991                                       10–8

---

*Background.*—Although surgical breast biopsy is a standard procedure, dependable needle biopsy would be preferable. Stereotactic automated needle core biopsy using a 14-gauge needle was compared to surgical biopsy in 102 patients with mammographically suspicious, nonpalpable lesions.

*Results.*—The gun biopsy and the surgical biopsy were in agreement in 96% of the cases, including 22 of 23 carcinomas (table). Two lesions were diagnosed correctly only by gun biopsy, and 2 were diagnosed cor-

---

Comparison of Histopathologic Results of Needle Core Biopsy and Surgical Biopsy
(Current Series)

| Needle Biopsy Results | Surgical Biopsy Results | | | | | | |
| --- | --- | --- | --- | --- | --- | --- | --- |
| | Cancer | FA | FCC | Normal | Other | Insufficient Tissue | Total |
| Cancer | 22 | 0 | 0 | 0 | 0 | 0 | 22 |
| FA | 0 | 13 | 0 | 2 | 0 | 0 | 15 |
| FCC | 0 | 0 | 57 | 0 | 1* | 0 | 58 |
| Normal | 1 | 0 | 0 | 4 | 0 | 0 | 5 |
| Other | 0 | 0 | 0 | 0 | 2 | 0 | 2 |
| Insufficient tissue | 0 | 0 | 0 | 0 | 0 | 0 | 0 |
| Total | 23 | 13 | 57 | 6 | 3 | 0 | 102 |

Note: K = .936 (values > .75 reflect strong agreement). *Abbreviations: FA*, fibroadenoma; *FCC*, fibrocystic change.
* Mammographic finding in this case corresponded to the surgical diagnosis (radial scar).
(Courtesy of Parker SH, Lovin JD, Jobe WE, et al: *Radiology* 180:403–407, 1991.)

rectly only by surgical biopsy. One of the lesions, which was close to the chest wall, retracted, causing the stereotactic calculations to be inaccurate and the lesion to be missed. Therefore, lesions close to the chest wall may not be suitable for stereotactic gun biopsy, and the needle must be viewed stereotactically in the lesion to avoid false negatives.

*Conclusions.*—Stereotactic 14-gauge needle gun biopsy can be an acceptable alternative to surgical biopsy in women with mammographically suspicious breast lesions. The advantages of needle biopsy include decreased cost, time, complications, and disfigurement.

---

**Recurrent Breast Cancer: Stereotaxic Localization for Fine-Needle Aspiration Biopsy**

Mitnick JS, Vazquez MF, Roses DF, Harris MN, Schechter S (Tisch Hosp, New York City; State Univ of New York, Brooklyn)
*Radiology* 182:103–106, 1992                                    10–9

*Introduction.*—Local tumor excision and irradiation is now an accepted alternative to mastectomy in the treatment of breast cancer. Previous studies have shown that follow-up mammography after local excision cannot distinguish between new benign calcifications and recurrent breast cancer. Whether stereotaxic localization for fine-needle aspiration biopsy is a reliable method of detecting recurrent breast cancer manifested as calcifications on mammography was investigated.

*Patients.*—Forty-three women aged 35–64 years who had been treated with lumpectomy and radiation therapy for breast cancer 1–8 years previously and whose follow-up mammograms showed new calcifications at

Correlation of Aspiration and Biopsy
Results in the 13 Patients Who
Underwent Surgical Biopsy

| Cytologic Findings | | Histopathologic Findings | |
|---|---|---|---|
| Diagnosis | N | Diagnosis | N |
| Adenocarcinoma | 6 | Adenocarcinoma | 6 |
| Suspicious | 0 | Suspicious | 0 |
| Atypical | 1 | DCIS | 1 |
| Benign | 5 | Benign | 5 |
| | | Scars (n = 3) | |
| | | Fat necrosis | |
| | | (n = 2) | |
| Inadequate | 1 | Scar | 1 |

*Abbreviation:* DCIS, ductal carcinoma in situ.
(Courtesy of Mitnick JS, Vazquez MF, Roses DF, et al: *Radiology* 182:103–106, 1992.)

or near the scar underwent fine-needle aspiration under stereotaxic guidance. None of the women had a palpable lesion. Surgical biopsy was performed when the aspirate was malignant, suggestive of malignancy, atypical, or inadequate. Patients whose aspirate was benign were followed by mammography at 6-month intervals.

*Results.*—The aspirates were malignant in 6 patients, atypical in 1, inadequate in 1, and benign in 35. Thirteen patients then underwent surgical biopsy, including 5 who had benign needle aspirates but wanted further assurance. Malignancy was confirmed in all 7 patients with malignant or atypical aspirates (table). All 7 new malignancies were within 2.5 cm of the original excisional site. Six patients with recurrence underwent mastectomy. One patient refused mastectomy and underwent a second wider excision.

*Conclusions.*—Stereotaxic fine-needle aspiration biopsy of the focus of mammographically detected new calcifications after breast-conserving surgery and irradiation may be a promising method for distinguishing benign from malignant microcalcifications.

▶ These 2 studies (Abstracts 10–8 and 10–9) deal with stereotactic biopsy techniques for primary mammographically suspicious lesions or possible recurrence. This technique, however, cannot be for the biopsy of lesions that are very close to the chest wall, because they may not be localized well with mammographic guidance.

Core needle biopsies may be particularly helpful in obviously benign lesions (e.g., fibroadenomas), or in mammographically obvious cancers. With the advent of ERICA in determining the estrogen-receptor status of tumors, as well as the ability to show calcifications radiographically in the 14-gauge core biopsy specimen, it is possible to expand the indications for core biopsy.

These 2 articles detail 2 primary uses: 1 in the initial diagnosis of breast cancer, and the other in possible recurrence of conservatively treated breast cancer. It is currently not recommended for diffuse lesions or very small lesions in which sampling errors may occur. The reader should also be cautioned in using this technique, because there is obviously a learning curve before this procedure is mastered. Very close cooperation between the primary surgeon, mammographer, and pathologist is essential to optimize the reproducibility of results with this procedure.—T.J. Eberlein, M.D.

**Evaluation of the Contralateral Breast: The Role of Biopsy at the Time of Treatment of Primary Breast Cancer**
Smith BL, Bertagnolli M, Klein BB, Batter S, Chang M, Douville LM, Eberlein TJ (Brigham and Women's Hosp, Boston, Mass)
*Ann Surg* 216:17–21, 1992                                    10–10

*Background.*—The appropriate assessment of patients with a history of breast cancer is still debated. In such patients, minimal assessment of the contralateral breast clearly includes frequent mammography and physical evaluations. Some surgeons have advocated including a blind biopsy as well at the time the primary breast carcinoma is diagnosed. It is not clear, however, whether such patients, in the absence of physical or mammographic evidence of malignancy, benefit from a truly blind biopsy of the contralateral breast.

*Methods.*—Ninety-five women undergoing blind contralateral breast biopsy were studied prospectively. The blind biopsy was done during surgery for a known primary breast tumor. Patients with palpable or mammographic abnormalities prompting biopsy were excluded.

*Findings.*—Only 2 infiltrating carcinomas were discovered, for a positive biopsy rate of 2.1% for invasive disease. Three additional biopsy specimens demonstrated lobular carcinoma in situ, a finding that does not usually change clinical management. In 1 patient with negative findings on biopsy of the contralateral breast, invasive carcinoma developed in that breast within 2 years. No subgroups at increased risk of a positive contralateral biopsy could be identified.

*Conclusions.*—Blind biopsy of the contralateral breast at the time of initial treatment of breast cancer is not an efficient way of detecting cancer in that breast. Alternative strategies for the management of patients with a history of breast cancer should be considered.

▶ In this prospective controlled series, retrospectively analyzed, only 2 infiltrating carcinomas were documented in benign contralateral biopsies. Of the 12 patients with invasive lobular histology, only 1 had lobular carcinoma in situ in the contralateral biopsy specimen. No invasive cancers were seen. Patients with mammographic or physical suggestions of abnormality, therefore, should undergo biopsy of the contralateral breast. Other patients, however, should have close follow-up examinations and a minimum of a yearly mammogram. This would seem to result in a reduction in mortality in women with contralateral breast cancer similar to that achieved in screening programs (1, 2).—T.J. Eberlein, M.D.

*References*

1. Shapiro S, et al: *J Natl Cancer Inst* 69:349, 1982.
2. Tabar L, et al: *Lancet* 1:829, 1985.

## Breast Cancer: Importance of Adequate Surgical Excision Prior to Radiotherapy in the Local Control of Breast Cancer in Patients Treated Conservatively

Ghossein NA, Alpert S, Barba J, Pressman P, Stacey P, Lorenz E, Shulman M, Sadarangani GJ (Albert Einstein College of Medicine, New York City; Cabrini

Med Ctr, New York City, Mt Sinai School of Medicine, New York City)
*Arch Surg* 127:411–415, 1992                                    10–11

*Background.*—Now that conservative treatment for localized breast cancer is well accepted, many researchers are looking for risk factors associated with an unacceptably high incidence of local failure. The extent of excision done for mammary carcinoma before radiotherapy was studied as a possible risk factor for local recurrence.

*Methods.*—In 503 patients, 323 tumors (62%) were excised with a minimal rim of tissue; 142 patients (27%) had wide excision; and 56 (11%) had quadrantectomy. All groups had comparable tumor stages and tumor sizes, and had received similar degrees of radiation therapy.

*Findings.*—Of the tumorectomy patients, 41% had involved margins. Only 14% in the wide excision group and 7% in the quadrantectomy group had involvement (table). Local failure in those who had tumorectomy was 15%; in those who had wide excision, 7%; and in those who had quadrantectomy, 5%. Among patients with T1 ductal carcinoma, only 4% with excisions greater than 5 cm had recurrences. Those with lesser excisions had a 20% recurrence rate (Fig 10–3).

*Conclusions.*—Biopsy specimen excision may result in minimal breast deformity and excellent cosmesis, but the incidence of local recurrence associated with it is unacceptably high. Such failure may place the patient at high risk of distant dissemination, especially when the recurrence develops shortly after initial treatment. Unless long-term randomized trials prove otherwise, minimal excisional biopsy before radiation therapy should be discouraged.

▶ This study documents a recurrence rate that is correlated with size of excision, regardless of specific pathology. As one would expect, margins were more frequently involved in the tumorectomy patients.

Incidence of Microscopically Involved Margin According to
Surgical Procedure and Specimen Size

| Procedure | Specimen Size (Largest Dimension, cm) | Margin Involved,* No. (%) | |
|---|---|---|---|
| Tumorectomy | 4 ± 1.5 | 129/316 (41) | ⎤ |
| Wide excision | 8 ± 3.3 | 19/139 (14) | ⎬ *P*<.001 |
| Quadrantectomy | 13 ± 5.5 | 4/56 (7) | ⎦ |
| **Total** | | **152/511 (30)** | |

* Ten specimens where margins were not specified were excluded.
(Courtesy of Ghossein NA, Alpert S, Barba J, et al: *Arch Surg* 127:411–415, 1992.)

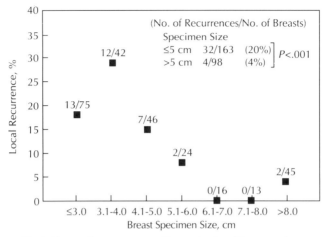

**Fig 10–3.**—The incidence of recurrence according to the size of breast specimen resected in 261 stage T1 (≤2 cm) infiltrating ductal carcinomas. (Courtesy of Ghossein NA, Alpert S, Barba J, et al: *Arch Surg* 127:411–415, 1992.)

In a related manuscript (1), the size of excision was particularly important in predicting local recurrence when an extensive intraductal component of the tumor was present. If the tumor did not have an extensive intraductal component, the size of the excision could be smaller and still insure adequate local control.

Thus the recommended procedure has been to attempt excision with negative margins. If microscopically positive margins for invasive cancer still exist, radiation therapy is performed. If the patient has involved margins and an extensive intraductal component to the tumor, however, wide excision or mastectomy may be indicated.—T.J. Eberlein, M.D.

*Reference*

1. Vicini FA, et al: *Ann Surg* 214:200, 1991.

## TREATMENT

### Cosmetic Results After Surgery, Chemotherapy, and Radiation Therapy for Early Breast Cancer

Abner AL, Recht A, Vicini FA, Silver B, Hayes D, Come S, Harris JR (Harvard Med School, Boston, Mass; William Beaumont Hosp, Royal Oak, Mich)
*Int J Radiat Oncol Biol Phys* 21:331–338, 1991                    10–12

*Objective.*—Chemotherapy is used increasingly along with radiotherapy to treat early-stage breast cancer. The effects of chemotherapy on the cosmetic outcome were examined in 1,624 patients with clinical stage I or II invasive breast cancer, 390 of whom received adjuvant chemotherapy.

*Management.*—In all, 170 patients were followed for 2 years or longer after receiving either cyclophosphamide-methotrexate-fluorouracil (CMF) or doxorubicin-based chemotherapy in conjunction with breast irradiation. Another 170 patients received only radiation. The groups were matched for tumor size and radiation technique. The median time of cosmetic follow-up was 5 years.

*Results.*—Patients given chemotherapy had fewer excellent cosmetic scores and more fair or poor results at follow-up than those given radiotherapy alone. Sequential radiotherapy and chemotherapy yielded excellent cosmetic scores more often than concurrent treatment did. Patients given CMF therapy and those given doxorubicin-based treatment had comparable cosmetic results.

*Conclusions.*—Chemotherapy appears to compromise the cosmetic outcome in women with early-stage breast cancer who also receive radiotherapy.

---

## Are Cosmetic Results Following Conservative Surgery and Radiation Therapy for Early Breast Cancer Dependent on Technique?

de la Rochefordière A, Abner AL, Silver B, Vicini F, Recht A, Harris JR (Harvard Med School, Boston, Mass)
*Int J Radiat Oncol Biol Phys* 23:925–931, 1992                    10–13

---

*Introduction.*—Survival rates are equivalent between breast-conserving treatment, consisting of conservative surgery plus radiation, and mastectomy. Given this, preservation of a satisfactory cosmetic appearance becomes a consideration. Several radiation factors are associated with a worsening of the cosmetic result, including doses to the whole breast of more than 50 Gy, fractions of more than 2 Gy/day, imprecise matching of fields in the axillary and/or supraclavicular region, and use of a large

Factors Influencing Cosmetic Outcome at 3 Years (1982–1985)

| | No. of patients evaluated at 3 yrs. | % excellent | *p*-value | % excellent/good | *p*-value |
|---|---|---|---|---|---|
| RT alone | 279 | 77 | 0.09 | 97 | NS |
| Seq. RT/CT | 57 | 65 | | 95 | |
| TTV ≤ 35 cm$^3$ | 85 | 86 | 0.0009 | 96 | NS |
| TTV = 36–85 cm$^3$ | 78 | 78 | | 97 | |
| TTV ≥ 86 cm$^3$ | 70 | 51 | | 94 | |
| T ≤ 2 cm, no CT | 141 | 84 | 0.03 | 99 | NS |
| T = 2.1–3 cm, no CT | 45 | 68 | | 91 | |
| T ≥ 3.1 cm, no CT | 21 | 62 | | 100 | |

*Abbreviations: Seq. RT/CT,* sequential radiotherapy/chemotherapy; *TTV,* total tissue volume resected; *T,* tumor size.

(Courtesy of de la Rochefordière A, Abner AL, Silver B, et al: *Int J Radiat Oncol Biol Phys* 23:925–931, 1992.)

volume boost. A retrospective study was carried out to evaluate cosmetic results as they relate to treatment technique.

*Methods.*—The analysis included 1,159 patients with stage I or II breast cancer who underwent conservative surgery and radiotherapy during a 15-year period. In all cases, treatment consisted of gross excision followed by radiation therapy, which included an implant or electron beam boost, with a total dose to the primary site of 60 Gy or more. Certain technical modifications were introduced after 1981, including limiting the dose to the whole breast, using a boost dose of no more than 18 Gy, providing a more accurate matching, and using sequential rather than concurrent radiation therapy/chemotherapy. An analysis was made of cosmetic results, as assessed by the examining physician, in patients treated before and after 1982. Further, factors associated with a worsened cosmetic outcome were explored.

*Results.*—The median follow-ups were 107 months for the earlier cohort and 67 months for the latter cohort. Whereas 59% of the earlier cohort had excellent cosmetic results, 74% of the latter cohort had such outcomes. The rates of acceptable—i.e., excellent or good—results were 84% and 94%, respectively. In the latter cohort a significant association was noted between the likelihood of achieving an excellent result and the volume of resected breast tissue and use of chemotherapy. There was no such relationship with number of fields or boost type (table).

*Conclusions.*—The described technique of breast-conserving surgery and radiation therapy—including 45–46 Gy of radiation to the breast and a 16–18 Gy boost to the primary site—is associated with a high rate of acceptable cosmetic results. Adjuvant chemotherapy, use of a third field, and boost type do not appear to affect cosmetic results. The use of sequential radiation and chemotherapy and wide resection do not reduce the likelihood of obtaining excellent results.

▶ These 2 related studies are from same research group. The first paper (Abstract 10–12) addresses a study of 170 patients who received polychemotherapy and were compared with 170 patients who received radiation alone. Breast cosmesis was adversely affected by polychemotherapy and concurrent radiation and polychemotherapy was associated with poorer cosmesis than sequential adjuvant therapies. Finally, whether doxorubicin was or was not one of the chemotherapeutic agents administered made no difference in the cosmetic outcome as long as the chemotherapy was given sequentially.

The second study (Abstract 10–13) describes newer treatment methods; lowering the dose of radiation to the entire breast, changing the boost dose, and using sequential rather than concurrent radiation therapy and chemotherapy. These radiation techniques are not standard and associated with much higher rates of cosmetic acceptability.

The optimum method of combining chemotherapy and radiation therapy, however, remains uncertain. Although chemotherapy appears to have little effect on the risk of local failure after breast-conserving surgery when radiation therapy is not used, it may appear to have a synergistic effect when radiation therapy is administered (1). Further studies regarding the specifics of sequencing these 2 modalities are required before more definitive conclusions can be drawn.—T.J. Eberlein, M.D.

*Reference*

1. Fisher B, et al: N Engl J Med 312:664, 1985.

---

**Salvage Mastectomy for Local and Regional Recurrence After Breast-Conserving Operation and Radiation Therapy**
Osborne MP, Borgen PI, Wong GY, Rosen PP, McCormick B (Mem Sloan-Kettering Cancer Ctr, New York City)
*Surg Gynecol Obstet* 174:189–194, 1992                    10–14

---

*Background.*—Rates of local and regional recurrence of breast cancer 5 years after breast-conserving surgery and radiation therapy reportedly vary from 5% to 22%. Patients with local and regional failure but no distant metastases are advised to have salvage mastectomy. Older series of patients treated with salvage mastectomy indicate that the postsalvage relapse rate 10 years after salvage surgery is about 50%. Findings in a more recent series of 46 patients were reviewed retrospectively.

*Patients and Findings.*—The women had been treated initially for breast carcinoma by tumor excision and radiation therapy. After local and regional recurrence without evidence of metastases, the patients underwent salvage mastectomy. They were treated between 1970 and 1990. All 46 patients had excision of the primary tumor, and 27 also had local excision with axillary dissection. A median radiation dose of 48 Gy was delivered to the breast. At the time of breast-conserving surgery, the disease stages was 0 in 7 patients, I in 13, II in 14, and III in 1. Local and regional relapse occurred at a median 28 months after initial therapy. In 35 patients, relapses occurred only in the breast. Salvage surgery con-

---

Influence of Time to Initial Relapse on Postsalvage Recurrence

| *Time to relapse after initial therapy** | *Median length of follow-up study after salvage** | *No. of pts.* | *Postsalvage relapse* | |
|---|---|---|---|---|
| | | | *No.* | *Per cent* |
| <24 . . . . . . . . . | 37 | 14 | 7 | 50 |
| 24 to 48 . . . . . | 26 | 20 | 5 | 25 |
| >48 . . . . . . . . . | 25 | 12 | 1 | 8 |

* In months.
(Courtesy of Osborne MP, Borgen PI, Wong GY, et al: *Surg Gynecol Obstet* 174:189–194, 1992.)

sisted of total mastectomy in 50%, modified radical mastectomy in 33%, and radical mastectomy in 17%.

*Outcomes.*—The median follow-up after salvage mastectomy was 28 months (range, 1 month to 18 years). The actuarial proportion free of disease at 5 years was 55%. The overall 5-year survival rate was 76%. The median time to relapse was 97 months. The median survival time was 103 months. Local recurrence after salvage surgery occurred in 15%. A possible correlation was found between the time to initial relapse and postsalvage outcome (table).

*Conclusions.*—The findings suggest that salvage mastectomy provides local control of recurrent breast carcinoma. Relapse-free survival time may be improved by systemic therapy after salvage surgery.

▶ Time to local recurrence does not predict outcome after salvage mastectomy. Invasive versus noninvasive histologic findings of the recurrent tumor, however, do seem to predict prognosis (1, 2).

If axillary dissection has been performed previously, it is not repeated, because radiation therapy usually accompanies the primary breast-conserving treatment. Immediate reconstruction should not be discouraged, and if performed, the use of autologous tissue trasfer is recommended.

Most single institutions have small numbers of patients with recurrent disease. These patients, however, have a significant risk for distant disease. Therefore, participation in multicenter trials of adjuvant therapy should be considered for patients treated with salvage mastectomy who have invasive histology in their recurrent tumors.—T.J. Eberlein, M.D.

*Rererences*

1. Recht A, et al: *Int J Radiat Oncol Biol Phys* 15:255, 1988.
2. Abner, A, et al: *J Clin Oncol* 11:44, 1993.

## AXILLARY DISSECTION

### Value of Axillary Dissection in Addition to Lumpectomy and Radiotherapy in Early Breast Cancer

Cabanes PA, Salmon RJ, Vilcoq JR, Durand JC, Fourquet A, Gautier C, Asselain B, for the Breast Carcinoma Collaborative Group of the Institut Curie (Institut Curie, Paris)

*Lancet* 339:1245–1248, 1992                                                    10–15

*Background.*—Axillary dissection of early breast cancer is still controversial. The side effects are substantial, and the value of this procedure in reducing recurrences and improving survival has not been proven unequivocally. A prospective, randomized study was undertaken to assess the value of axillary dissection along with lumpectomy in 658 patients with early breast cancer treated between 1982 and 1987.

*Methods.*—Lumpectomy alone was compared with lumpectomy plus axillary dissection. All patients had a unilateral tumor 3 cm or smaller in diameter and lymph node involvement or metastasses. Both groups received radiation therapy. The mean age, tumor/node/metastasis status, and presence of hormonal receptors were similar in both groups. Follow-up was for a median of 54 months.

*Findings.*—The patients had a 5-year survival rate of 94%. Those undergoing axillary dissection had a significant survival advantage. The rate of breast tumor recurrence was similar in the 2 groups, but those treated with axillary dissection had less frequent visceral metastases, supraclavicular metastases, and lymph node recurrences. Patient age, presence of positive nodes, histologic grading, and the presence of hormonal receptors were related to survival. The treatment-adjusted relative risk was 2.4.

*Conclusions.*—Axillary dissection is justified in the treatment of small breast cancers. It is still unclear, however, whether the better survival is the result of axillary clearance itself or of adjuvant treatment for lymph node involvement.

▶ This report from the Institute Curie showed similar breast cancer recurrence rates, whether or not axillary dissection was performed. In the dissection group, however, there were fewer visceral, supraclavicular, and lymph node recurrences. These results seem to parallel the findings of prophylactic lymph node dissection in melanoma. Biologically, it appears that there is a subgroup of patients for whom axillary dissection is therapeutic and results in a reduction of visceral and other metastases. The cancer in the majority of patients, however, will behave in the predicted manner as determined by the number of lymph nodes replaced with disease.—T.J. Eberlein, M.D.

---

## A Mathematical Model of Axillary Lymph Node Involvement Based on 1446 Complete Axillary Dissections in Patients With Breast Carcinoma

Kiricuta CI, Tausch J (Universität Würzburg, Würzburg, Germany)
*Cancer* 69:2496–2501, 1992                                    10–16

*Objective.*—The presence of axillary lymph node metastasis is the chief prognostic indicator in patients with breast cancer. The findings in 1,446 complete axillary dissections, done in 1983–1986 in patients with histologically proven breast carcinoma, were studied to develop a mathematical model for use in treating breast cancer conservatively.

*Methods.*—The sample size from level I needed to designate $N_0$ axillary status with 90% certainty was determined, as was the probability of residual axillary tumor occurring after sampling from level I. The maximum number of involved axillary nodes at levels I, II, and III expected after sampling from level I also was estimated.

TABLE 1.—Probability (%) of M Involved Axillary Lymph Nodes in
All Axillary Levels

| M | All sizes | T1 | T2 | T3 |
|---|---|---|---|---|
| 0 | 92.46 | 93.16 | 90.87 | 90.89 |
| 1 | 6.33 | 6.14 | 6.79 | 6.36 |
| 2 | 0.82 | 0.56 | 1.50 | 0.00 |
| 3 | 0.30 | 0.09 | 0.83 | 0.00 |
| 4 | 0.03 | 0.01 | 0.00 | 1.27 |
| 5 | 0.05 | 0.03 | 0.00 | 1.38 |
| 6 | 0.00 | 0.00 | 0.01 | 0.00 |
| 7 | 0.00 | 0.00 | 0.00 | 0.11 |
| 8 | 0.00 | 0.00 | 0.00 | 0.00 |
| 9 | 0.00 | 0.00 | 0.01 | 0.00 |
| 10 | 0.00 | 0.00 | 0.00 | 0.00 |

Sample size of 11 nodes from level I. No node was found to be involved by the pathologist for all tumor sizes (all sizes), $T_1$, $T_2$, and $T_3$ tumors.
(Courtesy of Kiricuta CI, Tausch J: *Cancer* 69:2496–2501, 1992.)

TABLE 2.—Probability (%) of M Involved Axillary Lymph Nodes in
All Axillary Levels

| M | All sizes | T1 | T2 | T3 |
|---|---|---|---|---|
| 0 | 72.26 | 75.67 | 65.51 | 63.48 |
| 1 | 16.21 | 15.67 | 17.27 | 17.76 |
| 2 | 6.48 | 4.83 | 10.45 | 0.00 |
| 3 | 2.61 | 2.05 | 3.69 | 4.52 |
| 4 | 1.00 | 0.90 | 1.01 | 4.12 |
| 5 | 0.57 | 0.34 | 0.68 | 6.75 |
| 6 | 0.35 | 0.22 | 0.57 | 1.13 |
| 7 | 0.20 | 0.09 | 0.29 | 2.07 |
| 8 | 0.11 | 0.07 | 0.19 | 0.09 |
| 9 | 0.15 | 0.12 | 0.24 | 0.03 |
| 10 | 0.02 | 0.00 | 0.05 | 0.01 |
| 11 | 0.02 | 0.02 | 0.02 | 0.03 |
| 12 | 0.01 | 0.01 | 0.02 | 0.00 |
| 13 | 0.01 | 0.00 | 0.02 | 0.00 |
| 14 | 0.00 | 0.00 | 0.00 | 0.00 |
| 15 | 0.00 | 0.00 | 0.00 | 0.00 |
| 16 | 0.00 | 0.00 | 0.00 | 0.00 |

Sample size of 5 nodes from level I. All were found to be uninvolved for all sizes, $T_1$, $T_2$, and $T_3$ tumors.
(Courtesy of Kiricuta CI, Tausch J: *Cancer* 69:2496–2501, 1992.)

*Results.*—The probability of axillary node involvement at all levels with a sample size of 11 nodes from level I is presented in Table 1 and with a sample of 5 nodes from level I in Table 2. The cutoff level for a $T_1$ primary tumor is 10 uninvolved axillary nodes.

*Implication.*—A confident designation of $N_0$ axillary status may be made if 10 nodes from level I examined in a patient with a $T_1$ primary are found to be uninvolved.

▶ The authors statistically reviewed 1,446 axillary dissections performed in a 3-year period. Using a very complex mathematical model, they determined the sample size, likelihood of residual tumor, and probability of maximum number of involved axillary nodes when level I nodes are sampled. This model uses tumor size as a basis for determining the necessary number of axillary nodes to be sampled. This model may also be used to estimate how many axillary lymph nodes could be involved it only a few nodes were sampled by the surgeon. The latter point has particular significance, not only in planning axillary lymph node radiation but in determining the need for other adjuvant treatments (e.g., chemotherapy and hormonal therapy) as well.

Although some individuals may believe that all patients should receive adjuvant therapy, therefore rendering axillary dissection superfluous, dissection is mandatory because it provides more complete staging information for protocol purposes. Level II dissections also reduce the risk of axillary recurrence, obviating the need for radiation therapy. Level I/II dissection of approximately 10–12 nodes is recommended because it provides adequate staging, reduces the risk of recurrence, and minimizes the risk of skip metastases.—T.J. Eberlein, M.D.

---

**Aggressive Axillary Evaluation and Adjuvant Therapy for Nonpalpable Carcinoma of the Breast**
Margolis DS, McMillen MA, Hashmi H, Wasson DW, MacArthur JD (Bridgeport Hosp, Bridgeport, Conn)
*Surg Gynecol Obstet* 174:109–113, 1992                              10–17

---

*Background.*—The use of mammography has increased the detection of nonpalable carcinomas of the breast. These small lesions can often be treated with limited resection, and some surgeons now omit axillary evaluation. Whether evaluation of axillary nodal involvement can safely be omitted in patients with small, nonpalpable lesions was investigated.

*Methods.*—During a 9-year (1979–1988), 128 biopsies were done in patients with nonpalpable carcinoma of the breast. Biopsies were performed with needle localization or roentgenography. Whatever the surgical treatment, all patients with axillary nodal involvement received chemotherapy; patients whose tumors were estrogen-receptor positive also were given tamoxifen citrate. All patients with axillary involvement were available for follow-up.

*Results.*—There were 84 invasive cancers and 44 in situ lesions. Axillary dissection was performed in 19 of the patients with in situ lesions; all results were negative. Positive axillary lymph nodes were found in 14 of 69 dissections performed in patients with invasive cancer. The average size of the lesions associated with positive lymph nodes was 1.11 cm, compared to 1.09 cm for lesions with negative nodes. After a mean follow-up of 4.5 years, the rate of recurrence in patients with nonpalpable primary tumors and positive axillas was 62%. Data from the Connecticut Tumor Registry for the years 1983–1986 showed axillary nodal involvement in 16% of breast tumors measuring 1 mm or less, the smallest carcinomas of the breast detectable with current technology.

*Conclusion.*—Small, nonpalpable lesions have a relatively favorable prognosis, but axillary dissection is necessary, whatever the size of the primary lesion. With nodal involvement, these small carcinomas can be as aggressive as larger tumors with positive nodes.

▶ This is a small series in which the authors recommend axillary dissection in all patients. Although this is mandatory for complete staging information and entrance onto protocol, we do not generally recommend axillary lymph node dissection for patients with small areas of ductal carcinoma in situ (DCIS). If the area of DCIS extends over 2 cm, the likelihood of positive axillary metastases increases, therefore justifying axillary dissection.—T.J. Eberlein, M.D.

---

**Factors That Influence the Incidence of Brachial Oedema After Treatment of Breast Cancer**
Segerström K, Bjerle P, Graffman S, Nyström Å(Univ Hosp, Umeå; Sweden; Univ Hosp, Lund, Sweden)
*Scand J Plast Reconstr Surg Hand Surg* 26:223–227, 1992          10–18

---

*Background.*—Lymphedema after mastectomy is a complex problem that probably results from a combination of factors rather than from any single cause. The relative importance of the known and possible provoking factors of lymphedema in breast cancer was examined in 136 consecutive patients (mean age, 65 years) who were studied a mean of 42 months after mastectomy.

*Methods.*—Of the 136 patients, 93 received radiotherapy after mastectomy, which consisted of modified radical mastectomy with axillary dissection. Radiotherapy was given in high doses with few fractions. Variables assessed for their effect on the development of brachial edema were age, Broca index, operation on the dominant or nondominant side, horizontal or oblique incision, history of previous arm infections, and irradiation. The presence of edema was assessed by the water displacement method.

*Findings.*—Edema developed in 89% of those patients who had a history of 1 or more arm infections on the operative side and in 60% of those who received radiotherapy. The incidence of arm edema was also correlated with obesity and an oblique surgical incision, and less so with age or operation on the dominant or nondominant side. Edema was more common in patients who received radiotherapy to the axilla.

*Conclusions.*—In patients who had a mastectomy, soft tissue arm infections, obesity, axillary irradiation, and oblique skin incisions are all significantly correlated with the development of brachial edema. In patients who receive radiotherapy, decreasing the number of fractions given at the same total dose level appears to substantially increase the late effects on normal tissue.

▶ This study touches upon some of the major strategies used to minimize swelling after axillary dissection. A transverse incision, rather than a vertical or oblique incision, is recommended. Radiation therapy is indicated only if a complete dissection has not been performed.

Another important technical consideration is to spare the fat around the axillary vein. Proper treatment of infections, should they occur, is also important. Venipuncture and blood pressure determination should definitely be avoided after axillary dissection.—T.J. Eberlein, M.D.

MISCELLANEOUS

### Optimal Mastectomy Timing
McGuire WL, Hilsenbeck S, Clark GM (Univ of Texas Health Science Ctr, San Antonio)
*J Natl Cancer Inst* 84:346–348, 1992                                        10–19

*Background.*—Based on the results of a retrospective study of 249 patients, researchers at Guy's Hospital in London recommended in May 1991 that premenopausal breast cancer patients have their surgery delayed until at least 12 days after their last menstrual period. Other studies, however, had not reported an association between the timing of mastectomy and rates of recurrence and survival. The literature was reviewed to determine whether the available data support the existence of an optimal timing for mastectomy.

*Findings.*—In September 1991, results similar to those noted at Guy's Hospital appeared in a study of 283 patients from Memorial Sloan-Kettering Cancer Center in New York. Women whose mastectomy was performed during days 7–14 of the menstrual cycle had a higher rate of recurrence. A review of the literature showed that each report of a significant result found a different prognostically favorable window. The probability of finding a significant outcome by chance increased dramatically when multiple windows were tested on a single dataset in order to select the best one. Data concerning 675 patients with breast cancer from the San Antonio Tumor Bank were examined according to 14 possible pairs of 14-day windows. At least 1 ostensibly significant time period was found in 28 of 100 trials.

*Conclusion.*—There are insufficient data at present to allow scheduling surgery according to the menstrual period. A definite answer to the question must carefully define the day of the menstrual cycle by hormonal measurements and take into account the statistical problems discussed.

▶ This article explains the difficulty in defining the day of the menstrual cycle and its associated hormonal measurements as a statistical problem in the prediction of local recurrence. Although several studies have failed to show a correlation, investigation at Guy's Hospital (1) and Memorial Sloan-Kettering (2) showed a correlation between recurrence rates and menstrual cycle. However, the 2 studies did not agree as to the exact timing of surgery.

Currently, if the patient wishes to delay her surgery, this preference is accommodated. No accommodation, however, is made for menstrual cycle timing in the routine care of a patient with breast cancer.—T.J. Eberlein, M.D.

*References*

1. Aitken D, Minton JP: *Surg Clin North Am* 63:1331, 1983.
2. Larson NE, Crampton AR: *Arch Surg* 106:475, 1973.

---

**Fear of Recurrence, Breast-Conserving Surgery, and the Trade-Off Hypothesis**
Lasry J-CM, Margolese RG (Jewish Gen Hosp, Montreal, PQ, Canada)
*Cancer* 69:2111–2115, 1992                    10–20

---

*Background.*—Although breast-conserving surgery presumably leads to a better body image, patients are expected to be more concerned about the risk of cancer recurring than when mastectomy is carried out. Previous studies have cast doubt on the assumption that conservation is associated with a greater fear of recurrence, but some have indicated that patients who have lumpectomy are more fearful of recurrence than those having mastectomy.

*Methods.*—Fear of disease recurrence was compared in patients randomized into the National Surgical Adjuvant Breast Project trial who underwent total mastectomy, lumpectomy alone, or lumpectomy followed by radiotherapy. A Fear of Recurrence index was based on the patient's own concern and her perception of her family's concern about disease reappearing.

*Findings.*—The type of treatment was not associated with differences in fear of recurrence, but patients who had multiple operations were more fearful of recurrence and also had a poorer body image, resembling those who underwent total mastectomy. Patients who had a radical operation did not fear recurrence less than those who had a lumpectomy.

*Interpretation.*—The reputed trade-off between breast conservation and fear of cancer recurring was not verified. There seems to be little reason to raise this issue in selecting a surgical treatment for breast cancer.

▶ In this study of 219 patients conducted by the National Surgical Adjuvant Breast Project, it is reassuring that breast-conserving surgery is not associated with an increased fear of recurrence. Individual patients may express reassurance at having a mastectomy, but this study refutes the theory that this is a widely held belief.

Mastectomy may be a better alternative in patients with multifocal disease, truly extensive disease, first- and second-trimester pregnancies, and certain medical problems such as collagen vascular diseases (making follow-up after radiation therapy more difficult), as well as schizophrenia and the lack of availability of radiation therapy.—T.J. Eberlein, M.D.

---

**Prognosis Following Local Recurrence in the Conservatively Treated Breast Cancer Patient**
Haffty BG, Fischer D, Beinfield M, McKhann C (Yale Univ, New Haven, Conn)
*Int J Radiat Oncol Biol Phys* 21:293–298, 1991                10–21

---

*Introduction.*—Patients with early-stage breast carcinoma can be treated successfully with lumpectomy and radiation therapy. Most cases of local failure can be effectively salvaged with mastectomy. The outcome in 433 conservatively treated patients was evaluated to define prognostic factors for survival after local recurrence.

*Methods.*—The patients had been treated between January 1962 and December 1984. No specific attempt was made to obtain free surgical margins in the lumpectomy specimen. Some patients received adjuvant chemotherapy and hormone therapy. The median follow-up was 8 years; all patients were followed for at least 5 years.

*Results.*—Of 50 ipsilateral breast recurrences during follow-up, 44 represented the sole site of initial treatment failure and 6 occurred simultaneously with or after distant metastases. The 5-year actuarial survival after breast-only recurrence was 59%. Multivariate regression analysis showed 2 independent and highly significant prognostic factors for survival: the site of local recurrence, and the extent of disease at the time of local recurrence. Recurrences within 4 years tended to be at the same site and predicted a worse prognosis.

*Conclusion.*—Patients with later (after more than 4 years) recurrences and those with recurrences elsewhere in the breast had a more favorable prognosis. Mammography is of value in following patients for local recurrence after conservative treatment of early-stage breast carcinoma. In this series, 12 or 14 patients with nonpalpable, mammographically detected breast recurrences underwent salvage therapy and are alive and disease free.

▶ This article raises several issues with regard to recurrence of breast cancer after conservative surgery and radiation therapy. Careful examination and frequent mammograms (every 6 months in the first 2 years) should be the standard of treatment. Early recurrence, invasive disease, and metastatic disease are all unfavorable prognostic signs.

Patients with no evidence of metastatic disease who are treated with mastectomy undergo immediate reconstruction with autologous tissue transfer, which results in superb cosmesis and excellent salvage survival.—T.J. Eberlein, M.D.

## Colorectal Cancer

### INTRODUCTION

Cancer of the colon and rectum is one of the more common malignancies in the United States. Although its incidence has not changed statistically in the past 50 years, (1), changes have occurred in the affected population and site of primary lesion. Black Americans have an increasing occurrence of the disease, so that rates now approximate those seen in the while population (2). Also, within the past decade the incidence of colorectal tumors has shifted from a predominance in the rectum to a predominance in the colon (3–5).

Mortality from colorectal cancer has decreased with improvements in anesthetic techniques and blood transfusion as well as antibiotics. Strategies to control large bowel tumors would include (1) identification and prevention of large bowel carcinogens with screening programs; (2) attention to pathologic features that may predict for recurrence and aid in identifying patients for suitable adjuvant trials; (3) use of new techniques for identifying micrometastatic disease; (4) treatment of primary bowel tumors as well as performance of suitable pre- and posttreatment adjuvant trials; and (5) identification of patterns and treatment of recurrent colorectal malignancies.

**Timothy J. Eberlein, M.D.**

*References*

1. Devesa SS, Silverman DT: *J Natl Cancer Inst* 60:545, 1978.
2. *The Third National Cancer Survey Advanced 3-Year Report,* 1969–1971 Incidence. Washington, D.C: 1974. US Dept of Health, Education, and Welfare publication NIH 74-637.
3. Cady B, et al: *Cancer* 33:426, 1974.
4. Axtel LM, Chiazze L: *Cancer* 19:750, 1966.
5. Rhodes JB, et al: *JAMA* 235:1641, 1977.

EPIDEMIOLOGY, PREVENTION, AND SCREENING

## Changing Patterns in Colorectal Carcinoma: A 25-Year Experience

Sariego J, Byrd ME, Kerstein M, Sano C, Matsumoto T (Hahnemann Univ, Philadelphia, Pa)
*Am Surg* 58:686–691, 1992                                                  10–22

*Objective.*—It is commonly believed that right-sided colorectal carcinomas have become more prevalent and left-sided carcinomas less prevalent in the past several decades, although there is debate as to whethr this is a true phenomenon. Similarly, the anticipated shift toward earlier diagnosis remains to be established. The pattern of colorectal carcinoma was determined as were any changes in that pattern over time, in patients admitted to a single university hospital in a 25-year period.

*Observations.*—The analysis included 1,584 of 1,959 patients with colon or rectal carcinoma seen from 1964 to 1990. Of these, 801 were men and 783 were women. Although most of the tumors were adenocarcinomas throughout the study period, the proportion of other tumors increased from less than 1% in patients seen before 1975 to 7% in the most recent 5-year period. The extent of disease was significantly related to the date of diagnosis, with the proportion of patients who had distant metastases decreasing from 34% to 26% from 1975 to 1990. The proportion of patients with regional nodal metastases decreased from 26% to 23%. There was a steady increase in right colon and rectal tumors, with a concomitant decrease in tumors of the left colon and transverse colon (table). The number of anal carcinomas also increased slightly. The trend toward more left colon and rectal tumors appearing with localized disease rather than metastases approached significance.

*Conclusions.*—There is a trend in colorectal carcinoma toward decreasing stage at the time of diagnosis and toward a "rightward shift" in tumor location, particularly in the past 15 years. The increasing use of

|  | Tumor Location | | | |
|---|---|---|---|---|
|  | Before 1975 | 1975–1979 | 1980–1984 | 1985–1990 |
| Right colon (ascending) (227) | 9.0% (54) | 8.4% (28) | 17.2% (56) | 27.1% (89) |
| Transverse colon (303) | 25.8% (154) | 24.7% (82) | 10.1% (33) | 10.4% (34) |
| Left colon (descending and sigmoid) (697) | 56.5% (338) | 34.3% (114) | 38.6% (126) | 36.3% (119) |
| Rectum (164) | 1.0% (6) | 14.8% (49) | 17.2% (56) | 16.2% (53) |
| Anal canal (20) | 0.2% (1) | 0.6% (2) | 2.2% (7) | 3.0% (10) |
| Undefined colon (173) | 7.5% (45) | 17.2% (57) | 14.7% (48) | 7.0% (23) |
| Total (1,584) | 100.0% (598) | 100.0% (332) | 100.0% (326) | 100.0% (328) |

(Courtesy of Sariego J, Byrd ME, Kerstein M, et al: *Am Surg* 58:686–691, 1992.)

surveillance colonoscopy and sigmoidoscopy probably account for this trend; the prognostic importance awaits longitudinal analysis.

▶ This article reports the findings of a very large study that documents a rightward shift in the incidence of colorectal cancer similar to the results of the National Surgical Adjuvant Breast Project (1). Although, traditionally, patients with right colon tumors have presented at later stages, there is a recent trend to detect lesions at an earlier stage, no doubt because of the increasing use of colonoscopy.—T.J. Eberlein, M.D.

*Reference*

1. Wolmark, N, et al: *Ann Surg* 198:743, 1983.

---

### Serum Cholesterol Level, Body Mass Index, and the Risk of Colon Cancer: The Framingham Study
Kreger BE, Anderson KM, Schatzkin A, Splansky GL (Natl Heart, Lung, and Blood Inst, Framingham, Mass; Natl Cancer Inst, Bethesda, Md)
*Cancer* 70:1038–1043, 1992                                   10–23

---

*Objective.*—There is some evidence that low serum cholesterol levels are related to an increased risk of colon cancer, especially in men. Studies of this topic, however, have given in-consistent results, and it has

---

Univariate Associations With Incidence of Colon and Rectal Cancer: The Framingham Study—Examination 2 Through October 1988 (Cox Regression, Stratified According to Age)

| | Relative hazard (95% confidence limits) per unit of change* | | | |
| | *Men* | | *Women* | |
| Risk variable | *Colon (56 cases)* | *Rectal (19 cases)* | *Colon (66 cases)* | *Rectal (20 cases)* |
|---|---|---|---|---|
| Cigarettes | 0.88 (0.60–1.29) | 1.56 (0.87–2.81) | 0.68 (0.36–1.30) | 1.66 (0.68–4.07) |
| Alcohol | 1.00 (0.97–1.04) | 0.99 (0.92–1.05) | 0.95 (0.87–1.04) | 0.92 (0.74–1.13) |
| Cholesterol | 0.85 (0.75–0.97)† | 0.97 (0.77–1.21) | 1.05 (0.94–1.16) | 0.99 (0.81–1.20) |
| SF 0–20 | 0.95 (0.91–0.98)‡ | 0.98 (0.92–1.05) | 1.03 (1.00–1.07)§ | 0.99 (0.93–1.06) |
| Body mass index | 1.07 (1.00–1.15)† | 0.91 (0.80–1.05) | 1.03 (0.98–1.07) | 0.99 (0.90–1.10) |
| Glucose intolerance | 1.14 (0.35–3.64) | ‖ | ‖ | ‖ |
| Hypertension | 0.88 (0.42–1.84) | 1.21 (0.35–4.13) | 1.10 (0.61–1.96) | 1.41 (0.50–3.96) |
| Parity | — | — | 1.09 (0.99–1.22) | 0.83 (0.65–1.07) |

* Units of change are 20 cigarettes/day, 1 oz of pure ethanol equivalent/wk, 20 mg (.52 mmol) of total cholesterol/mL, 15 mg of SF 0-20 lipoprotein/mL, 1 kg/m² of body mass index, yes (vs. no) for glucose intolerance and hypertension, and 1 live birth for parity.
† $P \leq .05$.
‡ $P \leq .01$.
§ $.1 > P > .05$.
‖ Too few cases to assess.
(Courtesy of Kreger BE, Anderson KM, Schatzkin A, et al; *Cancer* 70:1038-1043, 1992.)

been suggested that any apparent association may be explained by the presence of preclinical disease. Data from the Framingham Study cohort were examined to assess the relationship between cholesterol and colorectal cancer.

*Methods.*—The cohort included 5,209 persons of both sexes who were initially enrolled in 1948-1951 and followed ever since. The baseline information collected for each patient included lipoprotein fractions, total cholesterol levels, body mass index, alcohol intake, and various cardiovascular risk factors. One analysis excluded the first 5 years and 10 years after baseline measurements to remove the influence of subclinical malignancies.

*Results.*—The analyses showed an inverse relationship between colon cancer and serum cholesterol levels in men (table), even after eliminating

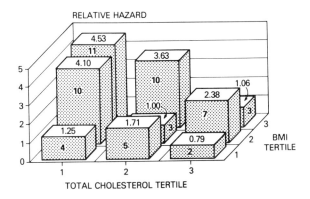

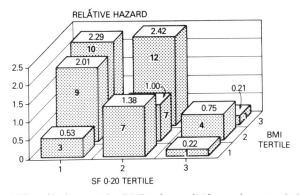

**Fig 10-4.**—Combined effect of body mass index (BMI) and serum lipids on colon cancer incidence in men. Relative hazard (numbers atop columns) is displayed with reference to the middle tertile (the "average" man) for both BMI and either total cholesterol or low-density lipoprotein (SF 0-20). On the sides of the columns are the numbers of cases in each combined category. The first 10 years of follow-up after baseline are omitted. In all instances, the combinations of high BMI and low serum lipid signal the greatest risk. (Courtesy of Kreger BE, Anderson KM, Schatzkin A, et al: *Cancer* 70:1038-1043, 1992.)

the first 10 years of follow-up (Fig 10–4). The Svedberg 0-20 fraction, corresponding to low-density lipoprotein levels, was the only lipoprotein fraction to show an association with cancer incidence. Body mass index was also directly related to the incidence of colon cancer in men.

*Conclusions.*—This study, using data from the Framingham cohort, finds that the combination of initial low serum cholesterol levels and obesity indicates a fourfold increased risk of colon cancer in men compared to persons with average values. If similar associations are found in other studies, the possible biological reasons should be determined, including dietary, metabolic, and genetic influences.

▶ This is a very interesting study using the Framingham study cohort of 5,209 men and women. Although the findings are epidemiologic in nature, if confirmed by other studies (for example, the National Surgical Adjuvant Breast Project), dietary, metabolic, and/or genetic influences can be identified and manipulated to alter the incidence of colorectal tumors.—T.J. Eberlein, M.D.

---

### Aspirin Use and Reduced Risk of Fatal Colon Cancer

Thun MJ, Namboodiri MM, Heath CW Jr (American Cancer Society, Atlanta, Ga)

*N Engl J Med* 325:1593–1596, 1991                                       10–24

*Background.*—There is growing evidence from animal and human epidemiologic studies that nonsteroidal anti-inflammatory drugs (e.g., aspirin) may have a protective effect against colon cancer. Data from an ongoing prospective cancer mortality study were used to test this hypothesis.

*Methods.*—The analysis included data on 662,424 adults enrolled since 1982 in the American Cancer Society's Cancer Prevention Study II. The average age at enrollment was 57 years. All of the participants were white persons who specified their frequency and duration of aspirin use at entry into the study. Mortality data were complete through 1988. Multivariate analysis was done on 598 patients and 3,058 matched controls to address the potential effects of other risk factors for colon cancer.

*Results.*—Deaths from colon cancer decreased with more frequent aspirin use among both men and women (table). For patients who took aspirin at least 16 times monthly for at least 1 year, thee relative risks were .60 for men and .58 for women. These risks were unchanged after exclusion of factors that might affect aspirin use and mortality, including arthritis, cancer, heart disease, and stroke at entry. Nor were the results significantly affected by adjustment for diet, obesity, physical activity, or family history. Acetaminophen use had no significant effect on risk.

*Conclusions.*—The frequent use of low doses of aspirin might reduce the risk of fatal colon cancer. No conclusions can be drawn as to the

Rates of Death From Colon Cancer, According to Frequency of
Aspirin Use, After Exclusion of Patients Who Had Selected
Illnesses at Enrollment

| ASPIRIN USE (TIMES/MO) | NO. OF DEATHS | PERSON-YEARS AT RISK | AGE-ADJUSTED DEATH RATE PER 100,000 | RELATIVE RISK (95% CI) * | P VALUE † |
|---|---|---|---|---|---|
| **Men** | | | | | |
| Excluding patients with colon cancer | | | | | |
| 0 | 284 | 642,110 | 44.7 | 1.00 | |
| <1 | 152 | 484,260 | 37.9 | 0.85 (0.67–1.07) | |
| 1–15 | 100 | 387,540 | 32.1 | 0.72 (0.52–0.99) | 0.0006 |
| ≥16 | 63 | 200,405 | 25.9 | 0.58 (0.36–0.93) | |
| Excluding patients with selected illnesses | | | | | |
| 0 | 171 | 487,932 | 40.0 | 1.00 | |
| <1 | 101 | 385,321 | 33.2 | 0.83 (0.62–1.12) | |
| 1–15 | 63 | 302,106 | 25.5 | 0.64 (0.40–1.01) | 0.0076 |
| ≥16 | 28 | 116,947 | 21.5 | 0.54 (0.26–1.13) | |
| **Women** | | | | | |
| Excluding patients with colon cancer | | | | | |
| 0 | 225 | 701,131 | 32.6 | 1.00 | |
| <1 | 139 | 669,575 | 26.8 | 0.82 (0.63–1.07) | |
| 1–15 | 87 | 504,234 | 23.6 | 0.72 (0.51–1.02) | 0.0056 |
| ≥16 | 61 | 264,277 | 19.8 | 0.61 (0.38–0.97) | |
| Excluding patients with selected illnesses | | | | | |
| 0 | 126 | 521,467 | 26.7 | 1.00 | |
| <1 | 98 | 531,469 | 25.9 | 0.97 (0.74–1.28) | |
| 1–15 | 54 | 396,956 | 18.6 | 0.70 (0.44–1.11) | 0.0512 |
| ≥16 | 32 | 175,409 | 17.7 | 0.66 (0.37–1.19) | |

Note: Patients with selected illnesses were those with cancer, heart disease, or stroke or who described themselves as sick at the time of the interview.
* In the analysis of risk, the groups with no aspirin use were the referent category. CI, confidence interval.
† P values denote the trend across categories of aspirin use.
(Courtesy of Thun MJ, Namboodiri MM, Heath CW Jr: *N Engl J Med* 325:1593–1596, 1991.)

mechanism of this effect, whether direct (e.g., by inhibition of prostaglandin synthesis) or indirect (e.g., by inducing bleeding in persons with polyps or early cancer leading to early diagnosis). Controlled trials in high-risk patients may be useful.

▶ This is an analysis of more than 662,000 men and women enrolled in a cancer prevention study through the American Cancer Society. Almost 600 cancer patients with more than 3,000 matched controls were studied in detail.

Although the association of aspirin use and a reduced risk of fatal colon cancer may initially appear incidental, this effect could possible be explained through suppression of cell proliferation or stimulation of an immune response by inhibiting prostaglandin synthesis.

It would be interesting to further study this question in greater detail; such prospective, randomized trials could be incorporated in the Physicians' Health Study or the Nurses' Health Study.—T.J. Eberlein, M.D.

### Can Hemoccult-II Replace Colonoscopy in Surveillance After Radical Surgery for Colorectal Cancer and After Polypectomy?

Jahn H, Joergensen OD, Kronborg O, Fenger C (Odense Univ Hosp, Odense, Denmark)

*Dis Colon Rectum* 35:253–256, 1992

10–25

*Purpose.*—Surveillance after radical surgery for colorectal cancer and removal of colorectal adenomas includes colonoscopy, which is hard on patients, physicians, and economic resources. A study of the Hemoccult-II (H-II) test was undertaken to investigate whether at least some post-operative colonoscopies could be replaced with this simple fecal occult blood test.

*Patients and Methods.*—Between 1983 and 1990, the H-II test was performed 1–2 weeks before 1,244 colonoscopies in 529 patients who had previously had curative resection and before 328 colonoscopies in 279 patients with previously detected colorectal adenomas. The H-II test was performed on 2 samples taken from each of 3 consecutive stools. The endoscopist was not told the results of the H-II test.

*Results.*—The H-II test was positive in 3 of 9 patients with local recurrences, in 2 of 13 paatients with new carcinomas, and in 31 of 186 patients with adenomas (table). The H-II was positive more often in patients with large and multiple adenomas, sigmoid adenomas, and adenomas with villous elements and moderate to severe dysplasia, but the sensitivity still was not more than 25% to 40%.

*Conclusions.*—The H-II test is not sensitive enough for the detection of new carcinomas and adenomas in patients being followed up after colorectal cancer surgery.

Findings During 1,572 Colonoscopies in Relation to Hemoccult-II Results

|  | Positive | Negative |
|---|---|---|
| Cancer |  |  |
| Local recurrence | 3 | 6 |
| New carcinoma | 2 | 11 |
| Adenoma | 31 | 155 |
| Hyperplastic and inflamma-<br>tory polyps | 16 | 123 |
| Other possible bleeding<br>sources | 12 | 119 |
| Normal colonoscopy | 50 | 1044 |
| Total | 114 | 1458 |

(Courtesy of Jahn H, Joergensen OD, Kronborg O, et al: *Dis Colon Rectum* 35:253–256, 1992.)

▶ This study is significant for patients with colorectal cancer because it documents that stool testing for guiac is inadequate as a follow-up means of detection of cancer. The findings confirm the utility of colonoscopy in diagnosing and treating premalignant and colorectal neoplasia, but they do not settle the controversial issue of frequency of follow-up examinations. Although some might suggest a complete examination postoperatively followed by yearly examinations, consideration must be given to the morbidity associated with colonoscopy, as well as the potential for increased utilization once gene markers are used to identify segments of the general population at higher risk for colorectal cancer.—T. J. Eberlein, M.D.

## Screening Sigmoidoscopy and Colorectal Cancer Mortality

Newcomb PA, Norfleet RG, Storer BE, Surawicz TS, Marcus PM (Univ of Wisconsin, Madison; Marshfield Clinic, Marshfield, Wis)
*J Natl Cancer Inst* 84:1572–1575, 1992                                    10–26

*Purpose.*—Sigmoidoscopy is the colorectal cancer screening method with the greatest promise for reducing mortality. It might accomplish this by identifying both cancers and precursor lesions, (e.g., polyps), so that they can be treated. There are few data regarding the effectiveness of sigmoidoscopy as a screening procedure, however. A retrospective, case-control study sought to determine whether colorectal cancer screening with sigmoidoscopy is effective in reducing mortality.

*Methods.*—The records of 66 patients (cases) from a prepaid community health plan who died of colon or rectal cancer during a 9-year period were examined, as were those of 196 randomly selected controls

Odds Ratio of Rectal Cancer and Colon Cancer According to Screening Tests for Early Detection

| Sites and screening tests | OR* | 95% CI | *P* |
|---|---|---|---|
| All sites | | | |
| Fecal occult blood test | 1.15 | 0.93-1.44 | .21 |
| Digital rectal examination | 1.01 | 0.88-1.17 | .85 |
| Sigmoidoscopy | 0.21 | 0.08-0.52 | <.001 |
| Rectum and distal colon | | | |
| Fecal occult blood test | 1.10 | 0.82-1.49 | .53 |
| Digital rectal examination | 0.97 | 0.80-1.17 | .75 |
| Sigmoidoscopy | 0.05 | 0.01-0.43 | .006 |
| Other colon sites | | | |
| Fecal occult blood test | 1.01 | 0.70-1.45 | .97 |
| Digital rectal examination | 1.20 | 0.88-1.63 | .24 |
| Sigmoidoscopy | 0.36 | 0.11-1.20 | .10 |

* Odds ratios (ORs) are calculated per test from conditional logistic regression models and adjusted for family history, other screening tests, and duration of enrollment.
(Courtesy of Newcomb PA, Norfleet RG, Storer BE, et al: *J Natl Cancer Inst* 84:1572–1575, 1992.)

matched for gender, age, and duration of enrollment in the health plan. Data on screening history were collected exclusively from combined clinic and hospital records.

*Results.*—Only 10% of the cases had a history of screening sigmoidoscopy, vs. 30% of the controls. Compared to patients who had never had screening sigmoidoscopy, a history of 1 examination decreased the risk of death considerably. The odds ratio was 2.1. This benefit seemed to apply only to tumors of the rectum and distal colon. No reduction in mortality was associated with either fecal occult blood testing or digital rectal examination (table).

*Conclusions.*—These findings indicate that screening sigmoidoscopy can significantly reduce mortality from cancers of the rectum and distal colon. The study is limited by its small size and issues related to the decision to undergo screening. The findings should be confirmed nonexperimentally in large, well-documented populations.

▶ This retrospective, case-controlled study has obvious limitations in reproducing its significance to the general population. However, it seems intuitive that screening may well reduce mortality. The major issues remain identification of the population at greatest risk and the performance of cost-effective screening.—T.J. Eberlein, M.D.

PATHOLOGIC FEATURES

**p53 Expression in Colorectal Tumors**
Purdie CA, O'Grady J, Piris J, Wyllie AH, Bird CC (Univ of Edinburgh, Edinburgh, Scotland)
*Am J Pathol* 138:807–813, 1991                                              10–27

*Background.*—The p53 gene behaves as a tumor suppressor, and mutation or deletion of this gene is associated with a number of cancers. The region of the chromosome that contains p53 is frequently deleted in colorectal cancer. The expression of p53 was examined in a series of colorectal carcinomas and polyps.

*Methods.*—The fixative, periodate lysine paraformaldehyde dichromate (PLPD), allowed immunohistochemical analysis of p53 by using the monoclonal antibody PAb1801 on a series of 86 colorectal carcinomas and 62 polyps. The staining pattern was correlated with well-recognized indicators of clinical outcome.

*Results.*—Almost half of the carcinomas were stained positively by the antibody, but less than 10% of the adenomas stained positively for p53. The few positive adenomas always demonstrated moderate to severe dysplasia. Metastatic polyps and small familial, adenomatous, polyposis-related adenomas did not stain. Those carcinomas that stained for p53 were not different from those that did not stain in terms of site, differentiation, Dukes' stage, DNA ploidy, or tumor histology. Expression of p53 was detected only in neoplastic nuclei. The staining in positive tumors was heterogeneous and frequently more marked at infiltrative margins. The intensity of staining was significantly reduced in mitotic cells.

*Conclusions.*—Expression of immunohistochemically detectable p53 was observed in adenomas around the time of transition to carcinoma. The most intense staining was detected at infiltrative margins. Therefore, p53 may be involved in malignant transformation but not necessarily in tumor progression.

### Increased p53 Protein Content of Colorectal Tumours Correlates With Poor Survival

Remvikos Y, Tominaga O, Hammel P, Laurent-Puig P, Salmon RJ, Dutrillaux B, Thomas G (Institute Curie, Paris, France)
*Br J Cancer* 66:758–764, 1992                          10–28

*Introduction.*—Patients with colorectal cancers commonly have allelic losses on the short arm of chromosome 17. These losses have greater prognostic significance than other common molecular events, e.g., loss of the long arms of chromosomes 18 and 5. The p53 antioncogene seems to be the most promising target of the various genes mapping to the commonly deleted sequence. The effect of the p53 content in cancer cells on the outcome of colorectal cancer was examined.

*Methods.*—Seventy-eight colorectal cancers stored in a tumor bank in a 4-year period were studied. The median length of patient follow-up was 42 months. Flow cytometry was used to measure nuclear-attached p53, and an emzyme-linked immunosorbent assay was used to assay soluble p53. Both methods used a monoclonal antibody thought to be specific for a conformation epitope seen only on the mutated protein.

*Findings.*—Significant levels of nuclear-attached p53 were found in 64% of the tumors; another 2 had levels of p53 only in their soluble fraction. Correlations were noted between p53 content and 17p loss, hyperdiploid DNA content, and tumor site, although not Dukes' stage. Survival was better in patients negative for p53, but this was no longer the case after exclusion of 14 stage D tumors (Fig 10–5). The small sample size prevented multivariate analysis. On flow cytometry the finding of nuclear protein distinguishing the mutation-specific epitope—recognized by pAb240—was the best discriminator of survival (table).

*Conclusions.*—A 67% rate of positivity for p53 was reported in this series of colorectal cancers. A high p53 content is associated with poor survival, with more than 80% of patients with p53-negative tumors surviving at 3 years versus less than half of those with p53-positive tumors. The precise prognostic significance of p53 content must be determined in a large, prospective study.

▶ The study by Purdie et al. (Abstract 10–27) describes a new fixative that allows immunohistochemical analysis of p53 in paraffin-embedded speci-

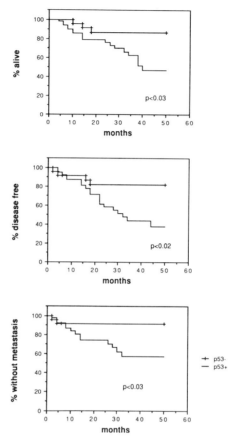

**Fig 10–5.**—Actuarial survival curves obtained according to the Kaplan-Meier method. The Mantel-Cox test was used for the differences between groups. *Upper panel,* overall survival (including stage D patients). *Middle panel,* disease-free survival. *Lower panel,* metastasis-free survival according to p53 content, for patients with stage A to C2 tumors. (Courtesy of Remvikos Y, Tominaga O, Hammel P, et al: *Br J Cancer* 66:758–764, 1992.)

mens. Unfortunately, because of the short time of clinical follow-up of patients studied in this investigation, there are no data that directly compare postoperative course and p53 staining. In a similar article (Abstract 10–28), a high p53 nuclear content was associated with poor survival when all the stage D tumors were included.

Both studies were relatively small, but they present important observations regarding colon tumors. Larger, prospective studies are currently being conducted to define the exact prognostic significance of p53.—T. J. Eberlein, M.D.

p53 Content and Survival at 3 Years

| p53 | | | % Disease free | % W/O metastasis | % Alive |
|---|---|---|---|---|---|
| Nuclear | 421/1801 | – | 73 | 80 | 84 |
| | | + | 33 | 59 | 46 |
| | | | $P < 0.02$ | $P < 0.1$ | $P < 0.005$ |
| | 240 | – | 83 | 92 | 88 |
| | | + | 35 | 54 | 45 |
| | | | $P < 0.005$ | $P < 0.02$ | $P < 0.007$ |
| Nuclear and soluble | 240 | – | 82 | 92 | 86 |
| | | + | 38 | 57 | 48 |
| | | | $P < 0.02$ | $P < 0.03$ | $P < 0.03$ |

(Courtesy of Remvikos Y, Tominaga O, Hammel P, et al: Br J Cancer 66:758–764, 1992.)

## Variables Correlated With the Risk of Lymph Node Metastasis in Early Rectal Cancer

Brodsky JT, Richard GK, Cohen AM, Minsky BD (Mem Sloan-Kettering Cancer Ctr, New York City)
*Cancer* 69:322–326, 1992                                  10–29

*Background.*—Local excision of rectal cancer is appropriate for selected tumors, but not for all. Knowledge of the pathologic variables that predict lymph node metastases (LNM) should be useful in the identification of those tumors that can be treated by excision alone and those that require a more aggresive approach.

*Methods.*—A retrospective analysis of data on 154 patients with pT1 or pT2 rectal cancer treated with radical resection was performed to determine the risk factors of LNM. Gross and microscopic pathologic characteristics of the primary tumor were examined as predictors of LNM. Comparisons were made using Fisher's test; significance was defined as a $P$ value of less than .05.

*Results.*—The incidence of LNM was 12% for $T_1$ and 22% for $T_2$ tumors. In the 12 well-differentiated cancers LNM was not detected. The incidence of LNM was significantly lower in tumors without lymphatic vessel invasion (LVI) or blood vessel invasion (BVI).

*Conclusions.*—Local excision is adequate for well-differentiated or moderately differentiated $T_1$ rectal cancers in the absence of LVI or BVI and for well-differentiated $T_2$ tumors. Poorly differentiated tumors, however, should receive more aggressive therapy to optimize patient survival.

▶ The risk of LNM found to correlate with tumor differentiation and lymphatic blood vessel invasion is reviewed in this article. These tumor pathologic features, which are incidentally not unlike breast cancer, would help in the selection of patients for conservative treatment of rectal cancer. These results also would identify patients who should be treated with more extensive lymph node dissections and/or adjuvant radiation and chemotherapy regimes.—T.J. Eberlein, M.D.

DIAGNOSTIC TECHNIQUES

### Radiolabeled Monoclonal Antibody Imaging (Immunoscintigraphy) of Colorectal Cancers: Current Status and Future Perspectives

Nabi HA, Doerr RJ (State Univ of New York, Buffalo; Buffalo Gen Hosp)
*Am J Surg* 163:448–456, 1992                                    10–30

*Introduction.*—In radioimmunoscintigraphy a radiolabeled antibody against a tumor or tumor byproduct is injected and followed by nuclear gamma camera imaging to localize primary carcinomas and metastases. The usefulness of this technique in patients with colon and rectal cancers has been established, particularly in those with suspected recurrences.

*Discussion.*—An important recent advance in radioimmunoscintigraphy is the development of methods to label antibodies with radiometals, including $^{111}$In. Clinical studies with 2 important monoclonal antibodies, the anticarcinoembryonic antigen (CEA) monoclonal antibody ZCE 025 and anti-TAG-72 monoclonal antibody B72.3, have been reported. The greatest potential gains from immunoscintigraphy are in patients with primary or resected colorectal carcinoma in whom there is a high clinical suspicion of recurrence and an elevated level of CEA. Immunoscintigraphy appears to have definite uses in the preoperative workup of patients with primary colorectal carcinomas. The technique can simultaneously detect lesions at multiple sites with sensitivity and specificity similar to those of CT. This use is limited in preoperative workups for liver metastases, although demonstration of 7 or more focal areas is highly suggestive of liver metastases from the bowel. Monoclonal antibody scanning may also be useful in detecting occult tumors in the lymph nodes and other abdominal and retroperitoneal soft tissues. Disease may thus be disclosed when results of all other tests, including CEA, are negative. A 100% rate of detection of recurrences has been shown in high-risk patients. The same study showed that repeated administration of murine monoclonal antibody ZCE 025 is safe and can detect recurrences at an early stage. Multicenter studies have indicated that immunoscintigraphy with $^{111}$In-labeled CYT-103 and ZCE 025 monoclonal antibodies is beneficial in 16% to 26% of cases.

*Summary.*—The use of radioimmunoscintigraphy with radiolabeled monoclonal antibodies in patients with colorectal cancers can significantly aid the preoperative evaluation of primary, recurrent, or occult cancers.

### Radioimmunoguided Surgery Using Iodine 125 B72.3 in Patients With Colorectal Cancer

Cohen AM, Martin EW Jr, Lavery I, Daly J, Sardi A, Aitken D, Bland K, Mojzisik C, Hinkle G (Mem Sloan-Kettering Cancer Ctr, New York City; Ohio State Univ, Columbus; Cleveland Clinic Foundation, Cleveland, Ohio; Univ of Pennsylvania, Philadelphia; Ochsner Clinic, New Orleans, La; et al)

*Arch Surg* 126:349–352, 1991

10–31

*Background.*—Accurate estimates of the extent of an abdominal tumor are essential for the effective management of primary or recurrent colorectal cancer. A preliminary study using the B72.3 murine monoclonal antibody labeled with iodine-125 ($^{125}$I) suggested that most tumor sites and many sites of occult disease may be detected in this way.

*Objective.*—A multicenter trial was undertaken in 104 patients with primary, suspected, or presumed recurrent colorectal cancer. Seventy-two of the patients had recurrent disease and 26 had primary colorectal cancer.

*Method.*—After receiving a potassium iodide solution for 2 days, the patients were skin tested with unlabeled antibody and then were given 1 mg of B72.3 antibody labeled with 74 × 10 Bq of $^{125}$I. A hand-held gamma-detecting probe was used to count all potential tumor sites after surgical exploration.

*Results.*—The gamma probe detected 75% of the tumor sites in patients with primary disease and 63% of the sites in those with recurrent cancer (table). Nine percent of the pathologically confirmed tumor sites were clinically occult and were identified by probe-directed biopsy specimens. Occult tumor was found in this way at 30 sites in 26 patients.

Tumor Localization Correlation

| RIGS† | Surgical Findings | Pathologic Findings | % |
|:-----:|:-----------------:|:-------------------:|:---:|
| + | + | + | 46.7 |
| + | + | − | 7.1 |
| + | − | + | 9.2 |
| + | − | − | 8.5 |
| − | + | + | 12.8 |
| − | + | − | 7.8 |
| − | − | + | 4.3 |
| − | − | − | 3.5 |

* Plus signs indicate positive finding for cancer; minus signs, negative test or finding for cancer.

† *Abbreviation:* RIGS, radioimmunoguided surgery. Sensitivity = 77%; predictive value + RIGS = 78%.

(Courtesy of Cohen AM, Martin EW Jr, Lavery I, et al: *Arch Surg* 126:349–352, 1991.)

*Discussion.*—The low energy of $^{125}$I and its 60-day half-life made it a useful label for tumor imaging. This method is able to identify milligram-sized tumor sites and, as used in this study, is relatively nontoxic. Finding occult disease has obviated radical resection in many instances or allowed appropriate extension of the operation.

▶ These 2 articles (Abstracts 10–30 and 10–31) document studies using the B72.3 murine monoclonal antibody labeled with $^{125}$I in the detection of occult colorectal tumor. This technique is capable of identifying quantities of tumor in milligrams, but it is not uniformly useful; it appears most useful and reproducible in a small set of medical centers. The lack of uniformity of the results probably is accounted for by the lack of antigen expression by the tumor, thereby denying positive tagging by the selected monoclonal antibody. Thus tagging to a different antigen or multiple antigens would presumably improve detection. Although this technique has been shown to be safe, more work is needed to identify another antigen to improve the rate of detection. In the meantime, this technique can be used to help identify occult metastases in the patient with a rising level of CEA.—T.J. Eberlein, M.D.

TREATMENT

### Improving Survival Rates for Patients With Colorectal Cancer
Jatzko G, Lisborg P, Wette V (Krankenhaus der Barmgerzigen Brüder, St Veit/Glan, Austria)
*Br J Surg* 79:588–591, 1992                                                        10–32

*Introduction.*—In patients undergoing surgery for colorectal carcinoma, extended resection margins are used to counter possible lymphogenous spread to a neighboring lymph drainage zone. For tumors located close to the border of such a zone, the neighboring zone is resected and the supplying blood vessels ligated at their origin. The results of this procedure in 575 patients with colorectal cancer were evaluated.

*Methods.*—The patients were operated on during a 7-year period. About half (284) had stage I or II tumors. One surgeon performed 91% of the operations. The surgical procedure was standardized, with no adjuvant therapy. The technique included meticulous application of the "no-touch" technique and linear or circular stapling for all anastomoses. The mesorectum was resected completely for rectal resection. None of the patients was lost to follow-up.

*Results.*—The 5-year survival rates for patients with stage I or II cancers exceeded 90%. The rate of metastases was higher, and survival lower, in patients with poorly differentiated tumors. Twenty-eight patients with colonic carcinoma had extension of the resection margins; none of them had tumor recurrence. At 5 years, 81% of patients with colonic carcinoma remained alive. Bowel continuity was maintained and abdominoperineal resection avoided in one third of the patients with carcinomas of the lower third of the rectum. That group had a tumor recurrence rate of 10.5%, compared with 14.3% in those undergoing abdominoperineal resection. The 5-year survival rate was also significantly better, 90% vs. 52%. At 5 years, 71% of patients with rectal carcinoma were still alive.

*Conclusions.*—In patients with cancer of the lower third of the rectum, high rates of sphincter preservation can be obtained without increasing tumor recurrence. In this study, tumor recurrence was not increased even with distal margins of less than 2 cm. High rates of local recurrence can be avoided by radical resection of the mesorectum; however, this resection may be limited by the high incidence of distant metastases in poorly differentiated tumors.

▶ This article reports the findings of a study of 575 patients, 91% of whom were managed by a single surgeon. The data are very useful as a result of meticulous technical detail. Most important, however, is the finding that, although tumor recurrence is not increased if the distal margin is less than 2 cm, local recurrence correlates with resection of the mesorectum and surrounding soft tissue. It should also be emphasized that poorly differentiated tumors of the lower third of the rectum were treated with abdominal peritoneal resection because of the possibility of submucosal spread. Also, patients with abdominal peritoneal resection had bulkier tumors compared to those not undergoing this procedure.—T.J. Eberlein, M.D.

## The Risk of Lymph Node Metastasis in Colorectal Polyps With Invasive Adenocarcinoma

Nivatvongs S, Rojanasakul A, Reiman HM, Dozois RR, Wolff BG, Pemberton JH, Beart RW Jr, Jacques LF (Mayo Clinic and Found, Rochester, Minn)
*Dis Colon Rectum* 34:323–328, 1991                                      10–33

*Background.*—When a colorectal polyp is found to contain a focus of invasive adenocarcinoma, appropriate management is uncertain. Some surgeons favor segmental bowel resection in all such cases, whereas others believe that polypectomy is adequate unless the tumor is undifferentiated, vessels are invaded, or the polypectomy is incomplete.

*Objective.*—The frequency of nodal metastasis was determined in 151 patients seen from 1979 to 1986 with invasive adenocarcinoma in a colorectal polyp who underwent bowel resection, alone or after polypectomy. The depth of invasion was recorded by a single pathologist using the system shown in Figure 10–6.

*Findings.*—Ten of 102 sessile polyps were associated with lymph node metastasis, as were 3 of 49 pedunculated polyps. Only polyps with level 4 invasion were associated with lymph node metastasis (table). Seven patients had residual tumor after polypectomy. There were no recurrences or metastases during a mean follow-up of 35 months.

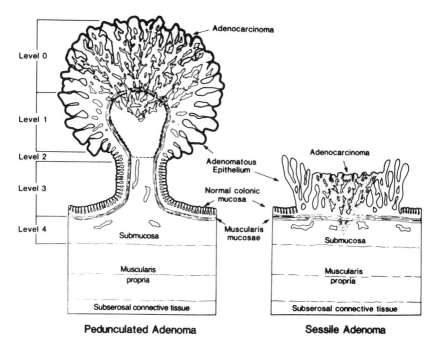

**Fig 10–6.**—Classification of polyps with invasive cacinoma. (From Nivatvongs S, Rojanasakul A, Reiman HM, et al: *Dis Colon Rectum* 34:323–328, 1991. Courtesy of Haggitt RC, Glotzbach RE, Soffer EE, et al: *Gastroenterology* 89:328–336, 1985.)

Positive Lymph Nodes in Pedunculated and Sessile Polyps
(Level 0 is Excluded)

| Level (Excluding Level 0) | Bowel Resection (No. of Patients) | Positive LN (No. of Patients) | % |
|---|---|---|---|
| ,1 | 22 | 0 | 0 |
| 2 | 3 | 0 | 0 |
| 3 | 13 | 0 | 0 |
| 4 (pedunculated) | 11 | 3 | 27 |
| 4 (sessile) | 102 | 10 | 10* |
| Total | 151 | 13 | 8.6 |

* Incidence of positive lymph nodes (LN) in pedunculated polyps was not different from sessile polyps. $P = .114$ (Fisher exact).
(Courtesy of Nivatvongs S, Rojanasakul A, Reiman HM, et al: *Dis Colon Rectum* 34:323–328, 1991.)

*Discussion.*—Nodal metastasis occurred in 9% of the patients with colorectal polyps containing invasive adenocarcinoma in this series. The risk of lymph node metastasis was high when invasion reached the submucosa of the bowel wall at the base of the stalk. Nodal metastasis also was associated with invasion of venous or lymphatic vessels. The extent and grade of carcinoma were not significant factors until invasion reached the base of the polyp.

**The Fate of Patients Following Polypectomy Alone for Polyps Containing Invasive Carcinoma**
Pollard CW, Nivatvongs S, Rojanasakul A, Reiman HM, Dozois RR (Mayo Clinic and Found, Rochester, Minn)
*Dis Colon Rectum* 35:933–937, 1992                    10–34

*Introduction.*—The surgical management of polyps containing invasive carcinoma in which the malignant cells have penetrated the muscularis mucosa through to the submucosa is uncertain. Results in 82 such patients treated by polypectomy were evaluated.

*Patients and Methods.*—Between 1979 and 1986, 82 patients with polyps containing invasive adenocarcinoma were treated by polypectomy alone. There were 46 men and 36 women (mean age, 70 years) with 48 pedunculated and 34 sessile polyps. Of the pedunculated polyps, 34 had invasion to the head, level 1; 13 had invasion to the stalk, level 3; and 1 had invasion to the base, level 4. All of the sessile polyps were level 4. Most of the polyps (79%) were in the rectum and sigmoid colon. About half (49%) were removed colonoscopically, 28% per anally, and 19% proctoscopically. Tubulovillous adenomas accounted for 41%, tubular adenomas for 32%, and villous adenomas for 22%. Patients were followed for a mean of 53 months.

*Outcomes.*—An adverse outcome was seen in 21% of the patients with sessile lesions, with 5 local recurrences and 2 distant metastases occurring up to 68 months postoperatively. None of the pedunculated polyps showed any sign of local recurrence or metastases. During follow-up, 28% of the patients had adenomatous polyps removed and 4% had malignant polyps removed.

*Conclusions.*—For level 1–3 pedunculated polyps, treatment with complete polypectomy appears to be safe as long as the carcinoma is not undifferentiated. More aggressive treatment is needed for sessile lesions and for level 4 pedunculated lesions. If these patients do not undergo bowel resection, they need long-term follow-up.

### The Care of Patients With Colorectal Polyps That Contain Invasive Adenocarcinoma: Endoscopic Polypectomy or Colectomy?

Kyzer S, Bégin LR, Gordon PH, Mitmaker B (Sir Mortimer B Davis–Jewish Gen Hosp, Montreal, PQ, Canada; McGill Univ, Montreal)
*Cancer* 70:2044–2050, 1992                                    10–35

*Introduction.*—Flexible endoscopic polypectomy has come to be the preferred procedure for management of most colorectal adenomatous polyps. There are insufficient data, however, to predict when this treatment will be sufficient in patients with invasive adenocarcinoma. A series of patients with invasive adenocarcinoma treated with endoscopic polypectomy was studied to determine the appropriateness of a policy of selective resection.

*Patients.*—During a 13-year period, 44 polyps with invasive adenocarcinoma were removed endoscopically from 42 patients. According to the classification of Haggitt, 27% of the polyps had level 1 invasion, 9% had level 2, 11% had level 3, and 39% had level 4. Fourteen percent were uncertain. About half of the patients (48%) had well-differentiated adenocarcinoma; and in the others it was moderately differentiated. No patient had poorly differentiated adenocarcinoma or lymphatic or vascular invasion. Twenty-three patients were deemed to have had complete excision, whereas none of 11 patients who underwent resection had residual adenocarcinoma. Twelve of 14 patients with inevaluable margins underwent resection; 1 was found to have residual adenocarcinoma. Residual tumor was found in only 2 of the 7 patients who had positive margins and underwent resection. When residual carcinoma was detected, the original lesion was always designated level 4 (table). At a mean follow-up of 66 months, no patient treated by polypectomy alone had recurrence.

*Conclusions.*—In patients with invasive adenocarcinoma discovered in a polypectomy specimen, only those with Haggitt level 4 lesions need to be considered for resection, provided there is no vascular or lymphatic invasion. With additional refinement, even many of these patients may not need surgery. Preparation of the polypectomy specimen for histologic examination is an important consideration.

▶ These 3 papers are grouped together because they address several important issues surrounding the management of patients with polyps showing invasive adenocarcinoma. In the first paper (Abstract 10–33), the authors studied 151 patients who underwent bowel resection after identification of polyps with adenocarcinoma. Importantly, patients with ulcerative colitis, familial polyposis, and other carcinomatosis lesions were excluded. In the complete group, only 8.6% of all patients with positive lymph nodes, whether pedunculated or sessile, had malignant invasion into the submucosa of the bowel wall below the stock of the polyp but above the muscularis propria (all sessile polyps with invasive carcinoma are in level IV). Although grade did

Treatment and Follow-Up Data in Relation to Levels According to Haggitt Classification

| Haggitt level | No. of polyps | Treatment | | Residual carcinoma* | Positive lymph nodes* | Dead of disease | Metastases | Follow-up (mo) |
| --- | --- | --- | --- | --- | --- | --- | --- | --- |
| | | *Polypectomy* | *Polypectomy + resection* | | | | | |
| ≥1 | 6 | 0 | 6 | 0/6 | 0/6 | 0 | 0 | 93 |
| 1 | 12 | 8 | 4 | 0/4 | 0/4 | 0 | 0 | 54 |
| 2 | 4 | 3 | 1 | 0/1 | 0/1 | 0 | 0 | 32 |
| 3 | 5 | 2 | 3 | 0/3 | 0/3 | 0 | 0 | 43 |
| 4 | 17 | 2 | 15 | 3/15 | 1/15 | 1 | 1 | 88 |

* Number of patients with residual carcinoma in the resected colon specimen/total number of patients undergoing colon resection. There were 29 polypectomy sites, but only 28 resected specimens because 1 patient had 2 polyps with invasive adenocarcinoma.
(Courtesy of Kyzer S, Bégin LR, Gordon PH, et al: *Cancer* 70:2044–2050, 1992.)

not appear to worsen the likelihood of lymph node metastases, lymphovascular invasion was highly associated with the risk of such an event.

Abstract 10–35 essentially draws the same conclusion: Invasive adenocarcinoma invading the surgical polypectomy specimen to level IV should be considered for resection.

Abstract 10–34 more directly addresses a group of patients treated with polypectomy alone for invasive adenocarcinoma. Again, the only recurrences developed in patients with sessile lesions (level IV). As long as the tumor was not undifferentiated, further treatment was not recommended. Once again, sessile polyps with invasive carcinoma (level IV) or pedunculated polyps with invasion into the submucosa of the bowel wall should be treated with resection.—T.J. Eberlein, M.D.

---

**Perioperative Blood Transfusion and Determinants of Survival After Liver Resection for Metastatic Colorectal Carcinoma**
Rosen CB, Nagorney DM, Taswell HF, Helgeson SL, Ilstrup DM, van Heerden JA, Adson MA (Mayo Clinic and Found, Rochester, Minn)
*Ann Surg* 216:493–505, 1992                                              10–36

---

*Background.*—For patients with colorectal carcinoma that metastasizes to the liver, resection is the only treatment that can achieve long-term survival; however, there is disagreement as to whether survival can be attributed to the operation itself or to selection. There have been several attempts to identify prognostic determinants for survival, with the significance of these determinants varying between studies. A retrospective study sought to determine the effect of perioperative transfusion on survival, to identify factors with prognostic value, and to estimate how many patients would be needed to demonstrate the efficacy of liver resection in a prospective, ranomized trial.

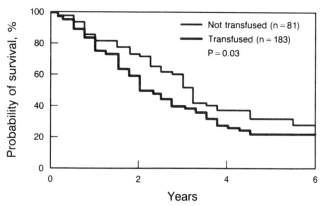

**Fig 10–7.**—Perioperative blood transfusion and probability of survival after liver resection. (Courtesy of Rosen CB, Nagorney DM, Taswell HF, et al: *Ann Surg* 216:493–505, 1992.)

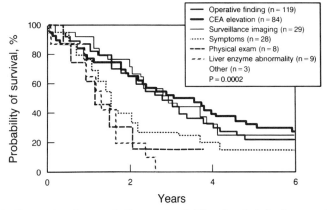

**Fig 10–8.**—Presentation of metastatic disease and probability of survival after liver resection. (Courtesy of Rosen CB, Nagorney DM, Taswell HF, et al: *Ann Surg* 216:493–505, 1992.)

*Methods.*—The analysis included 280 consecutive patients who underwent potentially curative liver resection for metastatic colorectal carcinoma during a 27-year period. Of these, 173 were men and 107 women (mean age, 59 years). All but 10 were followed for at least 5 years after operation or through 1990.

*Findings.*—At a median follow-up of 51 months, 64 patients were disease free; at a median of 35 months, 19 patients had recurrent disease. The overall 5-year survival rate was 25%, with a median survival of 2.8 years. The 60-day operative mortality rate was 4%. Most deaths were caused by clinically recurrent disease. Survival was significantly better in the 81 patients who did not receive blood from 1 week before to 2 weeks after surgery compared with the 183 patients who received at least 1 unit—32% vs. 21% at 5 years, excluding operative deaths (Fig 10–7).

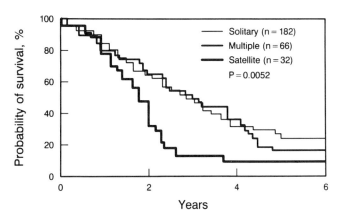

**Fig 10–9.**—Configuration of metastases and probability of survival after liver resection. (Courtesy of Rosen CB, Nagorney DM, Taswell HF, et al: *Ann Surg* 216:493–505, 1992.)

Survival was reduced in patients with extrahepatic disease, extrahepatic lymph node involvement, satellite configuration of multiple metastases, and initial detection by liver enzyme abnormalities; prognosis was better in patients with a synchronous presentation of metastatic and stage B primary disease (Fig 10–8 and 10–9). According to an exponential survival model, the number of patients needed in a prospective randomized trial would be 36 if 5-year survival without resection was 1%, 74 if 5%, 168 if 10%, and 428 if 15%.

*Conclusion.*—Perioperative blood transfusion may be adversely associated with survival in patients undergoing liver resection for metastatic colorectal carcinoma. The factors suggesting a poor survival included a satellite pattern of metastases and initial detection by clinical examination, or a liver enzyme abnormality. Unfortunately, any randomized trial of this treatment would be impractical, at least for a single center, because of the large sample required. Resection would appear to offer a better chance of survival in selected patients, but only if the tumor can be completely extirpated at operation.

▶ This series reported, as in other large series (1, 2), that extrahepatic disease, lymph node involvement, satellite configuration of the metastases, detection of metastases by clinical examination, or liver enzyme abnormality predicted a poor survival. The finding that perioperative transfusion, whole blood, and packed red blood cells were adversely associated with patient survival was not significant when other porgnostic determinants were considered in a multivariate analysis.

Blood transfusions increase suppressor cell activity, inhibit natural killer cell activity, and increase $\alpha_2$-macroglobulin (which causes lymphocyte suppression), and cause increased levels of prostaglandin $E_2$, which increases suppressor cell activity and inhibits interleukin-2 production. There may well be a biological explanation for this observation; however, in a more general clinical approach, surgeons recognize that clinical improvement in patient status is greatest when blood loss is minimized, thereby decreasing the need for fluid and blood product replacement, potential admission to the intensive care unit, and the other cardiopulmonary effects associated with a decreased blood volume.—T.J. Eberlein, M.D.

*References*

1. Hughes KS, et al: *Surgery* 103:278, 1988.
2. Nakamura S, et al: *Br J Surg* 73:727, 1986.

**High-Dose Preoperative Radiation and Radical Sphincter-Preserving Surgery for Rectal Cancer**

Marks G, Mohiuddin M, Eitan A, Masoni L, Rakinic J (Thomas Jefferson Univ Hosp, Philadelphia, Pa; Rambam Univ Hosp, Haifa, Israel; La Sapienza Univ,

Rome, Italy)
*Arch Surg* 126:1534–1540, 1991

*Introduction.* —In 1976 a selective program of high-dose radiation therapy and sphincter-preserving surgery for treatment of clinicopathologically unfavorable and low-lying rectal cancers was begun. The primary goals were to reduce local recurrence and to extend the scope of anal sphincter preservation.

*Patients and Methods.*—The 143 patients included 82 men and 61 women (mean age, 62 years). High-energy photon therapy, 40 to 60 Gy, was given for 4.5 to 6 weeks in doses of 1.8–2.5 Gy. After another 4.5 to 5 weeks, patients were reevaluated to determine the best sphincter-preserving procedure. The procedure was combined abdominal nontranssacral resection in 61 patients, transabdominal transanal resection in 50, and low anterior resection in 32. Patients were followed for a median of 50 months.

*Outcome.*—No patient died in the postoperative period. Perioperative and delayed complications occurred in 24% of patients, the most common being an anastomotic leak (Table 1). Local recurrence occurred in 13% of the 117 patients followed for at least 2 years (Table 2). The 5-year actuarial survival rate was estimated at 80%. Anorectal function was judged as acceptable in 91% of the patients.

*Conclusions.*—In patients with high-risk rectal cancers, including those in the distal third of the rectum, high-dose preoperative radiation therapy and sphincter-preserving surgery can offer good results. Survival was unexpectedly good, and control of local recurrence was achieved with acceptable morbidity and zero mortality.

Table 1.—Perioperative and Delayed Morbidity

| Cause of Morbidity | CATS Resection (n = 61) | TATA Resection (n = 50) | LAR (n = 32) | Total (N = 143) |
|---|---|---|---|---|
| Technical complications of surgery | 0 | 1 | 0 | 1 |
| Presacral hemorrhage | 0 | 0 | 1 | 1 |
| Sacral wound infection | 5 | 0 | 0 | 5 |
| Pelvic infections | 2 | 3 | 0 | 5 |
| Anastomotic complications | | | | |
| Disruptions | 2 | 0 | 1 | 3 |
| Leaks | 6 | 3 | 2 | 11 |
| Strictures | 2 | 1 | 0 | 3 |
| Pulmonary embolism | 0 | 1 | 0 | 1 |
| Deep-vein thrombosis | 0 | 1 | 0 | 1 |
| Adhesive small-bowel obstruction | 2 | 2 | 0 | 4 |
| Total | 19 | 12 | 4 | 35 |

*Abbreviations:* CATS, combined abdominotranssacral; TATA, transabdominal transanal; LAR, low anterior resection.

(Courtesy of Marks G, Mohiuddin M, Eitan A, et al: *Arch Surg* 126:1534–1540, 1991.)

Table 2.—Local Recurrence After High-Dose
Radiation Therapy in 117 Patients Followed Up for
24 Months or Longer

| Stage | No./Total (%) of Cases |
|---|---|
| Favorable | 0/35 |
| Unfavorable | |
| B2 | 5/43 (12) |
| C1 | 2/12 (17) |
| C2 | 8/27 (30) |
| **Total** | **15/82 (18)** |

(Courtesy of Marks G, Mohiuddin M, Eitan A, et al: *Arch Surg* 126:1534–1540, 1991.)

## Preoperative Irradiation and Surgery for Initially Unresectable Adenocarcinoma of the Rectum

Mendenhall WM, Souba WW, Bland KI, Million RR, Copeland EM III (Univ of Florida, Gainesville)
*Am Surg* 58:423–429, 1992                    10–38

*Objective.*—The management of incompletely resectable rectal adenocarcinoma is controversial and generally disappointing. The value of preoperative radiation therapy was assessed in 42 patients with rectal adenocarcinoma that was unresectable initally.

*Patients.*—The study group constituted about one fourth of the patients who had planned preoperative irradiation and surgery with cura-

Preoperative Irradiation and Surgery

| Study | Minimum Follow-Up | Number of Patients | Number Having Surgery | Number Having Complete Resection | Local Recurrence | 5-Year Survival Rate |
|---|---|---|---|---|---|---|
| University of Oregon (1960-1982) | Not stated | 35 | 20 (57%) | 18 (51%)* | 9/18 (50%)† | 12%‡ |
| Massachusetts General Hospital (1970-1976) | 3.5 years | 25 | 19 (76%) | 16 (64%) | 5/13 (38%)¶ | 28%§ |
| Tufts (1968-1977) | Not stated | 44‖ | 38 (86%) | 26 (59%) | 5/26 (19%) | Not stated |
| University of Florida Present Series (1970-1986) | 5 years | 42 | 41 (98%) | 21 (50%) | 10/21 (48%) | 6/42 (14%) |
| Uppsala University (1979-1985) | Not stated | 44 | 27 (61%) | 11 (25%) | Not stated | Not stated |
| University of Bergen (1976-1981) | Not stated | 55 | 42 (76%) | 15 (27%) | 1/15 ( 7%) | Not stated |

* Includes unspecified number of patients with positive margins.
† Seven of 9 patients had tumor at surgical margins.
‡ For overall group of 40 patients.
§ Actuarial survival.
¶ Three postoperative deaths excluded.
‖ Includes 4 sigmoid colon lesions and 1 transverse colon lesion.
(Courtesy of Mendenhall WM, Souba WW, Bland KI, et al: *Am Surg* 58:423–429, 1992.)

tive intent for previously untreated rectal adenocarcinoma between 1970 and 1986. All 42 were followed for 5 years or longer. Thirty-five patients had persistent disease or recurrence after treatment.

*Management.*—Five of the 42 patients had exploratory laparotomy before radiation therapy. Thirty patients received 4,500–5,000 cGy before operation; only 4 received less than 4,000 cGy. The 41 survivors (1 patient died of aspiration pneumonia) underwent surgery a mean of 4.5 weeks after radiation therapy was completed.

*Results.*—Cancer was resected in 37 patients, completely in 21 of them. Two patients died after operation. Five patients had significant postoperative complications. Pelvic disease was controlled in half of the patients with apparently complete resection of disease and in 7 others. The absolute 5-year survival rate was 14%, but it was 29% in those who had a complete resection.

*Discussion.*—Preoperative irradiation has yielded mixed results in patients with inoperable rectal adenocarcinoma (table). High-dose radiation therapy alone may palliate patients, but the chance of cure is small. The best approach may be preoperative irradiation and surgery, possibly combined with intraoperative radiation therapy. The role of chemotherapy also deserves to be considered.

---

**Does Preoperative Radiation Therapy Enhance the Probability of Local Control and Survival in High-Risk Distal Rectal Cancer?**

Mendenhall WM, Bland KI, Copeland EM III, Summers GE, Pfaff WW, Souba WW, Million RR (Univ of Florida, Gainesville)
*Ann Surg* 215:696–706, 1992                                    10–39

---

*Background.*—Reported local recurrence rates for adenocarcinoma of the rectum and rectosigmoid in patients treated with operation alone range from 18% to 30%. Since 1975, patients with clinically resectable rectal cancer treated at 1 hospital have been given preoperative radiation therapy to decrease the risk of local recurrence. The outcome in patients given irradiation before operation was compared with that in patients treated before 1975 with operation alone.

*Patients.*—Between 1975 and 1986, 148 patients with clinically resectable adenocarcinoma of the rectum and rectosigmoid underwent preoperative radiation therapy. All patients had at least 5 years of follow-up. Three different radiation protocols were used during the study period: 1975–1978, 3,100 cGy in 12 fractions or 3,500 cGy in 20 fractions; 1979–1983, 4,000–5,000 cGy at 180 cGy per fraction; and 1984–1986, 3,000 cGy in 10 fractions. The results in a subset of 132 patients with locally advanced lesions treated with preoperative radiation therapy and resection were compared with those in 132 patients with stages B2 and C cancers who underwent complete resection alone before 1976.

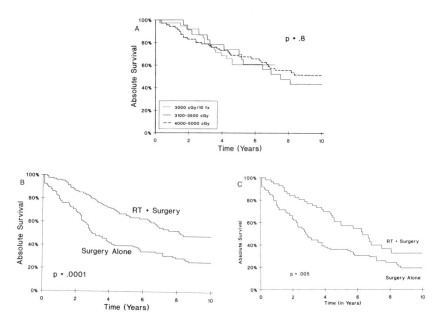

**Fig 10–10.**—Absolute survival. **A,** preoperative radiation therapy (132 patients). The absolute survival rates at 5 years were 3,100–3,500 cGy, 70%; 4,000–5,000 cGy, 67%; 3,000 cGy in 10 fractions, 61% (P = .798). **B,** preoperative radiation therapy and surgery (132 patients) compared with surgery alone (135 patients). Absolute survival at 5 years was 66% after preoperative radiation therapy and surgery and 40% after surgery alone (P = .0001). **C,** preoperative radiation therapy (56 patients with tethered or annular lesions) compared with surgery alone (98 patients with stage B2 and C lesions). Absolute survival at 5 years was 61% after preoperative radiation therapy and surgery compared with 36% after surgery alone (P = .0054). (Courtesy of Mendenhall WM, Bland KI, Copeland EM III, et al: *Ann Surg* 215:696–706, 1992.)

*Results.*—There were no statistically significant differences in survival between patients treated with the various irradiation schedules (Fig 10–10). Absolute survival at 5 years, however, was 66% after preoperative radiation therapy and resection and 40% after resection alone. This difference was statistically significant. Absolute survival at 5 years in patients with locally advanced lesions treated with preoperative radiation therapy and resection was 61%, compared with 36% in patients with stages B2 and C lesions treated with surgery alone. This difference was also statistically significant. Postoperative complication rates in the preoperatively irradiated patients and those who had surgery alone were similar.

*Conclusions.*—Preoperative radiation therapy in patients with resectable adenocarcinoma of the rectum and rectosigmoid significantly improves local recurrence rates and 5-year survival rates.

▶ These 3 studies address issues surrounding preoperative radiation therapy. The first article (Abstract 10–37) investigates high-dose radiation therapy and radical sphincter-preserving surgery for distal rectal cancers. By stringent patient evaluation, these authors were able to preserve anal function with little morbidity. As would be expected, the major morbidity associated with preoperative radiation resulted from an anastomotic leak and local recurrence, which was most prevalent in C2 lesions. The 80% 5-year actuarial survival is most likely attributable to skilled patient selection as well as radical surgical procedures after radiation. The authors do not comment on the downstaging of tumors as a result of the preoperative radiation therapy. Thus, in selected patients, preoperative radiation therapy can extend the indications for sphincter preservation.

In Abstract 10–38, the authors report data concerning 42 patients with unresectable rectal adenocarcinoma who were treated with preoperative radiation therapy followed by surgery. As was expected, control of pelvic disease was higher in patients who underwent complete resection, in contrast to incomplete or no resection. Incomplete resection remains controversial. It should be emphasized that it is very difficult to compare various regimens of preoperative radiation therapy because of variables in technique, patient selection, and data analysis. However, it would seem that, because adjuvant protocols involving radiation therapy and chemotherapy have been effective, the preoperative regimen should consist of a similar strategy, perhaps with or without intraoperative radiation therapy to diminish the risk of pelvic disease.

Abstract 10–39 questions whether preoperative radiation therapy extends survival in patients with resectable rectal cancers. Three separate regimens of radiation therapy were used, and no difference between these groups was found. Although group having radiation therapy and surgery reported improved survival when compared to similar historical patients treated without radiation, the reader should be cautioned against overinterpreting the results because of this historical control comparison. More important, however, is that local recurrence rates and overall survival were quite good. Several additional points deserve emphasis: First, to administer radiation therapy to the appropriate patient assumes familiarity with rectal ultrasound; second, with regard to accurately staging the tumor, it is difficult to comment about downstaging because patients treated before surgery are compared with those treated with surgery when knowledge of the extent of downstaging is available. In this series, however, 11% of the patients had no residual disease.

Clinical trials to explore this issue are necessary because postoperative radiation therapy reportedly decreases local recurrence but does not improve 5-year survival unless chemotherapy is added. Thus clinical trials looking at preoperative radiation therapy will be difficult to perform without the inclusion of chemotherapy.—T.J. Eberlein, M.D.

---

**Radiation Therapy and Fluorouracil With or Without Semustine for the Treatment of Patients With Surgical Adjuvant Adenocarcinoma of the Rectum**

Gastrointestinal Tumor Study Group (EMMES Corp, Potomac, Md)

*J Clin Oncol* 10:549–557, 1992                                    10–40

---

*Background.*—The Gastrointestinal Tumor Study Group (GITSG) demonstrated previously that postoperative radiation therapy and chemotherapy with fluorouracil (5-FU) and semustine (MeCCNU) decreased the recurrence rate of rectal cancer in the pelvis. However, MeCCNU was subsequently shown to be leukemogenic. Therefore, the importance of MeCCNU to the adjuvant regimen was reevaluated by the GITSG.

*Methods.*—Previously untreated patients with histologically proved adenocarcinoma of the rectum who had undergone curative resection were randomized to treatment with combination radiation therapy and 5-FU followed by either 1 year of 5-FU and MeCCNU or 6 months of escalating doses of 5-FU. Eleven of the 210 patients enrolled were excluded, leaving 199 eligible for the study.

*Results.*—In both treatment groups about half of the patients experienced severe treatment-related toxicity. There was 1 treatment-related death in each group. No episodes of leukemia were detected. The median follow-up was almost 6 years. Recurrent disease developed in about 50% of each group of patients. The probability of a 3-year disease-free survival was 54% in the group given combination therapy and 68% in the group given increasing doses of 5-FU. Approximately half of the patients in each group died during the course of the study.

*Conclusions.*—Significant differences between the 2 treatment groups in survival or recurrence were not observed. Therefore, it is concluded that MeCCNU is not an essential component of successful postoperative combined modality treatment of adjuvant rectal cancer.

▶ This report, a product of the GITSG, examined the necessity of including MeCCNU as a component of postoperative combination chemotherapy in treatment of rectal cancer. Escalating doses of 5-FU reportedly resulted in a lower risk of recurrent disease but equaled the toxicity in the MeCCNU-treated patients. This conclusion reflects a significant improvement in adjuvant rectal trials, the authors' data have been corroborated by another cooperative group (1).—T.J. Eberlein, M.D.

*Reference*

1. O'Connell M, et al: *Proc Am Soc Clin Oncol* 10:134, 1991.

RECURRENCE

### Patterns of Recurrence After Curative Resection of Carcinoma of the Colon and Rectum

Galandiuk S, Wieand HS, Moertel CG, Cha SS, Fitzgibbons RJ Jr, Pemberton JH, Wolff BG (Mayo Clinic and Found, Rochester, Minn; Creighton Univ,

Omaha, Neb)
*Surg Gynecol Obstet* 174:27–32, 1992                                          10–41

*Background.*—Carcinoma of the colon and rectum is common and is prone to frequent, and often fatal, recurrence. Tumor characteristics including location, Dukes' stage, grade, ploidy and perforation, obstruction, adherence or invasion of adjacent tissue, were examined to determine whether sites and timing of recurrence could be predicted.

*Methods.*—Data were collected from 818 patients who had undergone curative resection for Dukes' stage $B_2$ or C carcinoma of the colon and rectum and were being treated with 1 of 3 adjuvant protocols.

*Results.*—Of the 818 patients, 353 had disease recurrence. The median time to recurrence was 16.7 months. Dukes' C lesions, adhesion, perforation, or invasion were significantly associated with earlier recurrence. The most frequent recurrence sites were hepatic, pulmonary, local or regional, intra-abdominal, and retroperitoneal, in that order. When the primary site was rectal, there were more local or regional recurrences and fewer retroperitoneal recurrences than when the primary site was colonic. Stage C primary tumors led to fewer local or regional recurrences than stage B primary tumors, but were associated with a greater tendency to involve retroperitoneal or peripheral nodes. Colonic primary tumors that invaded or adhered to other organs had a lesser tendency toward pulmonary metastases. The degree of anaplasia and ploidy had a significant effect on recurrence rate, but not on timing or patterns of recurrence.

*Conclusions.*—In this series, Dukes' stage C and invasion or adhesion of adjacent organs were significantly associated with earlier recurrence. The most frequent recurrence sites were hepatic and pulmonary. This type of information may allow more precise follow-up evaluation and earlier detection of recurrence, allowing for more effective retreatment.

▶ This series included 818 patients in whom patterns of recurrence were examined. Earlier recurrence was associated with Dukes' C classification, adherence, or invasion of other organs. Perforation was also found to be associated with earlier recurrence.

Because surgeons most frequently follow patients with colorectal cancer, they tend to focus on intralumenal recurrence by performing colonoscopy and measuring the level of carcinoembryonic antigen. Only a small percentage of patients in this series had intralumenal recurrence. The vast majority of recurrences were distant liver and pulmonary metastases. This paper emphasizes the need for systemic adjuvant treatment of colorectal cancer.—T.J. Eberlein, M.D.

### Technical and Biological Factors in Disease-Free Survival After Hepatic Resection for Colorectal Cancer Metastases

Cady B, Stone MD, McDermott WV Jr, Jenkins RL, Bothe A Jr, Lavin PT, Lovett EJ, Steele GD Jr (New England Deaconess Hosp, Boston, Mass; Harvard Med School, Boston; Univ of Southern Maine, Portland)

*Arch Surg* 127:561–569, 1992                    10–42

*Introduction.*—The selection of patients for hepatic resection of metastatic colorectal cancer is a matter of controversy. Because few of these patients achieve long-term, disease-free survival, some question whether hepatic resection has any role at all. Preoperative and postoperative prognostic factors were sought in a review of 129 patients who underwent hepatic resection for colorectal cancer metastases, survived the operation, and had a curative resection.

*Methods.*—Technical factors examined included the margins of resection, specimen weight, use of cryotherapy, type of hepatic resection, and blood transfusion. Among the biological factors analyzed were the highest level of carcinoembryonic antigen (CEA) obtained before hepatic resection, the number of nodules of metastatic disease, the maximum diameter of the largest matastatic lesion, and the number of satellite lesions.

*Results.*—Neither patient age nor any clinical feature of the primary cancer correlated with the rate of disease-free survival. The disease-free interval from primary colon resection to hepatic resection ranged from 0 to 282 months (median, 17 months), and it was not related to survival. Increasing preoperative levels of CEA signaled a worsening prognosis. No disease-free survivors had preoperative levels of CEA above 200 ng/mL. The number of hepatic metastases and the weight of the specimen also were significant prognostic factors; no patient with 3 or more nodules or with a specimen weight of 1,000 g or more survived disease free beyond 48 months. Whereas patients with a negative margin had a 50% 5-year disease-free expectation, no patients with a positive microscopic margin survived disease free beyond 20 months. Patients with diploid metastases fared better than those with nondiploid metastases.

*Conclusions.*—Multivariate analysis found the most important favorable prognostic factor to be a surgical margin of 1 cm or greater. Nonhepatic recurrence, however, was unrelated to surgical margins. There is a need for improved patient selection criteria. Also, intraoperative liver examination by ultrasound during primary colon cancer resection is strongly recommended.

▶ This article examines a large series of patients undergoing hepatic resection for colorectal cancer. Several points of this manuscript require emphasis. Before hepatic surgery is contemplated, patients should be younger than 80 years and in good physical condition. Further, their primary tumor site should be controlled, with less than 4 metastatic nodules and no evidence of metastatic disease outside the liver; the CEA level should be less than 200 ng/mL. Intraoperative ultrasound is strongly recommended for its accuracy and reproducibility.

The most important factor in analysis of results in these patients, however, is the technical achievement of a 1 cm or greater surgical margin.

Despite advances made in both patient selection and the technique of hepatic resection, the overall rate of survival will not be greatly enhanced until better systemic therapy is available.—T.J. Eberlein, M.D.

MISCELLANEOUS

## Local Immunity and Metastasis of Colorectal Carcinoma

Kubota Y, Sunouchi K, Ono M, Sawada T, Muto T (Univ of Tokyo, Tokyo, Japan)

*Dis Colon Rectum* 35:645–650, 1992                                    10–43

*Background.*—Although the finding of tumor-infiltrating lymphocytes (TILs) may represent a host response against the tumor, decreases in a variety of in vitro and in vivo immunologic responses are seen in patients with cancer. Depression of these responses has been attributed to increased activity of suppressor cells e.g. prostaglandin. Prostaglandin $E_2$ ($PGE_2$), if it plays an important part as an immunosuppressive agent, could affect TILs at the tumor site and enhance metastasis. The effects of local immunity in the metastasis of colorectal carcinoma were studied.

*Methods.*—The subsets of TILs and $PGE_2$ were measured in resected specimens from patients with colorectal cancer. Fourteen patients had metastases and 32 did not. Immunohistochemical staining of frozen tissues was performed to evaluate the subsets of TILs, with the number of positive cells expressed as the number positive per $250 \times 250 \ \mu m^2$.

*Findings.*—Marked lymphocytic infiltration was more common in cancers without metastasis (table). Early cancers had larger numbers of T cells and natural killer cells, which decreased in parallel with the presence of metastasis. The $PGE_2$ level, measured by radioimmunoassay, was higher in blood from the draining vein than in blood from the feeding

Lymphocytic Infiltration and Metastasis

| | Lymphocytic Infiltration | | |
| --- | --- | --- | --- |
| | Little | Moderate | Marked |
| Metastasis | | | |
| (−) (n = 48) | 14 (29%) | 13 (27%) | 21 (44%) |
| (+) (n = 34) | 22 (61%) | 9 (25%) | 3 (8%) |

$\chi^2 = 14; P < .01.$
(Courtesy of Kubota Y, Sunouchi K, Ono M, et al: *Dis Colon Rectum* 35:645-650, 1992.)

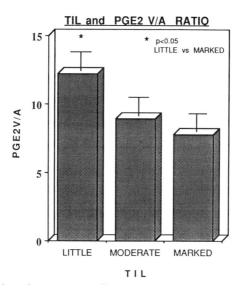

**Fig 10–11.**—Correlation between tumor-infiltrating lymphocyte (*TIL*) and prostaglandin E$_2$ vein/artery (*PGE$_2$ V/A*) ratio. The number of TIL was decreased in parallel with the increase of PGE$_2$ V/A ratio. (Courtesy of Kubota Y, Sunouchi K, Ono M, et al: *Dis Colon Rectum* 35:645–650, 1992.)

artery. Metastatic cancers had a higher PGE$_2$: draining vein/feeding artery ratio than nonmetastatic cancers. As this ratio increased, the number of TILs decreased (Fig 10–11).

*Conclusions.*—Tumor-infiltrating lymphocytes and PGE$_2$ may play an important role in the metastasis of colorectal carcinoma. The effect of PGE$_2$ may be to suppress local immunity and thus enhance metastasis.

▶ This article discusses the influence of the immune system on the rate of metastatic growth and looks at 2 specific immunologic markers. One is the lymphocytic infiltrate, which when present is associated with a lower rate of metastasis, and the other is the PGE$_2$ level, which when elevated may suppress local immunity, thus enhancing metastatic potential.

There are many reports in the literature of lymphocytic infiltrates, natural killer cell activity, delayed-type hypersensitivity, and so on associated with metastatic potential. Only through a more thorough understanding of the immune response to tumors will we be able to identify parameters that can be manipulated to adversely affect the metastatic potential of cancer.—T.J. Eberlein, M.D.

**Role of the Rectum in the Physiological and Clinical Results of Coloanal and Colorectal Anastomosis After Anterior Resection for Rectal Carcinoma**
Lewis WG, Holdsworth PJ, Stephenson BM, Finan PJ, Johnston D (The Gen

Infirmary, Leeds, England)
*Br J Surg* 79:1082–1086, 1992

*Introduction.*—Low anterior resection is generally done to preserve the anal sphincter and restore intestinal continuity in patients undergoing potentially curative resection for rectal cancer. Although this procedure improves quality of life over abdominoperineal resection, and survival is just as good, up to half of the patients have problems with anorectal function. The relationships between length of the residual anorectum, anorectal physiologic function, and clinical outcome were studied in 34 patients undergoing anterior resection for rectal carcinoma.

*Methods.*—The patients underwent anal sphincter function studies at a median of 13 months postoperatively. Ten patients who had undergone sigmoid colectomy for carcinoma without rectal excision also were studied. An independent clinical assessment of anal continence was performed, and these data were correlated with patient responses to a questionnaire regarding quality of life (table).

*Results.*—Patients who had a coloanal anastomosis had lower resting anal pressure and lesser rectal capacity than those who had a colorectal anastomosis. All patients had an intact rectoanal inhibitory reflex, but maximal anal pressure during this reflex was lower after coloanal anastomosis. In the group having coloanal anastomosis, the volume required for maximal sphincter inhibition also was lower. The median bowel frequency was 4 movements per day after coloanal anastomosis vs. 2 per day after colorectal anastomosis at 1 year postoperatively; the former group also had a greater degree of urgency of defecation.

*Conclusions.*—In patients undergoing anterior resection for rectal cancer, the length of rectum preserved has a significant impact on anorectal function and thus on quality of life. Rectal length affects the func-

---

Characteristics of Patients and Clinical Results

| | Coloanal anastomosis | Colorectal anastomosis | | |
| --- | --- | --- | --- | --- |
| | | <4 cm | ≥4 cm | >12 cm |
| No. of patients | 11 | 12 | 11 | 10 |
| Median age (years) | 65 (58–61) | 69 (43–77) | 66 (43–81) | 68 (48–79) |
| Sex ratio (M:F) | 5:6 | 7:5 | 5:6 | 4:6 |
| Median follow-up (months) | 11 (4–100) | 17 (5–76) | 13 (4–36) | 27 (9–54) |
| Median height of anastomosis above HPZ (cm) | 0 (0–2) | 3·5 (3–4) | 5 (4·5–6) | >12 |
| Median bowel frequency per 24 h | 4 (2–8) | 3 (1–10) | 2 (1–4) | 1 (1–4)* |
| Urgency (*n*) | 5 | 4 | 0† | 0† |
| Faecal leakage (*n*) | 8 | 8 | 2 | 0* |

Values in parentheses are ranges.
*Abbreviation:* HPZ, anal canal high-pressure zone.
* *P* < .01.
† *P* < .02 (vs. coloanal and < 4 cm, Fisher's exact test).
(Courtesy of Lewis WG, Holdsworth PJ, Stephenson BM, et al: *Br J Surg* 79:1082–1086, 1992.)

tional capacity of the neorectum and, thereby, the degree of anal sphincter inhibition during the neorectoanal inhibitory reflex. A colonic J pouch anastomosed to the upper anal canal may be considered for patients who need complete rectal excision. If possible, more than 4 cm of distal rectum above the anal canal high-pressure zone should be preserved for patients with tumors of the upper rectum.

▶ This is a physiological study of the rectum and its role in the results of coloanal and colorectal anastomoses after anterior resection. Surgeons strive for lower and lower anastomoses in an attempt to preserve the rectum; this paper objectively analyzes the impact of the length of rectum, as well as the neural and physiologic reflexes, after coloanal or colorectal anastomoses. In contrast to the assumption that anal continence is preserved when the internal anal sphincter and skeletal musculature of the pelvic floor remain intact during excision for carcinoma, this study introduces practical implications for carcinomas in the lower half of the rectum where complete rectal excision is necessary. A colonic J pouch anastomosis to the upper anal canal should be considered. For lesions in the upper half of the rectum, the patient's quality of life will be improved if more than 4 cm of distal rectum above the anal canal high-pressure zone can be preserved.

As noted in many previous reports concerning rectal surgery for adenocarcinoma, local recurrence can be avoided by obtaining adequate lateral circumferential margins and at least a 2-cm distal normal margin.—T.J. Eberlein, M.D.

## Tumor Biology and Basic Science

**Immunoregulation in Cancer-Bearing Hosts: Down-Regulation of Gene Expression and Cytotoxic Function in CD8+ T Cells**
Loeffler CM, Smyth MJ, Longo DL, Kopp WC, Harvey LK, Tribble HR, Tase JE, Urba WJ, Leonard AS, Young HA, Ochoa AC (Program Resources, Inc/DynCorp, Frederick, Md; Univ of Minnesota, Minneapolis; Natl Cancer Inst-Frederick Cancer Research and Development Ctr, Frederick, Md)
J Immunol 149:949–956, 1992
10–45

*Background.*—The causes of reduced immune responsiveness in tumor-bearing hosts are not well understood. No one has studied the impact of a decreased immune response in cancer patients on the clinical response in immunotherapy trials. Immunoregulation in cancer-bearing hosts was explored.

*Methods and Findings.*—There was a marked reduction in the treatment efficacy of adoptively transferred T lymphocytes obtained from murine hosts bearing tumor for more than 30 days compared with normal mice and mice with tumors for less than 21 days. An in vitro analysis of the functions of the T lymphocytes from the late tumor-bearing mice (TBM) demonstrated an apparently normal proliferative response to anti-CD3 and interleukin-2 (IL-2) with adequate lymphokine production

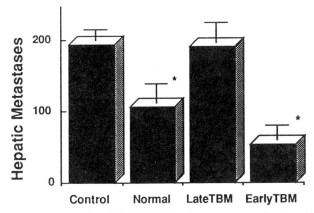

**Fig 10–12.**—Mice were treated with T-AK cells derived from non–tumor-bearing mice (normal) or mice bearing tumor for less than 21 days (early TBM) or more than 30 days (late TBM). Hepatic metastases were counted 12 days after tumor inoculation. Groups were compared using the Wilcoxon Rank sum test. *P < .001 vs. control; *bars* = SD. (Courtesy of Loeffler CM, Smyth MJ, Longo DL, et al: *J Immunol* 149:949-956, 1992.)

from CD4+ cells. There was a significant drop, however, in the cytotoxic function of CD8+ cells. The reduced cytotoxicity did not result from cell-mediated suppression. In CD8+ cells from late TBM, the expression of granzyme B mRNA was significantly delayed and lessened in magnitude. Culture supernatants from 2 unrelated tumor cell lines inhibited the cytotoxic activity of normal CD8+ cells in vitro. (Figs 10–12 and 10–13; table).

*Conclusions.*—The degree of immune responsiveness of T lymphocytes, particularly the CD8+ subset, appears to be an important part of the success of adoptive transfer of T-AK cells plus IL-2 in this animal model. It may also be important in human immunotherapy trials. Careful immunologic assessment of patients before they undergo immunotherapy may be able to identify those whose T cells have not been suppressed by a tumor product and who therefore may be more likely to respond to immunologic therapy.

▶ This study provides a significant example of the mechanism for lack of an immune response in tumor-bearing hosts. Specifically, these authors look at CD8+ effector T cells and show that they have diminished cytotoxic activity because of a delayed and decreased expression of granzyme B messenger RNA. It is not known, however, whether this decreased cytotoxicity is responsible for the lack of therapeutic efficacy of these cells in vivo, or whether it may simply reflect derangement of the immune response caused by the progressive tumor growth. Few reports associate in vitro lytic activity with in vivo therapeutic efficacy. However, CD8+ subsets of T cells are important elements in the success of adoptive transfer of T cells plus IL-2 in both animal and human immunotherapy trials. In human trials, most patients

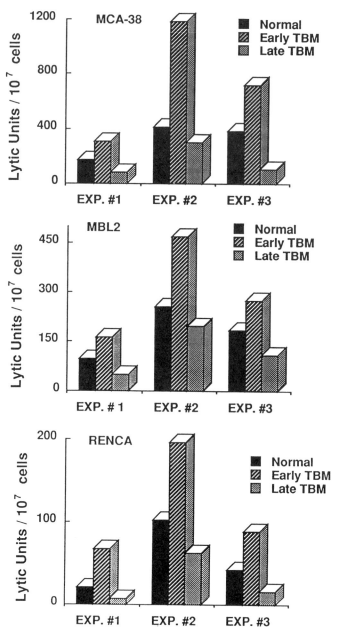

**Fig 10–13.**—Cytolytic activity of normal, early, and late TBM T-AK cells against MCA-38 (colon carcinoma), MBL2 (lymphoma), and RENCA (renal cell carcinoma) tumor cell lines. Enriched T cells were activiated with anti-CD3 100 units of rIL-2/mL. Lytic function was tested on day 2 of culture. (Courtesy of Loeffler CM, Smyth MJ, Longo DL, et al: *J Immunol* 149:949–956, 1992.)

Suppression of In Vitro Cytolytic Activity of Normal Lymphocytes
by Tumor Cell Supernatant

| Cells | Lytic U/$10^7$ cells | | |
|---|---|---|---|
| | Experiment 1 | Experiment 2 | Experiment 3 |
| Normals | 138 | 93 | 118 |
| Supernatant | | | |
| 10% | 126 | 116 | 126 |
| 30% | 99 | 89 | 66 |
| 50% | 83 | 48 | 21 |

Note: Suppression of cytolytic activity of normal lymphocytes by supernatant of MCA-38 cells in culture. Lymphocytes were activated with anti-CD3 and cultured with 100 units/mL of IL-2. Various concentrations of supernatant from MCA-38 tumor cultures were titrated into the cell cultures. Cultures were started at $1.5 \times 10^6$ cells/mL and cell counts and cytotoxicity assays were performed on day 3 of culture.

(Courtesy of Loeffler CM, Smyth MJ, Longo DL, et al: *J Immunol* 149:949–956, 1992.)

have had very advanced disease, and one would predict that response rates might improve if tumor burdens were lessened. Future trials will attempt to carefully evaluate patients immunologically before they undergo immunotherapy to identify both T cells and cytokines that may help to regulate the immune response and/or predict for response to therapy.—T.J. Eberlein, M.D.

---

**Passive Immunization Against Tumor Necrosis Factor Inhibits Interleukin-2–Induced Microvascular Alterations and Reduces Toxicity**
Edwards MJ, Abney DL, Heniford BT, Miller FN (Univ of Louisville, Ky)
*Surgery* 112:480–486, 1992                                    10–46

---

*Introduction.*—Interleukin-2 (IL-2) mediates the regression of some malignancies, but its therapeutic efficacy is limited by dose-dependent toxicity. The acute hemodynamic instabilty and vascular leak syndrome seen after IL-2 administration occur secondary to neutrophil-mediated events in the microcirculation. Because Il-2 has few direct effects on polymorphonuclear leukocytes, it was hypothesized that IL-2–induced toxicity is mediated by tumor necrosis factor-alpha (TNF) and would be inhibited by TNF neutralizing polyclonal antibody (IP-400).

*Methods.*—The cremaster muscles of anesthetized rats were prepared for in vivo microcirculatory observations using fluorescent microscopy. Fluorescein isothiocyanate was conjugated to bovine serum albumin (FITC-BSA). Relative interstitial fluorescence was quantitated as an index of macromolecular leakage. After surgical preparation and arterial FITC-BSA injection, the animals were injected with IL-2, TNF, or IL-2 plus IP-400. Vital signs, leukocyte-endothelial interactions, and interstitial fluorescence were measured every 30 minutes for up to 2 hours after injection.

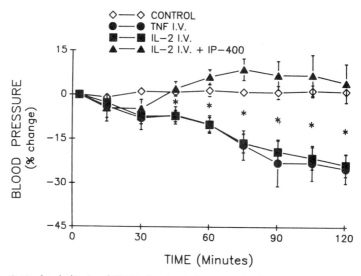

**Fig 10–14.**—Interleukin-2 and TNF induced a similar progressive decrease in mean arterial blood pressure (mm Hg) in 2 hours. Passive immunization against TNF with IP-400 effectively inhibited the IL-2-induced hypotension. *I.V.*, intravenously. *$P < .05$. (Courtesy of Edwards MJ, Abney DL, Heniford BT, et al: *Surgery* 112:480–486, 1992.)

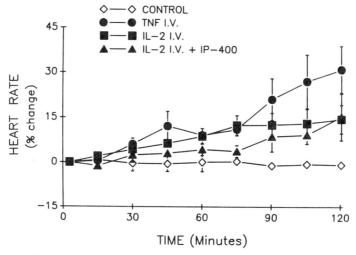

**Fig 10–15.**—Passive immunization against TNF with IP-400 did not significantly alter IL-2-induced tachycardia. Tumor necrosis factor also evoked progressive increase in heart rate. *I.V.* intravenously. (Courtesy of Edwards MJ, Abney DL, Heniford BT, et al: *Surgery* 112:480–486, 1992.)

*Results.*—Interleukin-2 and TNF injection acutely induced hypotension and tachycardia and increased macromolecular leakage and leukocyte-endothelial adherence (Fig 10–14). Tumor necrosis factor also induced progressive increases in heart rate. The addition of IP-400 to IL-2, however, effectively inhibited these events (Fig 10–15).

*Conclusions.*—Interleukin-2–induced acute microvascular alterations and hypotension are mediated by TNF. Passive immunization with IP-400 against TNF effectively inhibits the IL-2–induced vascular effects.

▶ This study addresses one of the side effects surrounding IL-2–based immunotherapy trials: microvascular alterations and hemodynamic instability. all of the high-dose IL-2 trials have been characterized by TNF production, which clearly contributes to IL-2 toxicity. However, the problem becomes more complex. There is obvious activation of neutrophils, prostaglandins, and other entities that also contribute to the toxicities associated with IL-2. In fact, neutrophil depletion before IL-2 treatment prevents the acute multiple organ edema of IL-2 therapy (1).

Tumor necrosis factor, however, is a major player in IL-2–induced hypotension and, indirectly, in hemodynamic instability. Reducing the dose and using a different molecule show that TNF is not produced under these conditions of immunotherapy and thus greatly aids in reduction of the toxicity (2).

Obviously, by reducing toxicity, immunotherapy trials may become more prevalent and therapeutically efficacious.—T.J. Eberlein, M.D.

*References*

1.  Welbourn R, et al: *Ann Surg* 214:181, 1990.
2.  Michie HR, et al: *Ann Surg* 208:493, 1988.

### Germline Mutations of the p53 Tumor-Suppressor Gene in Children and Young Adults With Second Malignant Neoplasms

Malkin D, Jolly KW, Barbier N, Look AT, Friend SH, Gebhardt MC, Andersen TI, Børresen A-L, Li FP, Garber J, Strong LC (Massachusetts Gen Hosp, Boston, Mass; Dana-Farber Cancer Inst, Boston; Children's Hosp, Boston; Harvard Med School, Boston; St Jude Children's Research Hosp, Memphis, Tenn; et al)
*N Engl J Med* 326:1309–1315, 1992                    10–47

*Background.*—Germline mutations in the p53 tumor-suppressor gene have been identified in families with the rare Li-Fraumeni syndrome. In this familial syndrome carriers of an autosomal dominant trait have a 50% probability of invasive cancer by age 30 years. Patients in families with Li-Fraumeni syndrome who survive their first cancer have a high frequency of second primary tumors. Because p53 mutations are common in nonfamilial cancers, the possibility that such mutations in the germline are associated with second primary cancers was examined in children and young adults outside kindreds known to have Li-Fraumeni syndrome.

*Methods.*—The multicenter study included 59 patients (median age, 14 years) with 2 primary malignant neoplasms. In 27 cases the second tumor arose within the radiation field of the first tumor. In the remaining 32 cases the patient had not received radiation therapy or the second tumor developed outside the radiation field. Blood was drawn from each patient for extraction of genomic DNA. Mutations of p53 were identified by the polymerase chain reaction in combination with denaturant-gel electrophoresis and sequencing.

*Results.*—Cancers in 50 patients were types associated with the Li-Fraumeni syndrome. In 25 cases both the first and second tumors had this association. Four patients (6.8%) had mutations of the p53 gene that changed the predicted sequence of amino acids. An analysis of leukoctye DNA from close relatives of 3 patients suggested inheritance of the mutations, although only 1 parent had cancer at the start of the study. Mutations in 3 cases were identical to those previously found in the p53 gene. The fourth mutation was the first germline mutation to be identified in exon 9, at codon 325. Pedigree analysis identified at least 16 other potential carriers of the p53 mutation, only 1 of whom has had cancer to date.

*Conclusions.*—Because 55 of these 59 patients did not have germline p53 mutations, their second cancer probably reflected an interaction between the underlying treatment and inactivation of numerous tumor-suppressor genes, along with other genetic factors. A knowledge of germline p53 mutations may help to prevent the development of a second cancer in young patients and to identify family members who would benefit from surveillance and early detection of tumors.

▶ This investigation examines the tumor suppressor gene p53 and its possible mutations. Early detection of such mutations would be useful not only in treating these patients but also in identifying family members who may be at high risk for the future development of tumors.

Aside from the study of gene alterations such as p53 or retinoblastoma genes, it may also be possible to learn about the genetic markers of tumor by applying genetic engineering. These genes may be replaced, therefore offering another avenue of therapy.

Gene expression, alteration, and mutation are essential to the study of breast, ovarian, and bladder cancers as well as retinoblastoma. By understanding these mechanisms, a new role in cancer therapy will be found for the molecular geneticist and molecular biologist.—T.J. Eberlein, M.D.

---

**Cellular Interactions in Effector Cell Generation and Tumor Regression Mediated by Anti-CD3/Interleukin 2-Activated Tumor-Draining**

## Lymph Node Cells

Yoshizawa H, Chang AE, Shu S (Univ of Michigan, Ann Arbor)
*Cancer Res* 52:1129–1136, 1992
10–48

*Background.*—Activating lymphoid cells with interleukin-2 (IL-2) provides a population of lymphokine-activated killer (LAK) cells that is able to lyse a broad range of tumor cells but not normal cells. Lymphocytes that infiltrate solid tumors can be expanded by incubation in IL-2 and, unlike LAK cells, exert preferential cytotoxic activity against autologous tumor cells. These TIL cells exert more potent antitumor activity than do LAK cells.

*Objective.*—The MCA 106 murine sarcoma was used to determine the T- cell phenotype of preeffector cells and the mechanisms by which these cells differentiate in vitro to acquire effector function. The progressive growth of these weakly immunogenic cells in draining lymph nodes stimulates the production of tumor-sensitized preeffector lymphocytes, which develop into specific immune effector cells after activation in vitro with anti-CD3 monoclonal antibody and IL-2.

*Observations.*—Tumor regression required the collaboration of both activated CD4+ and CD8+ cells. The presence of CD8+ cells alone was sufficient if exogenous IL-2 was available in vivo. At the stage of in vitro activation, however, adding IL-2 did not substitute for the presence of CD4+ cells. The latter cells were sensitized independently of CD8+ cells in draining lymph nodes. Sensitization of CD8+ cells occurred independently in the absence of a CD4+ cell response.

*Implications.*—In this model of adoptive immunotherapy, CD8+ cells probably act as immediate antitumor effector cells. Each of the T- cell subsets can be sensitized independently during tumor growth, thereby acquiring preeffector cell function.

▶ This work demonstrates the effectiveness of activation signal (anti-CD3) in conjunction with low-dose IL-2, which can activate tumor-draining lymph nodes and therefore render them effective in adoptive immunotherapy experiments. This is significant in the tumor-draining lymph node system because it has direct applicability to humans. It further obviates the need for repetitive tumor stimulation that would be almost impossible in most human cancer situations.

This study confirms observations made by others (1, 2). These previous reports showed that CD3 caused much greater proliferation of lymphocytes. The combination of CD3 and low-dose IL-2 render the cells highly cytotoxic and very effective in adoptive immunotherapy.—T.J. Eberlein, M.D.

*References*

1. Schoof DD, et al: *Cancer Res* 50:1138, 1990.
2. Massaro AF, et al: *Cancer Res* 50:2587, 1990.

## Anti-Neoplastic Effects of Interleukin-4

Redmond HP, Schuchter L, Bartlett D, Kelly CJ, Shou J, Leon P, Daly JM (Univ of Pennsylvania, Philadelphia)
*J Surg Res* 52:406–411, 1992                                    10–49

*Objective.*—The effects of interleukin-4 (IL-4), a cytokine with potential antineoplastic effects, were examined on host antitumor responses in a murine model.

*Methods.*—Female C57/B16 mice were randomized to in vitro or in vivo study groups. The 20 animals assigned to in vitro studies received Lewis lung carcinoma or saline control. At 10 days post inoculation, the animals were killed and peritoneal macrophages and splenocytes were harvested for assessment of antitumor function with and without IL-4 coculture. The 20 mice in the in vivo studies received Lewis lung implants and were randomized 21 days later to receive IL-4 or saline daily. Tumor volume and survival were evaluated.

*Results.*—Treatment with IL-4 optimized alteration in cellular function and was associated with a decrease in tumor volume and improved median survival. When administered to cultured cells from the tumor-bearing study group, IL-4 enhanced superoxide anion generation as well as the mixed lymphocyte response and cytotoxic lymphocyte generation, and decreased tumor necrosis factor release but did not alter peritoneal macrophage tumor necrosis factor-independent antitumor responses. After 10 days of treatment, in vivo administration of IL-4 significantly decreased tumor growth. The median length of host survival was significantly prolonged in this group of mice.

*Conclusion.*—the T cell cytokine IL-4 has potent antitumor properties, both in vitro and in vivo, and appears to enhance both T-cell-dependent and T-cell-independent mechanisms.

▶ This investigation looks at one of the newer, somewhat less studied interleukins, IL-4; it shows that treatment with IL-4 optimizes cellular function and diminishes tumor burden.

Interleukin-4, however, has also been associated with a decreased immune response. This is particularly true in diseases such as leishmaniasis and systemic candidiasis in animals that have a high proportion of Th2 helper cells. These helper cells are unique in that they produce large amounts of IL-4 and do not produce IL-2 or gamma-interferon. Treatment with anti-IL-4 antibodies enhance the immune response and eradicate the systemic disease.

Therefore, depending on the specific system and conditions of experimentation, study of the interleukins can be exceedingly complex. Until the mechanisms are definded, knowledge of the immune response to human cancers will be incomplete.—T.J. Eberlein, M.D.

**Bryostatin 1-Activated T Cells Can Traffic and Mediate Tumor Regression**
Tuttle TM, Bethke KP, Inge TH, McCrady CW, Pettit GR, Bear HD (Virginia Commonwealth Univ, Richmond; Arizona State Univ, Tempe)
*J Surg Res* 52:543–548, 1992                                                    10–50

*Background.*—Adoptive immunotherapy is clinically limited by lack of autologous tumor cells for activating and expanding tumor-specific T cells. Drugs that bypass the T-cell receptor may substitute for tumor antigen in stimulating the growth of such cells. Bryostatin 1 activates protein kinase C, but unlike phorbol esters it is not a tumor promoter and has strong antitumor activity.

*Study Design.*—The ability of Bryostatin 1 in conjunction with the calcium ionophore ionomycin, to activate lymphocytes was tested using cells from popliteal lymph nodes draining a methylcholanthrene (MCA)-105 footpad sarcoma. The methylcholanthrene-203 sarcoma also was used; both are MCA- induced tumors of C57B1/6 origin.

*Observations.*—Adoptive transfer of Bryostatin/ionomycin-stimulated node cells eradicated the pulmonary metastases of MCA-105. The concomitant administration of interleukin (IL)-2 was not necessary. After intrasplenic injection of tumor cells, splenectomy, and intravenous injections of Bryostatin/ionomycin-stimulated node cells, these cells induced the regression of liver metastases. Adoptive transfer of stimulated MCA-105 node cells also cured mice of MCA-105 intra-dermal tumors but did not promote regression of MCA-203 tumors.

*Conclusions.*—The T cells from tumor-bearing mice that are exposed briefly to Bryostatin 1 and ionomycin are able to eliminate metastases without the need for IL-2 at the same time. The activated cells, however, are cultured in IL-2. Trials are warranted to learn whether these activated T cells are helpful in treating human cancers.

▶ In this study the authors attempt to bypass the need for tumor stimulation in order to sensitize a lymphocyte, and they also attempt to bypass the need for exogenous IL-2 administration. This alternative pathway is accomplished by using Bryostatin 1 and ionomycin. Bryostatin 1 stimulates protein kinase C and has other immunomodulatory properties. Bryostatin-1-activated T cells are able to traffic to and mediate regression of metastatic disease as well as provide long-term immunologic protection. Clinical trials using this approach are forthcoming.—T.J. Eberlein, M.D.

## In Vivo Activity of Tumor Necrosis Factor (TNF) Mutants: Secretory But Not Membrane-Bound TNF Mediates the Regression of Retrovirally Transduced Murine Tumor

Karp SE, Hwu P, Farber A, Restifo NP, Kriegler M, Mulé JJ, Rosenberg SA
(Natl Cancer Inst, NIH, Bethesda, Md; Cytel Corp, San Diego, Calif)
*J Immunol* 149:2076–2081, 1992                     10–51

*Background.*—Tumor necrosis factor (TNF) exists in 2 forms, membrane-bound and secretory variants. Murine tumor cells transduced by a retrovirus containing the cDNA encoding wild-type human TNF regress when injected into immunocompetent mice. The regression process is T-cell-mediated.

*Objective and Methods.*—An attempt was made to determine whether membrane-related or secreted TNF is responsible for tumor regression. A cloned murine fibrosarcoma (205 F4) was transduced with retrovirus encoding modified human TNF genes. The cloned tumor lines of 1 retroviral transduction expressed only membrane-bound TNF, but a second retrovirus led to the expression only of secretary TNF.

*Observations.*—The TNF produced by tumor cells transduced by both retroviral vectors was functional in vitro, as evident from direct lysis of the TNF-sensitive target L929 (murine fibroblasts). When tumor cells were injected subcutaneously into sygeneic mice, tumors expressing membrane-bound TNF grew progressively. Those expressing secretory TNF grew for 10 days and then regressed; all of these animals were free of tumor at 28 days. Regression of tumor was prevented by injecting an anti-TNF antibody.

*Conclusion.*—The secretory form of TNF is required for regression of TNF-transduced tumors.

▶ This investigation demonstrates how the understanding of a specific cytokine (in this case, TNF) and its specific effects on cells can be used in designing future clinical trials. The authors transduced TNF using retroviral vectors into tumor cells. The secretory variant of TNF-transduced tumor cells caused tumor regression, which was prevented by an anti-TNF antibody.

Antitumor gene therapies currently under development involve both the attempt to either magnify the host immune response to a tumor or alter the tumor to make it more susceptible to the host immune system. Further trials will be conducted in both animals and eventually in humans as the mechanisms for various gene markers and cytokines become understood. Not only will gene therapy be useful as a potential therapeutic modality, it will also help to identify mechanisms by contributing genetic material and restoring expression or the ability to produce certain proteins and cytokines. These kinds of studies will have far-reaching effects in the design of future human clinical immunotherapy trials.—T.J. Eberlein, M.D.

## Gastric Cancer

### INTRODUCTION

Gastric cancer is an extremely virulent disease in the United States. Although the incidence has declined in Western countries, it continues to be a major health problem. The incidence of proximal tumors (those of the cardia and gastroesophageal junction) has increased at a rapid rate, especially in white males (1). On a global basis, particularly in the Pacific basin, this disease is among the most common malignancies.

Two major thrusts have been undertaken to eradicate this disease. The first comprises attempts at more radical and accurate surgical staging procedures as well as resection techniques. The second is the development of better systemic therapies, because it appears that metastatic disease, either at presentation or very shortly after primary resection, is a major problem.

The articles thus chosen for review address several of these issues.

**Timothy J. Eberlein, M.D.**

*Reference*

1. Blot W, et al: *JAMA* 265:1287, 1991.

---

### Results of Surgery on 6589 Gastric Cancer Patients and Immuno-chemosurgery as the Best Treatment of Advanced Gastric Cancer
Kim J-P, Kwon OJ, Oh ST, Yang HK (Seoul Natl Univ Hosp, Seoul, Korea)
*Ann Surg* 216:269–279, 1992                                        10–52

*Background.*—Gastric cancer is the most common malignancy and the primary cause of cancer death in Korea. Despite the availability of en-

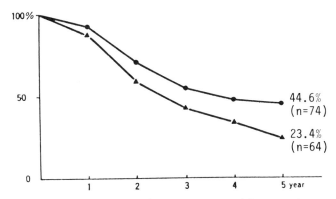

**Fig 10–16.**—Survival curve of the immunochemosurgery group and the surgery-alone group in stage II stomach cancer. *Circles,* immunochemosurgery; *triangles,* surgery alone. (Courtesy of Kim J-P, Kwon OJ, Oh ST, et al: *Ann Surg* 216:269–279, 1992.)

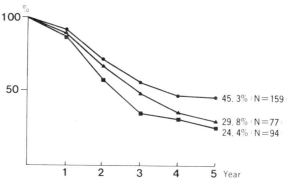

**Fig 10–17.**—Survival curve of immunochemosurgery group, surgery and postoperative chemotherapy group and surgery-alone group in stage III stomach cancer (330 cases, 1981–1985). *Circle,* immuno-chemosurgery, 45.3% (n = 159); *triangle,* surgery and postoperative chemotherapy, 29.8% (n = 77); *square,* surgery alone, 24.4% (n = 94). (Courtesy of Kim J-P, Kwon OJ, Oh ST, et al: *Ann Surg* 216:269–279, 1992.)

doscopy for early diagnosis, more than 70% of the patients have stage III or IV disease at the time of diagnosis. Between 1970 and 1990, of the 6,589 patients operated on for gastric cancer at the Seoul National University Hospital, 76.6% had advanced disease. The overall 5-year survival rate of patients with resectable gastric cancer was 46.6%; the 5-year survival rate of patients with stage III disease was only 30.6%. Two trials were carried out to evaluate the therapeutic efficacy of postoperative immunochemosurgery in patients with advanced but resectable gastric adenocarcinoma.

*Trial 1.*—Of 138 patients who underwent radical subtotal gastrectomy for stage III gastric cancer, 64 received no further anticancer therapy after operation and 74 received postoperative chemotherapy consisting of 5-fluorouracil, mitomycin C, and cytosine arabinoside, and immunotherapy with OK 432, a *Streptococcus pyogenes* preparation. The 5-year survival rates were 44.6% among patients who received postoperative immunochemo-surgery and 23.4% among patients who underwent gastrectomy only (Fig 10–16). The difference was statistically significant.

*Trial 2.*—Of 330 patients with histologically confirmed stage III gastric cancer, 159 received postoperative chemotherapy plus immunotherapy, 77 were given postoperative chemotherapy only, and 94 were given no further anticancer therapy after gastrectomy. The 5-year survival rates were 45.3% for patients who received postoperative immunochemo-surgery, 29.8% for those who were given postoperative chemotherapy only, and 24.4% for those who received no further postoperative anticancer treatment (Fig 10–17).

*Conclusions.*—Radical curative resection of gastric carcinoma, which includes subtotal gastric resection, dissection of regional and perigastric lymph nodes, and removal of omentum with adjacent tissues, combined with early postoperative chemotherapy and immunotherapy is the best approach to the treatment of advanced resectable gastric cancer.

## A Comprehensive Multi-Institutional Study on Postoperative Adjuvant Immunotherapy With Oral Streptococcal Preparation OK-432 for Patients After Gastric Cancer Surgery

Nio Y, for the Kyoto Research Group for Digestive Organ Surgery (Kyoto Univ, Kyoto, Japan)

*Ann Surg* 216:44–54, 1992                                                               10–53

*Background.*—Previous studies have shown that immunotherapy with OK-432, a penicillin-treated preparation of *Streptococcus pyogenes*, is effective against gastric cancer. When injected subcutaneously, intramuscularly, or intradermally, however, OK 432 causes side effects that often require interruption of treatment. The effects of orally and intradermally administered OK 432 immunotherapy on survival were compared in patients who underwent gastric resection for cancer.

*Patients.*—Of 1,011 patients with previously untreated primary gastric cancer, 819 underwent curative gastrectomy and 192 had a palliative procedure. Of the 819 patients who had curative surgery, 273 were randomized to postoperative treatment with orally administered OK 432, 274 were randomized to orally administered placebo, and 272 were randomized to intradermally administered OK 432 immunotherapy. Of 192 patients who underwent palliative operations, 62 were treated orally OK 432, 64 were given placebo orally, and 66 received OK 432 intradermally. Treatment was continued for 2 years in survivors. Forty-one patients (4.1%) were excluded from the data analysis because of misregistration.

*Results.*—The 5-year survival rates after curative surgery were 69% in placebo-treated patients, 75% in those treated postoperatively with OK

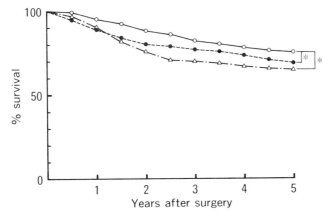

**Fig 10–18.**—Survival curves of patients after curative surgery. *Filled circles,* placebo group (n = 262); *open circles,* oral OK-432 group (n = 256; *triangles,* intradermal OK-432 group (n = 203). *P < .05, generalized Wilcoxon test. (Courtesy of Nio Y, for the Kyoto Research Group for Digestive Organ Surgery: *Ann Surg* 216:44–54, 1992.)

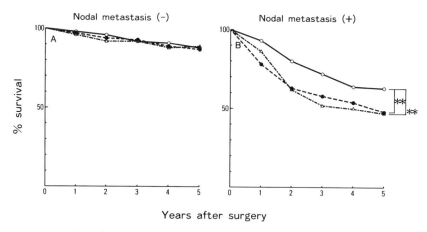

**Fig 10–19.**—Survival curves and nodal involvement in patients of the curative surgery stratum. **A,** nodal metastasis (−). *Filled circles*, placebo group (n = 145); *open circles*, oral OK-432 group (n = 131); *triangles*, intradermal OK-432 group (n = 116). **B,** nodal metastasis (+). *Filled circles*, placebo group (n = 116); *open circles*, oral OK-432 group (n = 124); *triangles*, intradermal OK-432 group (n = 147; **P < .01, generalized Wilcoxon test. (Courtesy of Nio Y, for the Kyoto Research Group for Digestive Organ Surgery: *Ann Surg* 216:44–54, 1992.)

432 orally, and 65% in those treated intradermally (Fig 10–18). The beneficial effect of the oral form of OK 432 was pronounced among patients with stage II, III, or IV gastric cancer, especially in those with regional node involvement (Fig 10–19). Furthermore, the survival rate in patients who underwent curative gastrectomy without splenectomy and were treated orally with OK 432 was significantly higher than that in

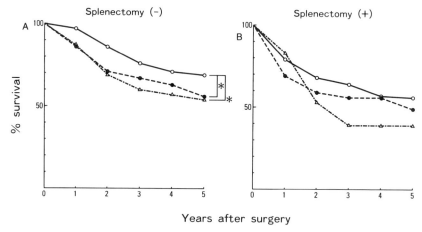

**Fig 10–20.**—Survival curves and splenectomy in patients of the curative surgery stratum. **A,** splenectomy (−). *Filled circles*, placebo group (n = 116); *open circles*, oral OK-432 group (n = 122); *triangles*, intradermal OK-432 group (n = 129). *P < .05, generalized Wilcoxon test. **B,** splenectomy (+). *Filled circles*, placebo group (n = 32); *open circles*, oral OK-432 group (n = 28); *triangles*, intradermal OK-432 group (n = 38). (Courtesy of Nio Y, for the Kyoto Research Group for Digestive Organ Surgery: *Ann Surg* 216:44–54, 1992.)

splenectomized patients so treated, indicating that the spleen has an important role in OK 432 immunotherapy (Fig 10–20). Survival rates among patients who underwent palliative surgery and were treated with placebo, OK 432 orally, or OK 432 intradermally did not differ significantly.

*Conclusions.*—Immunotherapy with orally administered OK 432 after curative resection for gastric cancer significantly improves survival. Immunotherapy with intradermal doses of OK 432 appears to have no clinical benefit.

▶ The first paper (Abstract 10–52) describes a personal series of more than 6,000 gastric cancer patients with an amazing .34% operative mortality. In this study the authors address both problems seen in the management of gastric cancer: local disease and systemic recurrence. They have therefore combined a very radical resection that includes omental and regional perigastric lymph node dissection with an early combination of chemotherapy and/or immunotherapy. The chemotherapy consisted of 5-FU, the most active agent against gastric cancer, as well as mitomycin-C combined with cytosine arabinoside and immunotherapy using OK 432, a streptococcal pyrogen preparation. Cutaneous sensitivity to dinitrochlorobenzene, lymphoblastogenesis, and antibody-dependent cellular cytotoxicity were all improved in the immunochemosurgery patients. It appears that this immunotherapy may help to revive depressed immunity in the patient with advanced cancer and alleviate the adverse effects of postoperative chemotherapy. The second trial, which was even larger, compared postoperative chemotherapy plus immunotherapy to chemotherapy alone and no further therapy. Again, those in the immunochemosurgery arm had the best 5-year survival rate.

Abstract 10–53 is a multi-institutional study of 819 patients who underwent curative surgery and received oral doses of placebo or OK 432 or intradermal doses of OK 432 immunotherapy. Orally administered OK 432 was particularly effective in stages II, III, and IV gastric cancer, especially in those patients who had regional lymph node involvement. This was particularly true if the patient did not undergo splenectomy. All of the patients in this second trial received mitomycin intraoperatively and then fluoropyrimidines daily for 2 years, which may have interfered with the subdermal administration of OK 432.

In any event, the importance of the immune system in eradication of micrometastatic disease in gastric cancer is emphasized by these 2 studies. Further trials with different combinations of chemotherapy and immunotherapies such as OK 432 are needed.—T.J. Eberlein, M.D.

**Pathology and Prognosis of Gastric Carcinoma: Findings in 10,000 Patients Who Underwent Primary Gastrectomy**
Nakamura K, Ueyama T, Yao T, Xuan ZX, Ambe K, Adachi Y, Yakeishi Y, Matsukuma A, Enjoji M (Kyushu Univ, Fukuoka, Japan)
*Cancer* 70:1030–1037, 1992                                    10–54

*Background.*—Gastric carcinoma is the most common cause of death from malignant disease in Japan. Mass screening trials that include fiberoptic endoscopy and double-contrast radiography, combined with more aggressive surgery for resectable tumors, has led to the earlier detection and more effective treatment of gastric carcinoma. Tumor stage at the time of operation is the most important prognostic factor. Factors that influence the prognosis for patients with gastric carcinoma were examined further.

*Patients.*—Between 1962 and 1989, 10,000 Japanese patients underwent primary gastrectomy. Of 7,031 patients with gastric cancer, 3,163 had early disease and 3,868 had advanced disease. Follow-up data were available for 5,458 patients (78%) with gastric carcinoma.

*Results.*—The annual incidence of gastrectomy for gastric carcinoma increased steadily throughout the study period. For the period 1985–1989, the rate of carcinoma detected early exceeded that of advanced carcinoma. The overall 5-year survival rates were 46% for advanced carcinoma and 89% for early carcinoma. The overall 10-year survival rates were 35% for advanced disease and 77% for early disease (Figs 10–21 and 10–22). Among patients with advanced carcinoma, age older than 70 years, total gastrectomy, tumors involving the entire stomach, tumor size greater than 10 cm in diameter, a macroscopic diffusely infiltrative pattern, adenosquamous histologic type, positive resection mar-

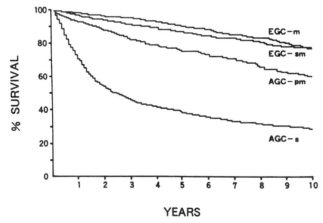

**YEARS**

**Fig 10–21.**—Survival rates according to depth of invasion. AGC, advanced gastric carcinoma; EGC, early gastric carcinoma; *m*, mucosa; *sm*, submucosa; *pm*, muscularis propria; *s*, serosa. (Courtesy of Nakamura K, Ueyama T, Yao T, et al: *Cancer* 70:1030–1037, 1992.)

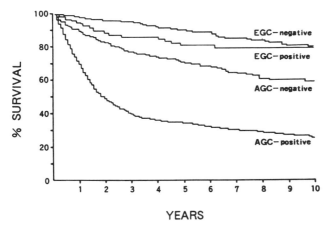

**Fig 10–22.**—Survival rates according to lymph node status. AGC, advanced gastric carcinoma; EGC, early gastric carcinoma. (Courtesy of Nakamura K, Ueyama T, Yao T, et al: *Cancer* 70:1030–1037, 1992.)

gins, and lymph node metastasis were significantly correlated with poorer survival. None of these factors was prognostic of poor survival among patients with early gastric carcinoma, except for age older than 70 years. The presence of lymph node metastases in patients with early gastric cancer was not associated with a poor prognosis.

*Conclusions.*—Early detection and aggressive dissection of resectable tumors, combined with proper histopathologic examination of surgical specimens, remains the most effective approach to the treatment of gastric carcinoma.

▶ This paper analyzed data collected in a 27-year period from more than 7,000 patients with gastric carcinoma. Its major point is that aggressive surgical resection, even in patients with lymph node metastasis but otherwise early gastric cancer, could result in acceptable survival rates. These authors emphasize intraoperative frozen section biopsy, assurance of tumor-free margins of resection, the status of enlarged lymph nodes, and identification of the histologic tumor type. Aggressive surgical resection in the patient population remains a controversial issue in the United States that will be settled only in a multi-institutional, randomized trial.—T.J. Eberlein, M.D.

### FAMTX Versus Etoposide, Doxorubicin, and Cisplatin: A Random Assignment Trial in Gastric Cancer

Kelsen D, Atiq OT, Saltz L, Niedzwiecki D, Ginn D, Chapman D, Heelan R, Lightdale C, Vinciguerra V, Brennan M (Mem Sloan-Kettering Cancer Ctr, New York City; Cornell Univ Med College, New York City; North Shore Univ Hosp Community Clinical Oncology Program, Manhasset, NY)
*J Clin Oncol* 10:541–548, 1992          10–55

*Background.*—Nonrandomized trials of high-dose methotrexate, high-dose fluorouracil, doxorubicin, and leucovorin (FAMTX) and of etoposide, doxorubicin, and cisplatin (EAP) for treatment of gastric cancer have been reported. Both regimins resulted in high overall response rates, substantial complete response rates, and major myelosuppressive toxicity. The use of these 2 chemotherapeutic combinations was compared in 60 previously untreated patients with advanced gastric cancer in a prospective, stratified, randomized study. All had histologically proved gastric cancer that was not potentially curable by other means.

*Method.*—The patients were randomly and equally assigned to receive EAP or FAMTX at dosages and treatment schedules identical to those in the original investigations. The study design initially called for a group of 130 patients; however, patient entry was halted when interim analysis revealed significant differences in toxic effects.

*Results.*—Response rates were similar: 33% for FAMTX and 20% for EAP. Complete remission was achieved in 3 patients given FAMTX but in none given EAP. The median survival was 6 months in the group given EAP and 7.3 months in the group given FAMTX. At 12 months, 7% the EAP-treated group and 17% of the FAMTX-treated group remained alive. Signs of myelosuppression, including leukopenia, anemia, and thrombocytopenia, were significantly greater after EAP treatment. Although there was no difference in the number of admissions for toxicity, the group given EAP required a median of 8 days of hospitalization per month for treatment-related toxicity versus 5 days for the group given FAMTX. Four patients given EAP died of myelosuppression-related sepsis, compared with none given FAMTX.

*Conclusions.*—In patients with gastric cancer, the FAMTX chemotherapeutic regimen is at least as effective as EAP and causes significantly less myelosuppressive toxicity. Although it is still an investigative regimen, further trials of FAMTX have begun in both adjuvant and advanced disease settings. A higher-intensity dose of fluorouracil may be possible if myelosuppression can be reduced.

▶ This prospective, stratified, randomized study compared high-dose methotrexate, high-dose fluorouracil, doxorubicin, and leucovorin (FAMTX) with the combination of etoposide, doxorubicin and cisplatin (EAP) in patients with gastric cancer. The FAMTX regimen yielded slightly higher response rates and several complete responses. Myelosuppression was significantly greater with EAP. Perhaps combination trials with granulocyte colony-stimulating factor (CSF) or granulocyte macrophage-CSF may permit higher doses of fluorouracil, further improving response rates.—T.J. Eberlein, M.D.

## Regional Lymph Node Metastasis in Gastric Cancer: Evaluation With Endoscopic US

Akahoshi K, Misawa T, Fujishima H, Chijiiwa Y, Nawata H (Kyushu Univ, Fukuoka, Japan)

*Radiology* 182:559–564, 1992                                   10–56

*Objective.*—The value of endoscopic ultrasonography (EUS) in assessing regional node metastasis was examined in 83 patients with gastric cancer confirmed by endoscopic biopsy between 1986 and 1990. The histopathologic and sonographic findings were compared in 1,519 resected lymph nodes.

*Findings.*—Metastatic adenopathy was identified in 31% of patients. Endoscopic ultrasonography detected 42 round or elliptical echoic structures that were hypoechoic to surrounding tissues; metastasis was confirmed histologically in 40 of these specimens. Regional node metastasis was correctly diagnosed with EUS in 14 of 26 affected patients. The absence of metastasis was correctly identified in all but 2 of 57 patients. The study had an overall accuracy of 83% and positive and negative predictive values of 87.5% and 82%, respectively. Detection increased with the maximal diameter of the involved node and with the ratio of the metastatic area to the cross-sectional area of the involved node.

*Conclusions.*—With EUS, lymph nodes that could not be brought well into focus could not be clearly identified. The new technique probably will prove useful in diagnosing regional node metastasis, and it may help in staging gastric cancer before treatment.

▶ This study of 83 patients with gastric cancer assessed the new technique of EUS to evaluate regional lymph node metastasis. Because detection of regional lymph node metastasis is important in staging gastric cancer for protocol inclusion, and because transcutaneous ultrasound and CT are accompanied by wide degrees of inaccuracies, this methodology holds promise.

Although this is not the first report of EUS, it is one of the most detailed because it compares EUS with pathologic lymph node status. The technique had a poor detection rate except for perigastric lymph nodes with metastases near the primary lymph nodes that could not be brought adequately into focus of the ultrasound beam and could not be identified clearly. It may prove clinically useful for staging gastric cancer before therapy. In the future, however, further refinements will be necessary to improve its diagnostic accuracy.—T.J. Eberlein, M.D.

### Preoperative Staging of Gastric Cancer: Comparison of Endoscopic US and Dynamic CT

Botet JF, Lightdale CJ, Zauber AG, Gerdes H, Winawer SJ, Urmacher C, Brennan MF (Mem Sloan-Kettering Cancer Ctr, New York City; Cornell Univ, New York City)
*Radiology* 181:426–432, 1991                                    10–57

*Objective.*—Fifty consecutive patients seen in from 1986 to 1988 with confirmed gastric adenocarcinoma underwent preoperative staging by endoscopic ultrasonography (EUS). Dynamic CT of the chest and abdomen also was done preoperatively in 33 patients. The imaging findings were compared with the pathologic results according to the tumor/node/metastasis system.

*Findings.*—The EUS findings of tumor depth were concordant with the pathologic findings in 92% of $T_1$ and $T_2$ tumors, 97% of $T_3$ tumors, and 86% of $T_4$ tumors. With respect to node status, the sonographic findings agreed with the pathologic findings in 91% of $N_0$ lesions, 68% of $N_1$ lesions, and 82% of $N_2$ tumors. The findings of tumor depth on dynamic CT agreed with the pathologic findings in 42% of the 33 patients studied.

*Conclusion.*—Endoscopic US may be an important method of clinically staging gastric cancer for both clinical and research purposes.

▶ Fifty consecutive patients were studied by preoperative staging with EUS or dynamic computed CT. In this study, EUS was significantly superior to dynamic CT in examination of the tumor as well as for lymph node status. When ultrasound and CT were combined, accordance for overall stage was significantly improved.

Once again, EUS, particularly if improved technically, will aid in the preoperative staging and evaluation of patients, especially those selected for neoadjuvant therapies. Obviously, EUS has limited efficacy in the detection of future metastases.—T.J. Eberlein, M.D.

### Management of Small Soft-Tissue Sarcoma of the Extremity in Adults

Geer RJ, Woodruff J, Casper ES, Brennan MF (Mem Sloan-Kettering Cancer Ctr, New York City)
*Arch Surg* 127:1285–1289, 1992                                10–58

*Objective.*—In the grading of soft tissue sarcomas of the extremities, tumor size is considered but its value is not emphasized. For tumors measuring no more than 5 cm in size, there is debate as to the extent of resection and the necessity for adjuvant therapy. A prospective database was reviewed to study the significance of small soft tissue sarcomas of the extremities.

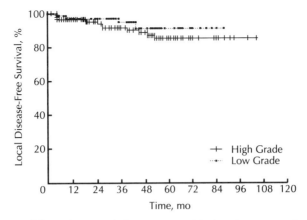

**Fig 10–23.**—Local disease-free survival of 114 patients with high-grade tumors vs. 60 with low-grade tumors. *P* = .39. (Courtesy of Geer RJ, Woodruff J, Casper ES, et al: *Arch Surg* 127:1285–1289, 1992.)

*Patients.*—The database included 1,747 adults with primary or recurrent soft tissue sarcoma treated at a single center during an 8-year period. Of these, 214 had localized lesions of the extremities measuring 5 cm or less, and 174 of the 214 were seen for primary management. Patients were characterized by demographic data, tumor characteristics, treatment and outcome. They were followed for a median of 48 months.

*Outcomes.*—Most of the 174 patients (87%) had excisional biopsy, and 91% had limb-sparing operations. Two thirds of the tumors were classified as high grade. Seventeen patients had local recurrences, with no significant differences between high-grade and low-grade tumors (Fig 10–23). The overall 5-year survival was 94%; neither survival nor local recurrence-free survival was affected by grade, depth, location, type of operation, or sex (table). In 7% of the patients with high-grade tumors, distant metastases developed, compared to none of those with low-grade tumors. The rates of 5-year survival and local recurrence-free survival were unimproved by postoperative adjuvant chemotherapy or radiation therapy.

*Conclusions.*—A 94% 5-year survival was reported in patients with small soft tissue sarcomas of the extremities. No new prognostic factors were identified, although high-grade tumors were associated with an increased risk of distant metastases. Because of their favorable prognosis, these patients should not be included in trials of adjuvant therapy.

▶ This manuscript reports the results of a study from the Memorial Sloan-Kettering Cancer Center of patients with small soft tissue sarcomas of the extremity. The main implication of this work is to emphasize the importance of adequate surgical management of these small tumors. Whereas high-grade tumors are associated with an increased risk of distant metastases, in general, these tumors have extremely good prognoses. Thus the inclusion of these patients into adjuvant treatment trials would seem inappropriate.

Five-Year Local Recurrence-Free Survival and Survival by
Risk Factors

| Risk Factor | No. of Patients | Local Disease-Free Survival, % | P | Survival, % | P |
|---|---|---|---|---|---|
| Age, y | | | | | |
| <50 | 110 | 98 | <.01 | 97⌐ | |
| ≥50 | 64 | 65 | | 86⌐ | .09 |
| Sex | | | | | |
| M | 97 | 80 | .06 | 94⌐ | |
| F | 77 | 93 | | 93⌐ | .71 |
| Depth | | | | | |
| Superficial | 98 | 98 | .68 | 95⌐ | |
| Deep | 76 | 76 | | 92⌐ | .51 |
| Location | | | | | |
| Proximal | 82 | 91 | .12 | 98⌐ | |
| Distal | 92 | 82 | | 89⌐ | .17 |
| Grade | | | | | |
| High | 114 | 84 | .39 | 91⌐ | |
| Low | 60 | 90 | | 100⌐ | .15 |
| Operation | | | | | |
| Amputation | 15 | 93 | .48 | 84⌐ | |
| Limb sparing | 159 | 85 | | 95⌐ | .16 |
| Margin | | | | | |
| Positive | 15 | 56 | .01 | 100⌐ | |
| Negative | 159 | 88 | | 93⌐ | .42 |
| Chemotherapy | | | | | |
| Yes | 44 | 89 | .25 | 89⌐ | |
| No | 70 | 78 | | 91⌐ | .51 |
| Radiation | | | | | |
| Yes | 42 | 77 | .08 | 92⌐ | |
| No | 117 | 92 | | 93⌐ | .70 |

(Courtesy of Geer RJ, Woodruff J, Casper ES, et al: *Arch Surg* 127:1285–1289, 1992.)

Patients who have positive margins should undergo further surgery, because adjuvant therapy is of dubious benefit in this patient population.—T.J. Eberlein, M.D.

## Sarcomas

### Comparison of Amputation With Limb-Sparing Operations for Adult Soft Tissue Sarcoma of the Extremity

Williard WC, Hajdu SI, Casper ES, Brennan MF (Mem Sloan-Kettering Cancer

Ctr, New York City)

*Ann Surg* 215:269–275, 1992

10–59

*Introduction.*—In the past 2 decades, fewer patients with soft tissue sarcoma have undergone amputation at the study institution. Local control of disease has improved with advances in radiation therapy and chemotherapy. In addition, evidence that amputation improves survival is lacking. The efficacy and future role of amputation in extremity soft tissue sarcoma were investigated.

*Methods.*—A prospective sarcoma database established at Memorial Sloan-Kettering Cancer Center in July 1982 was analyzed in a retrospective fashion for the period from July 1982 to January 1990. Data on the 649 patients were updated by a mailed questionnaire or telephone contact. Therapy for each patient was selected on an individual basis; 92 underwent amputation (18 as a salvage procedure) and 557 had an extremity-sparing procedure. The median follow-up for all patients was about 23 months.

*Findings.*—The group having amputation included significantly more patients with high-grade tumors, tumors requiring chemotherapy, tumors 5 cm or larger, or 10 cm or larger tumors that invaded a major nervous or vascular structure. Significantly more patients in the group having extremitysparing had liposarcomas; synovial sarcomas and chondrosarcoma were more common in patients who underwent amputation. Tumors of the upper arm and thigh had more extremity-sparing procedures, whereas lower leg and foot tumors were more likely to lead to amputation. In patients with larger tumors and in those with high-grade lesions, survival was significantly poorer after amputation. Amputations resulted in significantly better local control, but patients in this group were more likely to have metastatic spread, consistent with their large, high-grade tumors. Patients who had local recurrence after an extremity-sparing procedure had a better rate of survival than those who had no recurrence after an amputation. Patients with high-grade tumors 10 cm or larger had improved rates of survival with chemotherapy, regardless of the type of operation.

*Conclusion.*—Patients selected for amputation had the worst risk factors. Despite stratification for risk factors, amputation offered no advantage over extremity-sparing procedures. Amputations are recommended only for patients whose tumor cannot be grossly resected with an extremity-sparing procedure while still preserving a useful extremity. Better systemic treatment, not more radical surgery, is needed to improve survival in these patients.

### The Changing Role of Amputation for Soft Tissue Sarcoma of the Extremity in Adults

Williard WC, Collin C, Casper ES, Hajdu SI, Brennan MF (Mem Sloan-Kettering Cancer Ctr, New York City)
*Surg Gynecol Obstet* 175:389–396, 1992                    10–60

*Background.*—The use of amputation in soft tissue sarcoma of the extremities has been questioned on the grounds that it offers little survival benefit, whereas proponents believe that it is the only real alternative for control of this potentially fatal disease. Use of amputation for soft tissue sarcoma of the extremities at Memorial Sloan-Kettering Cancer Center has declined in the past 2 decades. A retrospective analysis attempted to determine the reason for this change, its effect on local recurrence and survival, and its future role.

*Methods.*—Two separate databases were reviewed. The first included 408 patients who underwent a surgical procedure for soft tissue sarcoma of an extremity from 1968 to 1978. These patients were followed for a median of 8 years; 131 underwent an amputation. The other database consisted of 649 patients treated from 1982 to 1990; 92 had an amputation. The median follow-up in this group was 32 months. The 223 patients who had amputations were compared for differences in risk factors, indications for amputation, and effect on recurrence and survival.

*Findings.*—The groups were relatively homogeneous, although the group treated earlier had more tumors 5 cm or larger and more liposarcomas and rhabdomyosarcomas; the group treated later had more chon-

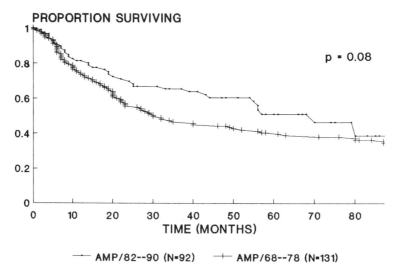

**Fig 10–24.**—Comparison of survival by treatment from 1968 to 1978 versus from 1982 to 1990. AMP, amputation. (Courtesy of Williard WC, Collin C, Casper ES, et al: *Surg Gynecol Obstet* 175:389–396, 1992.)

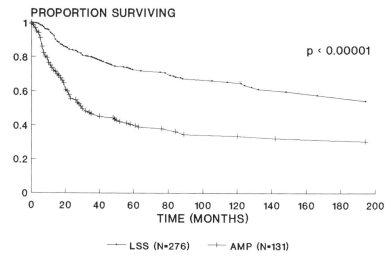

**PROPORTION SURVIVING**

p < 0.00001

TIME (MONTHS)

⎯ LSS (N=276)   ⟍ AMP (N=131)

**Fig 10–25.**—Survival differences in patients with limb-sparing operation versus amputation for soft-tissue sarcoma of the extremity during the period 1968 to 1978. (Courtesy of Williard WC, Collin C, Casper ES, et al: *Surg Gynecol Obstet* 175:389–396, 1992.)

drosarcomas. In both periods, patients considered for amputation had the worst prognostic factors, namely, high-grade and large tumors. The proportion of patients having an amputation decreased from 32% to 14% but the overall survival rate in the 2 groups of amputees were unchanged. There was an associated decrease in local recurrence, however (Fig 10–24). Patients without local recurrence had significantly improved survival. In the group treated earlier, the overall survival rate was significantly better in patients undergoing a limb-sparing procedure (Fig 10–25).

*Conclusions.*—The decreasing use of amputation in the treatment of soft tissue sarcoma of the extremities is associated with a significant decrease in local recurrence but no change in survival. Unless limb-sparing operations are clearly inappropriate for tumor control or extremity function, they should be considered as an alternative to amputation. In selected patients, amputation remains an appropriate procedure. This study provides the best evidence that local recurrence itself does not significantly affect survival.

▶ The first study (Abstract 10–59) makes an important contribution to knowledge about the biology of sarcomas. In the past, these tumors were treated with radical amputation. As improved radiotherapeutic techniques became available, however, compartment excision or gross excision with negative margins became possible and preferred. In this series from Memorial Hospital, as one might expect, amputations were associated with the most severe risk factors such as large high-grade tumors or neurovascular involvement. Amputations resulted in significantly better local control; however, distant metastases were much more prevalent in this group when compared to the group having limb-sparing surgery. Thus it appeared logical that the poorer risk factors, i.e., large-size or high-grade tumors, or nerve or vessel involvement, predisposed the patient to systemic disease. The findings also point to the obvious problem in the treatment of soft tissue sarcomas; a real need for more effective systemic therapy.

Controversy exists in the treatment of soft tissue sarcomas with regard to the impact of local recurrence. Some would argue that local recurrence predisposes the patient to systemic metastases (1), whereas others have achieved excellent salvageability after resection of local recurrence of soft tissue sarcomas (2, 3).

The second study (Abstract 10–60) simply compares the amputations performed from 1968 through 1978 and from 1982 through 1990 at Memorial Sloan-Kettering Cancer Center. These authors document a decreased incidence of amputation in the latter study period. This was associated with a significant decrease in local recurrence after amputation but no change in survival when compared to the earlier group. This latter point provides the best evidence that local recurrence per se has no significant impact on survival.

Through techniques such as biochemical profiles using nuclear magnetic resonance and molecular biological markers, one may be able to predict not only the incidence of micrometastases at the time of presentation but also the potential response to systemic agents.—T.J. Eberlein, M.D.

*References*

1. Emrich LJ, et al: *J Clin Epidemiol* 42:105, 1989.
2. Huth JF, Eilber FR: *Semin Surg Oncol* 4:20, 1988.
3. Singer S, et al: *Arch Surg* 127:548, 1992.

**Prognostic Factors in 227 Patients With Malignant Fibrous Histiocytoma**
Pezzi CM, Rawlings MS Jr, Esgro JJ, Pollock RE, Romsdahl MM (Univ of Texas MD Anderson Cancer Ctr, Houston)
*Cancer* 69:2098–2103, 1992                                                    10–61

*Objective.*—Prognostic factors that could help to guide clinical management were sought in a series of 227 patients seen from 1970 to 1983 with localized malignant fibrous histiocytoma who underwent surgical treatment.

*Patients and Treatment.*—The mean age was 54 years. More than 60% of the patients had tumors on the extremities. Tumors were resected with a minimal margin of 2 cm of normal tissue. One forth of the patients had surgery alone, whereas most of the others received radiotherapy as well. Adjuvant chemotherapy was begun in the 1970s.

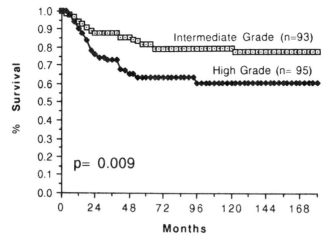

**Fig 10–26.**—Overall survival according to tumor grade. (Courtesy of Pezzi CM, Rawlings MS Jr, Esgro JJ, et al: *Cancer* 69:2098–2103, 1992.)

*Findings.*—The overall survival rate was 50%; 38 patients died of other causes. Local recurrences developed in 28% of the patients, and 22% had distant disease without local recurrence. The lungs were the most common site of distant disease, followed by the skeleton. Survival declined with increasing size of the primary tumor and with increasing tumor grade (Fig 10–26). Survival of patients with both intermediate- and high-grade tumors was influenced by tumor size.

*Conclusion.*—The major prognostic factors for malignant fibrous histiocytoma are tumor size and grade of the primary tumor.

▶ This study from the MD Anderson Cancer Center examines a group of patients with malignant fibrous histiocytoma. Using this uniform pathologic diagnosis, the authors show that tumor size and histologic grade are the 2 most important factors not only for predicting prognosis but also for predicting the outcome of treatment of soft tissue sarcomas.

Because of the uniformity and large numbers in this study, subset analysis was possible; it showed that small tumors of high grade had excellent prognosis. Similarly, intermediate-grade tumors had a better prognosis than high-grade tumors. Subset analyses in a uniform population make it possible to exclude patients who have good prognoses (Small tumors, high-grade or intermediate-grade tumors) from systemic chemotherapy trials and confine trials to those patients who have a high risk of systemic disease and poor survival (patients with large and high-grade tumors).—T.J. Eberlein, M.D.

### Long-Term Salvageability for Patients With Locally Recurrent Soft-Tissue Sarcomas

Singer S, Antman K, Corson JM, Eberlein TJ (Brigham and Women's Hosp, Boston, Mass; Dana Farber Cancer Inst, Boston)

Arch Surg 127:548–554, 1992                                    10–62

*Background.*—Local recurrence usually correlates with shorter survival in patients with soft tissue sarcomas. Efforts to prevent local recurrence and improve survival have centered on surgical strategies, radiation therapy, and chemotherapy. The records of 39 patients were reviewed to determine factors related to tumor recurrence.

*Methods.*—Between 1971 and 1988, 39 patients were seen with locally recurrent soft tissue sarcomas. The mean age of the 23 men and 16 women was 51 years; the mean follow-up after local recurrence was 9 years. Data were collected on the characteristics of the primary tumor, type of resection, type of adjuvant therapy, and characteristics of local recurrence.

*Results.*—The mean time to local recurrence was 22 months. More than half (59%) had high grade tumors. There was a wide range of tumor size, from smaller than 5 cm (28%) to larger than 10 cm (41%). Most patients had been treated with wide local excisions (85%); 70% had positive margins. Of those treated with wide local excision, 61% had truncal sarcomas and 39% had extremity sarcomas. Twenty-one of the 39 patietns with local recurrence had no evidence of metastatic disease and underwent resection of the recurrent sarcoma with curative intent. Fourteen remained free of disease at a mean follow-up of 112 months, and 7 died of locally recurrent or metastatic disease. Those in whom salvage was achieved were more likely to have had extremity rather than truncal tumors, to have undergone excisional biopsy, and to have had some form of postoperative adjuvant therapy. A major factor in local recurrence was evidence of positive margins.

*Conclusions.*—Local recurrence in soft tissue sarcomas was associated with high-grade tumors and the presence of positive or close margins at excision. Aggressive treatment of local recurrence only, including radical compartment excision with or without postoperative radiation therapy, was successful in two thirds of these patients. Excisional biopsy of tumors larger than 3 cm may compromise the definitive excision.

▶ The authors document the long-term salvageability in patients who have local recurrence of soft tissue sarcomas. As in previous studies, local recurrence in this patient population was most often associated with high-grade tumors. However, close or positive margins was also a major risk factor. Two thirds of the patients could be salvaged long term after treatment of the local recurrence.

This article stresses several technical issues. Many of the local recurrences developed in patients who had undergone attempts at gross excisional biopsy of very substantial tumors. This often compromises a more definitive surgical procedure. Emphasis is also placed on obtaining negative margins at the time of primary surgery, and, if possible, a compartmental excision should be performed, especially if the tumor is high grade. The use of radiation therapy for high-grade tumors is recommended.—T.J. Eberlein, M.D.

---

### A Prospective Study of the Value of Core Needle Biopsy and Fine Needle Aspiration in the Diagnosis of Soft Tissue Masses

Barth RJ Jr, Merino MJ, Solomon D, Yang JC, Baker AR (Natl Cancer Inst, Bethesda, Md)
*Surgery* 112:536–543, 1992                                                10–63

---

*Background.*—Biopsy of large soft tissue masses is necessary before definitive surgery. Both core needle biopsy (CNBX) and fine-needle aspiration (FNA) can be done in the office with the use of local anesthesia, but neither procedure may provide enough tissue to distinguish between a benign and malignant tumor or to estimate the grade of sarcoma.

*Objective.*—Thirty-eight large soft tissue masses were sampled by both CNBX and FNA biopsy in 37 patients. In 27 instances it was possible to compare the biopsy diagnosis with the histologic diagnosis made from a resection specimen. Sixteen of the 27 lesions were malignant.

*Findings.*—Core needle biopsy correctly diagnosed 10 of the 11 benign lesions and all 16 malignant lesions. In addition, sarcoma grade was correctly estimated in all instances. Fine-needle aspiration biopsy correctly classified only 4 benign lesions but accurately diagnosed 12 of 14 malignancies. The accuracy of the 2 procedures is compared in the table.

*Recommendations.*—Core needle biopsy is the preferred means for diagnosis of large soft tissue masses. Its reliability, however, depends on both careful biopsy technique and an experienced pathologist. In highly

| | CNBX | | FNA | |
|---|---|---|---|---|
| *Parameter* | *n* | *%* | *n* | *%* |
| Sensitivity | 16/16 | 100 | 12/14 | 86 |
| Specificity | 10/11 | 91 | 4/11 | 36 |
| Accuracy | 26/27 | 96 | 16/25 | 64 |
| Positive predictive value | 16/16 | 100 | 12/12 | 100 |
| Negative predictive value | 10/10 | 100 | 4/4 | 100 |

Diagnostic Accuracy of CNBX and FNA

Note: *Sensitivity,* correctly malignant/all patients with malignancies; *specificity,* correctly benign/all patients with benign conditions; *accuracy,* correctly malignant plus correctly benign/all biopsies; *postive predictive value,* correctly malignant/correctly malignant plus falsely malignant; *negative predictive value,* correctly benign/correctly benign plus falsely benign.

(Courtesy of Barth RJ Jr, Merino MJ, Solomon D, et al: *Surgery* 112:536-543, 1992.)

selected cases, FNA biopsy may be useful in the diagnosis of soft tissue masses.

▶ In this prospecitve series, albeit relatively small, the value of CNBX and FNA was assessed in the diagnosis of soft tissue sarcoma. Whereas CNBX was beneficial, especially in the large-grade sarcomas, emphasis is placed on the technique and abilities of the pathologists.

Pathologists extensively familiar with sarcomas prefer incisional biopsies. This obviously makes selection of the tumor mass more accessible and therefore avoids obtaining necrotic or inadequate samples. The suggestion is made, however, that an open biopsy risks contamination and therefore should be performed with a definitive surgical procedure in mind so that placement of the incision is optimal, homeostasis is secured, and unnecessary dissection is avoided. This study describes another series from Memorial Sloan-Kettering Cancer Center in which the significance of small (less than or equal to 5 cm) soft tissue sarcomas of the extremities only is examined. Several points deserve emphasis. No new prognostic factors were identified in this series. Overall survival of patients with these tumors is superb, thus their inclusion in adjuvant treatment trials is not recommended.

As in previous studies, high-grade tumors led to an increased risk of metastatic disease. Furthermore, unless margins are positive, adjuvant therapies are not beneficial. Obviously, if margins are positive with a small tumor, further surgical limb-sparing surgery may be possible. If radiation therapy is administered, brachytherapy techniques often are ideal in this setting.—T.J. Eberlein, M.D.

## Melanomas

### Patient Characteristics, Methods of Diagnosis and Treatment of Melanoma in the United States

Sutherland CM, Chmiel JS, Henson DE, Cunningham MP, Peace BB, Winchester DP (Tulane Univ, New Orleans, La; Northwestern Univ, Chicago; Natl Cancer Inst, Bethesda, Md; St Francis Hosp, Chicago; HCA Coliseum Med Ctr, Macon, Ga; et al)
*Surg Gynecol Obstet* 175:129–134, 1992                    10–64

*Purpose.*—The American College of Surgeons conducted a survey to evaluate patient characteristics and trends in the diagnosis and treatment of melanoma. Survey forms were mailed to hospital cancer programs, registries, and committees to obtain data on patients with melanoma diagnosed in 1981 and in 1987. Included in the analysis were primary melanomas of the skin, eye, mucous membrane, unspecified other sites, and metastases with unknown primary sites. For the 1981 study, 681 hospitals provided data on 5,004 patients, and for the 1987 study, 844 hospitals furnished data on 6,900 patients.

*Results.*—In both series, most melanomas occurred in the skin and in Caucasian patients. In 1987 compared to 1981, patients were signifi-

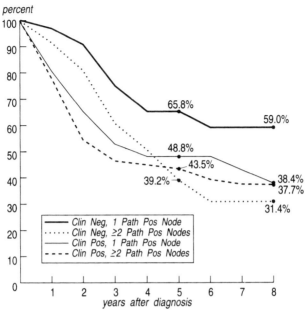

**Fig 10–27.**—Melanoma specific mortality by clinical node status and number of pathologic nodes for skin melanoma. *Clin,* clinical; *Neg,* negative; *Path,* pathologically, and *Pos,* positive. (Courtesy of Sutherland CM, Chmiel JS, Henson DE, et al: *Surg Gynecol Obstet* 175:129–134, 1992.)

cantly older at first diagnosis, and symptoms at initial diagnosis had declined. Patients with level I or II melanomas comprised 35.5% of Clark's level reported in 1981 and 41.3% of melanomas in 1987, indicating a significant shift to thinner levels of Clark's invasion. Breslow's thickness was available for 33.4% of patients in 1981 and for 27.1% in 1987, making this information difficult to interpret. Analysis of the cases with known Breslow's thickness suggested a slight shift toward thinner lesions in 1987. Analysis of 1981 survival and disease recurrence data showed the importance of clinical node status for patients with clinical stage I or II melanoma. The 8-year survival for patients with clinically negative node status and only 1 pathologically positive node was 59%, compared with 31.4% for clinically positive patients with at least 1 pathologic positive node and 38.4% for clinically negative patients with 2 or more positive nodes. The survival curves, however, were not obtained by random allocation to treatment and were not balanced by other prognostic factors (Fig 10–27). Thus the difference in survival should not be used as an argument for prophylactic node dissection. Compared with 1981, in the 1987 series there was a substantial decrease in the margins of excision, which is appropriate for thinner, less invasive melanomas. The 1987 data also showed an overall decline in the number of diagnostic studies performed.

*Comment.*—Although the decrease in the number of symptoms and invasion depth is encouraging, it is alarming that microstaging by Clark's level and Breslow's thickness was still not available for a substantial number of patients by 1987.

▶ This study, conducted by the American College of Surgeons, compared more than 11,000 patients in 1981 and 1987 and documents a slight decline in Breslow thickness. The importance of Clark's level, Breslow thickness, and nodal status in predicting survival was identified. Unfortunately, no definitive recommendation could be made with respect to lymph node dissection, because the patients were not randomly allocated and other prognostic factors were not taken into account. The study documents the current trend toward a decrease in the margin of excision for primary melanomas.

It is somewhat distressing that, even by the second study period of 1987, a substantial number of patients did not have Clark's level and Breslow thickness documented in their pathology reports. This lack of documentation obviously limits not only staging but also makes interpretation of survival more difficult.—T.J. Eberlein, M.D.

---

**Cutaneous Malignant Melanoma, Scotland, 1979–89**
MacKie R, Hunter JAA, Aitchison TC, Hole DN, McLaren K, Rankin R, Blessing K, Evans AT, Hutcheon AW, Jones DH, Soutar DS, Watson ACH, Cornbleet MA, Smyth JF (Glasgow Univ, Glasgow Scotland; Edinburgh Univ, Edinburgh, Scotland; Greater Glasgow Health Board; Raigmore Hosp, Inverness, Scotland; Aberdeen Univ, Aberdeen, Scotland; et al)
*Lancet* 339:971–975, 1992                                               10–65

---

*Background.*—In 1979 the Scottish Melanoma Group (SMG) was established to evaluate mortality from and the incidence, features, pathologic data, and management of cutaneous malignant melanoma in Scotland. The incidence and mortality over 11 years as they relate to anatomical site and pathologic types were reviewed.

*Methods and Findings.*—All 1,354 male and 2,459 female Scottish residents with primary cutaneous malignant melanoma diagnosed between 1979 and 1989 were included. The incidence per 100,000 population per year was 3.4 in 1979 for men and 6.6 for women (Fig 10–28). In 1989 those rates had risen to 7.1 and 10.4, respectively, representing an overall increase of 82% during the 11-year study period. The highest rates of increase were in lesions of the superficial spreading histogenetic type, arising on the leg in females and the trunk in males. After public education programs were begun in 1985, the proportion of all melanomas less than 1.5 mm thick increased significantly (Fig 10–29). Mortality data were available for 1,661 patients with a minimum follow-up of 5 years. The overall 5-year survival rate was 71.6%—77.6% for women and 58.7% for men. Women's survival advantage persisted even after adjustment for thickness, ulceration, and histogenetic type.

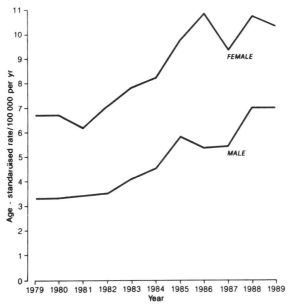

**Fig 10–28.**—Incidence of melanoma in Scotland, 1979–1989. Standardized to the Scottish 1981 population. (Courtesy of MacKie R, Hunter JAA, Aitchison TC, et al: *Lancet* 339:971–975, 1992.)

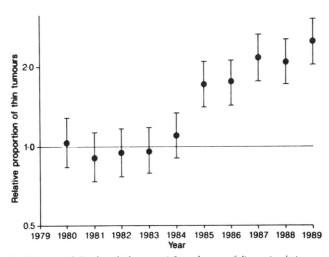

**Fig 10–29.**—Tumors with Breslow thickness < 1.5 mm by year of diagnosis relative to proportion in 1979. Adjusted for age, sex, tumor type, and site. Bars = 1 SD. (Courtesy of MacKie R, Hunter JAA, Aitchison TC, et al: *Lancet* 339:971–975, 1992.)

*Conclusions.*—A decade of data collection in Scotland enabled a detailed profile of the changing pattern of the incidence of and mortality from cutaneous melanoma. The information gathered will be useful in designing public education programs aimed at primary and secondary prevention of melanoma.

▶ This study from the Scottish Melanoma Group documents several epidemiologic trends. The first is an increase in the incidence of melanoma in both sexes, and the second is an increase in public education programs. Further, the proportion of thin melanomas has increased significantly even after adjustment for thickness, ulceration, and histogenic type.

Although this study does not address issues of treatment, it does emphasize the importance of public education programs and public awareness in the diagnosis and overall survivability from melanoma.—T.J. Eberlein, M.D.

---

**Relationship Between Immune Response to Melanoma Vaccine Immunization and Clinical Outcome in Stage II Malignant Melanoma**
Bystryn J-C, Oratz R, Roses D, Harris M, Henn M, Lew R (New York Univ, New York City; Univ of Massachusetts, Worcester)
*Cancer* 69:1157–1164, 1992                                          10–66

---

*Introduction.*—The incidence of malignant melanoma is doubling every 10 years in the United States. Although more than 90% of the patients have localized disease at diagnosis, residual deposits of tumor after surgery result in disease recurrence and death. A promising treatment for such patients is active specific immunotherapy with a melanoma antigen vaccine. Whether there is a relationship between induction of a delayed-type hypersensitivity (DTH) response to melanoma vaccine immunization and disease recurrence was investigated.

*Methods.*—Between October 1983 and February 1989, 108 consecutive patients with surgically resected stage II malignant melanoma were treated with the vaccine. All had histologically confirmed regional metastases but no evidence of distant disease. Between 4 weeks and 10 weeks after surgery, patients were immunized with a partially purified, polyvalent, melanoma antigen vaccine. The delayed-type hypersensitivity response to skin tests to the vaccine was measured before treatment and at the fourth vaccination. The mean follow-up was 28 months.

*Results.*—The 94 evaluable patients had a median disease-free survival (DFS) of 30 months. The estimated DFS at 3 years was 48%. Vaccine treatment induced a strong (31%) or moderate (25%) DTH response in slightly more than half of the patients; 44% had no response. The level of DTH response was related to the median duration of DFS (72 months, 24 months, and 15 months, respectively). Multivariate analysis demonstrated that the relationship between an increase in the DTH response and a prolonged DFS was independent of disease severity or overall immune competence.

*Conclusion.*—The vaccine produced no toxic side effects except for transient urticaria and stimulated a strong or moderate cellular immune response in 58% of these patients. Vaccine treatment may be able to slow the progression of melanoma in responders.

▶ This study documents the induction of a delayed-type hypersensitivity response to melanoma vaccine immunization. Although overall survival was not affected, the DFS was prolonged. This is another example of the immune system's role in the treatment and prognosis of melanoma. In this particular setting, the vaccine causes stimulation of the immune system; however, until the specific mechanisms are identified with regard to involvement of cells, cytokines, and/or antibody interactions, these types of observations will remain inconclusive, yet worthy of further study.—T.J. Eberlein, M.D.

# 11 Vascular

## Introduction

The recent publication of results from 2 large collaborative trials has clarified the role of carotid endarterectomy in patients with carotid artery stenosis. Both the NASCET study (Abstract 11-1) and the European carotid trial (Abstract 11-2) have demonstrated significant benefit from carotid endarterectomy in patients with severe (70% to 99%) symptomatic carotid stenosis. Randomized trials of surgical and medical therapy in patients with lesser degrees of symptomatic carotid stenosis or with asymptomatic carotid disease remain to be completed. Until that time, the study by Norris et al. (Abstract 11-3), which shows an approximate 2.5% risk per year ipsilateral stroke risk associated with asymptomatic carotid stenosis > 75% appears to support the use of carotid endarterectomy in selected asymptomatic patients, when the procedure can be done with a combined stroke and mortality < 1% to 2%.

The perception has been that aortic reconstruction procedures are associated with an increased risk of cardiac complications. In contrast, the report by Krupski et al. (Abstract 11-4) demonstrates that cardiac morbidity is essentially equivalent after aortic and infrainguinal operations. Techniques by which this risk may be reduced remain elusive, as shown by the report of Rivers et al. (Abstract 11-5), which documents no decrease in cardiac or noncardiac events in patients having epidural anesthesia compared with general anesthesia. Use of preoperative dipyridamole thallium cardiac scans potentially can identify patients who are at risk for perioperative cardiac complications as reported by Cambria et al. (Abstract 11-6). However, use of extensive preoperative cardiac testing and aggressive cardiac intervention in patients undergoing vascular reconstructive procedures remains essentially unproven. More importantly, proper selection of patients for arterial reconstruction based on careful natural history studies such as that by Brown et al. (Abstract 11-7), which reports that patients with aortic aneurysm less than 5 cm in diameter are unlikely to die of aneurysm rupture, and use of intraoperative techniques that limit postoperative complications, such as routine reimplantations of patent inferior mesenteric arteries, as described by Seeger et al (Abstract 11-8), are most likely to improve perioperative mortality.

The study of Fowl et al. (Abstract 11-9) demonstrates that measurement of ankle/brachial indices in patients with claudication can identify those individuals at risk for progressive disease who might benefit from early lower extremity revascularization. Similarly, Kowlek's study (Abstract 11-10) demonstrates that patients with juvenile-onset diabetes mellitus should undergo aggressive attempts at revascularization when limb-threatening ischemia is present. Surgical arterial reconstruction continues to be the primary therapy for patients with peripheral vascular disease, and the report by Tunis et al. (Abstract 11-11) demonstrates that use of transluminal angioplasty has not reduced the need for peripheral bypass surgery. Transluminal angioplasty has also been shown by Whittemore et al. (Abstract 11-12) to be of little benefit in the treatment of vein graph stenosis. The etiology of vein graft stenosis remains somewhat unclear; however, unsuspected, preexisting saphenous vein disease, as described by Panetta et al. (Abstract 11-13), may be an important predisposing factor. The technical aspects of arterial reconstruction remain important considerations when treating patients with lower extremity occlusive disease, as evidenced both by the study by Ricco (Abstract 11-14), which demonstrates improved results of iliofemoral bypass compared with femoral crossover bypass and by the report by Reifsnyder et al. (Abstract 11-15), which indicates a relatively high incidence of wound complications after in situ saphenous vein bypass.

Use of color-flow duplex scanning has been particularly useful in the diagnosis in calf vein thrombosis, as shown by Mattos et al. (Abstract 11-16) however, unfortunately, this modality was not used in the study by Lohr et al. (Abstract 11-17), in which aggressive treatment of calf vein thrombi was recommended. With the increased accuracy of that color flow duplex scanning offers, a more conservative approach of careful follow-up of calf vein thrombi and treatment only when extension into the popliteal vein occurs remains a good alternative. Finally, the use of routine arteriography for all penetrating extremity injuries is being shown to be unnecessary. However, as Frykberg et al. (Abstract 11-18) point out, experience in the interpretation of the physical signs of arterial injury and good patient follow-up are critical to the success of this strategy.

James M. Seeger, M.D.

---

### Beneficial Effect of Carotid Endarterectomy in Symptomatic Patients With High-Grade Carotid Stenosis

North American Symptomatic Carotid Endarterectomy Trial Collaborators
*N Engl J Med* 325:445–453, 1991                                            11-1

---

*Background.*—Until the mid-1980s, the use of carotid endarterectomy increased dramatically, although there was no strong evidence of benefit. Use of this procedure has decreased in recent years. A United States and Canadian prospective randomized trial was performed to determine whether carotid endarterectomy reduces the risk of stroke in patients with a recent adverse cerebrovascular event and ipsilateral carotid stenosis.

*Methods.*—Fifty North American centers participated in the study. All study patients had had a hemispheric or retinal transient ischemic attack or nondisabling stroke within 120 days of entry to the study. Severity of carotid stenosis, as measured by angiogram, was used to stratify the patients into 2 groups: high-grade stenosis, defined as stenosis of 70% to 99%; and medium-grade stenosis, defined as stenosis of 30% to 69%. There were 659 patients in the high-grade stenosis group. All patients received medical care, including antiplatelet therapy, and 328 were randomized to receive carotid endarterectomy. Each case in which an endpoint was reached was studied in blinded, independent fashion. Follow-up was complete.

*Results.*—By 24 months after randomization, life-table estimates of the cumulative risk of ipsilateral stroke were 26% in the medically treated group and 9% in the surgically treated group. This reflected an absolute risk reduction of 17% and a relative risk reduction of 65%. For major or fatal ipsilateral stroke, the cumulative risk was 13.1% in the medically treated group and 2.5% in the surgically treated group. This corresponded to an absolute risk reduction of 10.6% and a relative risk reduction of 81%. Even when all strokes and deaths were included, surgical treatment still carried a 10.1% reduction in absolute risk. Evidence for the efficacy of surgery for patients with high-grade stenosis was so strong that randomization of this group was halted. The study of medium-grade stenosis was continued.

*Conclusion.*—For patients who have ipsilateral high-grade stenosis after hemispheric and retinal transient ischemic attacks or nondisabling strokes, carotid endarterectomy appears to be a highly beneficial treatment.

▶ This is probably the most important paper published to date on carotid endarterectomy. Vascular surgeons will do well to become extremely familiar with every part of this pivotal publication.—J.M. Porter, M.D.

---

**MRC European Carotid Surgery Trial: Interim Results for Symptomatic Patients With Severe (70–99%) or With Mild (0–29%) Cartoid Stenosis**
European Carotid Surgery Trialists' Collaborative Group
*Lancet* 337:1235–1243, 1991                                               11–2

---

*Background.*—Patients who have had a nondisabling carotid territory ischemic stroke, transient ischemic attack (TIA), or retinal infarct, and are found to have stenosis at or near the bifurcation of the carotid artery on angiography, were randomized to surgery. Interim results are given of a multicenter, randomized trial designed to determine the operative and long-term risks of disabling stroke and the duration of nondisabled survival for patients with mild, moderate, or severe stenosis.

*Methods.*—During the past 10 years 2,518 patients at 80 centers were entered into the European Carotid Surgery Trial. All had a carotid territory nondisabling stroke or TIA, or a retinal infarct within the 6 months preceding randomization, and all had stenosis of the relevant carotid artery. Mild stenosis was defined as 0% to 29%; moderate stenosis was defined as 30% to 69%; and severe stenosis was defined as 70% to 99%. The patients were randomized to receive immediate surgery or no surgery. The mean follow-up to date is 3 years for 2,200 patients available for analysis of strokes lasting more than 7 days.

*Results.*—Moderate stenosis was seen in almost half the randomized patients. For this group, no conclusions could be drawn regarding the risk-benefit ratio of surgery, and full recruitment continues. Mild stenosis was seen in 374 patients. Even without surgery, these patients had little risk of ipsilateral stroke at 3 years; thus, the benefits of surgery were outweighed by the early risks. Severe stenosis was seen in 778 patients. In this group, the late benefits of surgery significantly outweighed its early risks. Overall, 7.5% of the patients with severe stenosis had a stroke or died within 30 days of surgery. During the next 3 years, however, patients who underwent immediate surgery had an extra 2.8% risk of ipsilateral stroke compared with 16.8% for controls. The surgery group also had a small reduction in the incidence of other strokes. The total risk of surgical death, ipsilateral stroke, or any stroke was 12.3% for the immediate surgery group compared with 21.9% for the control group. Disabling stroke or death occurred within 30 days of surgery in 3.7% of the patients. An extra 1.1% of surgery patients had a disabling stroke or died within 3 years compared with 8.4% of controls. The overall risk of any disabling or fatal stroke, including surgical death, was 6% in the surgery group compared with 11% in controls. In controls, however, the risks appeared to diminish after the first year, suggesting that delaying surgery by just a few months may make the overall difference nonsignificant.

*Conclusion.*—For patients with severe stenosis, carotid endarterectomy can avoid most ipsilateral ischemic strokes for the next few years. There is no apparent benefit of surgery in patients with mild stenosis, and recruitment continues in patients with moderate stenosis.

▶ This study stretches the definition of "randomized trial" to the limit. If the attending physician was "reasonably certain" after angiography that surgery was indicated, then the patient was declared ineligible for the trial. Thus, there is a major sampling error. In spite of this and other flaws in the study, it does corroborate the results of the NASCET trial, showing a clear advantage for carotid endarterectomy in symptomatic patients with 70% or greater internal carotid artery stenosis.—F.W. LoGerfo, M.D.

**Vascular Risks of Asymptomatic Carotid Stenosis**
Norris JW, Zhu CZ, Bornstein NM, Chambers BR (Univ of Toronto; Repatria-

tion Gen Hosp, Melbourne)
*Stroke* 22:1485–1490, 1991                                                11–3

*Background.*—Considerable evidence suggests that the asymptomatic neck bruit is a risk factor for later stroke, myocardial infarction, and death. Nevertheless, the risk of stroke is low. However, because most patients with bruit do not have significant carotid stenosis, an evaluation of the outcome of patients with proven carotid stenosis appears to be more important.

*Methods.*—A total of 696 patients with vascular laboratory-determined asymptomatic carotid stenosis seen over a mean period of 41 months were followed. The mean patient age was 64 years. Patients were followed clinically and by carotid Doppler ultrasound examinations.

*Findings.*—Seventy-five patients had transient ischemic attacks, and 29 had a stroke. A total of 132 patients had ischemic cardiac events during follow-up. Five patients died of stroke, and 59 died of cardiac causes. The annual rate of stroke was 1.3% in patients with 75% or less carotid stenosis and 3.3% in those with more marked stenosis. Patients with severe stenosis had an 8.3% annual rate of cardiac events, and an annual morbidity of 6.5%.

*Conclusion.*—Even moderate carotid stenosis increases the risk of cardiac ischemia and vascular death. The risk of stroke is increased in the presence of more than 75% stenosis, even in the absence of symptoms.

▶ This report by neurologists indicates that patients with diameter reduction of carotid stenosis greater than 75% have a combined transient ischemic attack and stroke rate of 10.5% per year, for a cardiac event rate of 8.3% per year and a death rate of 6.5% per year. It is crystal clear that symptomatic peripheral arterial disease, be it lower extremity or carotid, defines a patient population that is at extreme risk for morbid cardiovascular events, indeed a patient population approaching the end of life.—J.M. Porter, M.D.

## Comparison of Cardiac Morbidity Between Aortic and Infrainguinal Operations

Krupski WC, Layug EL, Reilly LM, Rapp JH, Mangano DT, Study of Perioperative Ischemia Research Group (Dept of Veterans Affairs Med Ctr; Univ of California, San Francisco)
*J Vasc Surg* 15:354–365, 1992                                            11–4

*Objective.*—Perioperative cardiac ischemic events were compared in a series of 53 patients having major abdominal vascular operations and in a group of 87 patients having infrainguinal vascular surgery. The respective average operating times were 421 and 459 minutes.

*Methods.*—Thirty-eight patients had dipyridamole-thallium cardiac scintigraphy preoperatively. The electrocardiogram and transesophageal

TABLE 1.—Perioperative Ischemia

| | | No. of patients with abnormalities (% studies performed) | | |
| Study | No. of patients studied | Infrainguinal n = 87 | Aortic n = 53 | p value* |
|---|---|---|---|---|
| **Preoperative** | | | | |
| Standard 12-lead ECG† | 140 | 60 (69) | 28 (53) | 0.08 |
| Continuous 2-Lead ECG (Holter Monitor)‡ | 93 | 22 (37) | 8 (24) | 0.3 |
| Dipyridamole-thallium scan§ | 38 | 7 (33) | 6 (35) | 0.8 |
| **Intraoperative** | | | | |
| Continuous 12-lead ECG‖ | 133 | 22 (26) | 12 (23) | 0.8 |
| Continuous 2-lead ECG (Holter monitor) | 139 | 32 (40) | 16 (31) | 0.4 |
| Transesophageal echocardiography | 133 | 8 (10) | 13 (26) | 0.02 |
| **Postoperative** | | | | |
| Continuous 2-lead ECG (Holter monitor)¶ | 133 | 46 (57) | 16 (31) | 0.005 |

* Infrainguinal vs. aortic.
† Indicates any abnormality, (e.g., myocardial infarction, arrhythmias, bundle branch block, and the like).
‡ Indicates ST segment changes suggestive of ischemia.
§ Reversible defect observed.
‖ Indicates ST segment changes suggestive of ischemia.
¶ Severe ischemia as defined by a 2-mm deviation of the ST segment from the baseline for ≥ 30 min.
(Courtesy of Krupski WC, Layug EL, Reilly LM, et al.: J Vasc Surg 15:354–365, 1992.)

echocardiogram were used to detect myocardial ischemia during surgery, and Holter monitoring was repeated 4 days postoperatively. The outcome events included cardiac death, nonfatal myocardial infarction, unstable angina, ventricular tachycardia, and congestive heart failure.

*Results.*—More patients in the infrainguinal group had diabetes, angina, and heart failure, but preoperative ECG and thallium scan abnor-

TABLE 2.—Postoperative Adverse Cardiac Outcomes

|  | *Infrainguinal* | *Aortic* | *p value** |
|---|---|---|---|
| Unstable angina† | 1 (1%) | 0 (0%) | 0.7* |
| Myocardial infarction† | 3 (3.5%) | 0 (0%) | 0.6* |
| Cardiac death† | 3 (3.5%) | 1 (2%) | 0.9* |
| Ventricular tachycardia | 7 (8%) | 6 (11%) | 0.7 |
| Heart failure | 9 (10%) | 8 (15%) | 0.6 |
| Total outcome events | 23 (26%) | 15 (28%) | 1.0 |

* Fisher's exact test.
† Total grave cardiac outcomes 8% vs. 2%, P = .3.
‡ Infrainguinal vs. aortic.
(Courtesy of Krupski WC, Layug EL, Reilly LM, et al: *J Vasc Surg* 15:354–365, 1992.)

malities were similarly frequent in the 2 surgical groups. Echocardiography demonstrated intraoperative ischemia in 26% of the patients having aortic surgery and in 10% of those having infrainguinal procedures (Table 1). Outcome events were similarly frequent in the 2 groups (Table 2). Holter monitoring more often demonstrated postoperative ischemia in patients having infrainguinal operations.

*Conclusion.*—Patients requiring infrainguinal vascular reconstruction have cardiac disease more often than those who require aortic surgery, and they have a risk of cardiac events that is at least as great.

▶ The widespread perception is that major aortic surgery has a high likelihood of perioperative cardiac complications which, based on the magnitude of surgery, should certainly be greater than that expected after lower extremity vascular repair. It seems clear, however, that by the time significant lower extremity arterial ischemic symptoms develop, they almost invariably have severe associated coronary disease. This study documents (by a variety of methods) that adverse cardiac outcomes are at least as likely to occur after lower extremity arterial repair as after aortic operations.—J.M. Porter, M.D.

**Epidural Versus General Anesthesia for Infrainguinal Arterial Reconstruction**
Rivers SP, Scher LA, Sheehan E, Veith FJ (Albert Einstein College of Medicine, Montefiore Med Ctr, New York)
*J Vasc Surg* 14:764–770, 1991                                            11–5

*Introduction.*—Epidural anesthesia is often the preferred approach for patients undergoing infrainguinal bypass surgery, especially those at risk of cardiovascular and pulmonary complications from general endotracheal anesthesia.

TABLE 1.—Cardiac Complications

| | 30-day mortality rate | Nonfatal postoperative MI | Reversible cardiac events* | Total |
|---|---|---|---|---|
| EPI n = 96 | 5 (5%) | 6 (6%) | 13 (14%) | 24 (25%) |
| GET n = 117 | 4 (3%) | 8 (7%) | 21 (18%) | 33 (28%) |

Abbreviations: MI, myocardial infarction; EPI, epidural; GET, general epidural intubation.
* Includes angina, arrythmia, and pulmonary edema that resolved without sequelae.
(Courtesy of Rivers SP, Scher LA, Sheehan E, et al: J Vasc Surg 14:764–770, 1991.)

*Methods.*—A total of 174 consecutive patients who underwent 213 infrainguinal bypass operations in 1986–1990 were studied prospectively. The mean patient age was 69 years. More than 90% of the operations were performed for limb salvage. Nearly one third of the patients had secondary revascularization. Epidural anesthesia was used in 96 procedures, and general endotracheal anesthesia was used in 117.

*Results.*—Cardiac complications were not substantially less frequent in patients who had epidural anesthesia (Table 1). Other systemic complications were more frequent in the epidural group (Table 2). In 69 patients at especially high risk (American Society of Anesthesiologists class IV and V or a Goldman score above 10), there was no significant difference in outcome in the 2 anesthetic groups (Table 3).

*Conclusion.*—If infrainguinal arterial reconstruction is indicated, it should not be postponed or avoided when a patient requires or requests general anesthesia.

▶ What seems intuitively correct does not always withstand scientific scrutiny. These prospective studies (Abstracts 5–9 and 5–13) show that, despite theoretical advantages, neither epidural anesthesia for leg bypass, nor epidural in combination with light general anesthesia for aortic reconstruction, is superior to general anesthesia alone. Nevertheless, epidural anesthesia may be preferable in select patients with severe pulmonary insufficiency (1). A reduction in postoperative hypercoagulability associated with epidural anes-

TABLE 2.—Miscellaneous Systemic Complications

| | EPI | GET |
|---|---|---|
| Venous thromboembolic | 1 | 2 |
| Renal failure | 2 | 0 |
| Stroke | 2 | 0 |
| Spinal headache | 1 | N/A |
| | 6 (6%) | 2 (2%) |

Courtesy of Rivers SP, Scher LA, Sheehan E, et al: J Vasc Surg 14:764–770, 1991.

TABLE 3.—Results

*Patients at high risk*

| | 30-day mortality rate | Nonfatal postoperative MI | Reversible cardiac events |
|---|---|---|---|
| EPI n = 31 | 1 | 5 | 5 |
| GET n = 33 | 3 | 1 | 9 |
| Total n = 64 | 4 | 6 | 14 |

*Abbreviations:* MI, myocardial infarction; *EPI,* epidural; *GET,* general intubation.
(Courtesy of Rivers SP, Scher LA, Sheehan E, et al: *J Vasc Surg* 14:764–770, 1991.)

thesia had recently been described in vascular surgical patients; this interesting observation requires confirmation (2). The potential benefits of *postoperative* epidural analgesia were not addressed in either report and deserve further study.—J. Mills, M.D.

*References*

1. Mason RA, et al: *J Cardiovasc Surg* 31:442, 1990.
2. Tuman K J, et al: *Anesth Analg* 73:696, 1991.

### The Impact of Selective Use of Dipyridamole-Thallium Scans and Surgical Factors on the Current Morbidity of Aortic Surgery

Cambria RP, Brewster DC, Abbott WM, L'Italien GJ, Megerman JJ, LaMuraglia GM, Moncure AC, Zelt DT, Eagle K (Massachusetts General Hosp; Harvard Med School, Boston)
*J Vasc Surg* 15:43–51, 1992                                              11–6

*Background.*—Cardiac evaluation before vascular surgery remains a controversial issue. It is suggested that dipyridamole-thallium scanning be carried out selectively before surgery on the aorta, on the basis of clinical markers of coronary artery disease.

*Methods.*—The use of thallium scanning was reviewed in 202 patients having elective aortic reconstruction (151 for abdominal aortic aneurysm and 51 for aortoiliac occlusive disease).

*Results.*—Preoperative dipyridamole-thallium scanning was done in 29% of the patients. As a result, 11% of the patients had coronary angiography and 9% underwent coronary bypass grafting/percutaneous coronary angioplasty before aortic surgery. There was 1 cardiac death, 4% of patients had nonfatal myocardial infarction or unstable angina, and 6% experienced pulmonary complications. The factors associated with postoperative death or cardiopulmonary problems included an operating time longer than 5 hours, the presence of aortoiliac occlusive disease, and a history of ventricular ectopy. Both prolonged surgery and intraoperative myocardial ischemia predicted major cardiac complications.

*Conclusion.*—Thallium scanning guided by clinical markers of coronary artery disease will identify those patients requiring aortic reconstruction in whom invasive management of coronary disease before reconstruction is appropriate.

▶ These authors advocate selective use of dipyridamole-thallium cardiac scanning in preoperative vascular patients. They performed the test in 29% of their patients and found a 9% incidence of preoperative coronary grafting. Interestingly, their perioperative clinical outcome was virtually identical to that reported in Abstract 5–4. It appears that the Oregon group and the Massachusetts General group are reaching substantially different conclusions based on the same data.—J.M. Porter, M.D.

---

### The Selective Management of Small Abdominal Aortic Aneurysms: The Kingston Study
Brown PM, Pattenden R, Gutelius JR (Queen's Univ, Kingston, Ont)
*J Vasc Surg* 15:21–27, 1992                                    11–7

---

*Background.*—The correct management of abdominal aortic aneurysms with a maximal diameter less than 5 cm remains uncertain, especially in those patients who are medically fit. The Kingston Abdominal Aortic Aneurysm Study, unlike other studies, is prospective, and it includes all patients seen with small aneurysms.

*Methods.*—A total of 268 patients entered the study between 1976 and 1988 and were monitored through 1990 (mean, 42 months). The

TABLE 1.—Deaths in the Aneurysm Study Group
Follow-up Patients

| | |
|---|---|
| Myocardial infarction | 15 |
| Respiratory failure | 8 |
| Stroke | 5 |
| Malignancy | 5 |
| Renal failure | 3 |
| Suicide | 1 |
| Unknown | 1 |
| Rupture | 1 |

(Courtesy of Brown PM, Pattenden R, Gutelius JR: *J Vasc Surg* 15:21-27, 1992.)

TABLE 2.—Comparison of Surgical Rates Related to Size at Entry

| Aneurysm size | Surgery | Continued follow-up |
|---|---|---|
| Less than 4.0 cm at entry | 31 patients (24%) | 98 patients (76%) |
| 4.0 cm or greater at entry | 83 patients (60%) | 56 patients (40%) |

(Courtesy of Brown PM, Pattenden R, Gutelius JR: *J Vasc Surg* 15:21–27, 1992.)

criteria for surgery included an increase in aneurysm size to 5 cm, expansion of more than .5 cm in 6 months, and the development of aneurysmal symptoms or significant aortoiliac occlusive disease.

*Results.*—Surgery was done on 114 patients, in whom the aneurysm increased by a mean of .9 cm annually. The remaining 154 patients were monitored without operation. There was 1 rupture in this group. The average annual increase in aneurysmal diameter in unoperated patients was .24 cm. Myocardial infarction was the most common cause of death in the monitored group (Table 1). Aneurysms measuring 4 cm or more at the outset more often required surgical treatment (Table 2). Men and women had comparable expansion rates (Table 3).

*Recommendation.*—These findings support a policy of observation for abdominal aortic aneurysms that have a maximum diameter less than 5 cm.

▶ We are beset on one side by the apparent increase in the incidence of aneurysms, the increased incidence of ruptured aneurysms, and a very high death rate from ruptured aneurysms. On the other side, we are told that small

TABLE 3.—Expansion Rates Stratified to Sex of Patient

| Surgical group | Follow-up group | Overall mean expansion |
|---|---|---|
| Men | | |
| 0.88 cm/yr | 0.25 cm/yr | 0.53 cm/yr |
| (98 patients) | (121 patients) | (219 patients) |
| Women | | |
| 0.80 cm/yr | 0.24 cm/yr | 0.42 cm/yr |
| (16 patients) | (33 patients) | (49 patients) |

(Courtesy of Brown PM, Pattenden R, Gutelius JR: *J Vasc Surg* 15:21–27, 1992.)

aneurysms less than 5 cm in maximum diameter should not be operated on. Clearly, every ruptured aneurysm population study done to date has shown that nearly 5% of ruptures occurred in aneurysms with a diameter less than 5 cm. Elective aneurysm mortality in America is probably between 3% and 5%. If we operated on 100 patients with small aneurysms to prevent rupture in 5, 3–5 patients would not survive aneurysm surgery; therefore, there would be no net gain. These are important numbers with which every vascular surgeon should be familiar.—J.M. Porter, M.D.

## A Preliminary Study of the Role of Duplex Scanning in Defining the Adequacy of Treatment of Patients With Renal Artery Fibromuscular Dysplasia

Edwards JM, Zaccardi MJ, Strandness DE Jr (Univ of Washington, Seattle)
J Vasc Surg 15:604–611, 1992                          11–8

*Background.*—Fibromuscular dysplasia (FMD) of the renal arteries is a recognized cause of hypertension that has a characteristic arteriographic appearance. It often is difficult to determine the functional significance of FMD lesions, particularly when both renal arteries are involved. Duplex scanning is an accurate means of detecting and quantifying renal artery stenosis.

*Methods.*—Nine patients with FMD of the renal artery were managed by either angioplasty or surgery. Eighteen arteries were treated, 4 of them more than once. Transluminal angioplasty was done 16 times, and 2 arteries that failed to improve underwent bypass surgery.

*Results.*—Fourteen of 18 treatments led to a reduction in blood pressure. In all these cases, the renal-aortic ratio decreased below the level at which greater than 60% stenosis is diagnosed. In the failures, velocity at the site of narrowing did not improve after intervention. Hemodynamic improvement was noted in patients who improved clinically.

*Conclusion.*—Duplex scanning is able, along with the clinical response, to help determine the cause of failure when a patient with FMD fails to improve after angioplasty or operative treatment.

▶ Well-performed duplex scanning can provide important information about visceral artery stenosis, both before and after surgery. It has become the initial diagnostic test of choice in centers with experienced and skilled vascular laboratory technologists.—J.M. Porter, M.D.

## Natural History of Claudicants With Critical Hemodynamic Indices

Fowl RJ, Gewirtz RJ, Love MC, Kempczinski RF (Univ of Cincinnati)
Ann Vasc Surg 6:31–33, 1992                          11–9

*Background.*—Earlier studies lacking hemodynamic data suggested that intermittent claudication of the lower extremity is a benign disorder. In more recent studies, the prognosis was much worse when ankle/brachial indices were low.

*Methods.*—An examination of records of nearly 1,500 patients having arterial studies in the lower extremity yielded 23 patients in whom 25 extremities had an ankle/brachial index of .35 or less, an ankle or transmetatarsal pulse volume of 3 mm or less in amplitude, and no history of ischemic rest pain or gangrene. The patients were followed up for a mean of 45.2 months.

*Results.*—Thirteen of the 25 extremities did not have limb-threatening symptoms, and claudication improved in 3 instances. The other 12 extremities had rest pain, ischemic ulceration or, in 3 extremities, gangrene. Eight of these limbs underwent revascularization, and only 1 ultimately required major amputation. One patient had primary above-knee amputation for extensive gangrene.

*Conclusion.*—All patients with intermittent claudication and critical ischemia require close follow-up, because perhaps half will have limb-threatening ischemia necessitating surgical treatment. Early surgery may be considered for patients who are considered unlikely to comply with regular follow-up.

▶ This is another important natural history study of claudication, this time in patients with critical hemodynamic indices. Of considerable interest is the observation that, during a mean follow-up of 45 months, half the patients with an initial ankle/brachial index equal to or less than .35 stabilized or improved, whereas half of these patients regressed. Did you know that almost all of the natural history information on claudication obtained before 1980 was based on questionnaires without vascular lab or patient examinations? A widely held belief that 80% to 90% of claudicants stabilize or improve with time and that only 10% to 20% deteriorate is erroneous. Detailed vascular laboratory studies reveal that the behavior of claudication is significantly related to the ankle/brachial index at the time of the initial evaluation. At least 50% of the patients with a claudication ankle/brachial index less than .5 will eventually require interventional therapy (1).—J.M. Porter, M.D.

*Reference*

1. Cronenwett JL, et al: *Arch Surg* 119:430, 1984.

### Peripheral Vascular Bypass in Juvenile-Onset Diabetes Mellitus: Are Aggressive Revascularization Attempts Justified?

Kwolek CJ, Pomposelli FB, Tannenbaum GA, Brophy CM, Gibbons GW, Campbell DR, Freeman DV, Miller A, LoGerfo FW (Harvard Med School, Boston)
*J Vasc Surg* 15:394–401, 1992                                             11–10

*Objective.*—Individuals with diabetes mellitus account for as many as two thirds of patients having lower limb amputation. The results of 67 bypass procedures in 60 patients with juvenile-onset diabetes mellitus were evaluated. The procedures constituted 5.5% of all bypasses done in patients with diabetes during the 6-year review period. The mean age was 44 years.

*Surgery.*—All but 9% of the operations were done for limb salvage. Most were primary infrainguinal bypasses using saphenous vein. Six procedures were revision surgery procedures, and 4 were inflow procedures.

*Results.*—Nearly one third of the patients had morbidity, but there were no postoperative deaths. The actuarial patency rate after primary vein graft surgery was 66% at 2 years, and the limb salvage rate was 83.4%. Seventeen primary infrainguinal bypass grafts that were done using saphenous vein failed, leading to 9 major limb amputations. Five of 8 failed grafts were successfully revised.

*Conclusion.*—Patients with juvenile-onset diabetes mellitus require arterial bypass surgery at a much younger age than other patients; nevertheless, a successful outcome may be anticipated.

▶ Type I diabetics, especially cigarette smokers, are among the most difficult patients with leg ischemia that we encounter. Although the results obtained by this excellent group are admirable, they are considerably inferior to those obtained by the same group in other patients. It is important for vascular surgeons to recognize the substantial difficulties presented by these patients, and for both the patients and surgeon to have realistic expectations from surgery.—J.M. Porter, M.D.

### The Use of Angioplasty, Bypass Surgery, and Amputation in the Management of Peripheral Vascular Disease

Tunis SR, Bass EB, Steinberg EP (Johns Hopkins Univ, Baltimore)
*N Engl J Med* 325:556–562, 1991                                           11–11

*Introduction.*—Although percutaneous transluminal angioplasty has become a popular alternative to peripheral bypass surgery in selected patients with peripheral vascular disease of the lower extremities, its effect on management of peripheral vascular disease and patient outcome has not been clearly defined. The extent to which angioplasty is used and the impact of this procedure on the surgical management of peripheral vascular disease were determined.

*Methods.*—Study data were derived from the records of hospital discharges in Maryland between 1979 and 1989. Information was obtained on all angioplasty procedures, peripheral bypass operations, and lower extremity amputations performed for peripheral vascular disease during this period.

*Findings.*—Between 1979 and 1989, the estimated annual rate of angioplasty for peripheral vascular disease of the lower extremities increased from 1 to 24 per 100,000 Maryland residents. The adjusted annual rate of peripheral bypass surgery increased as well, from 32 to 65 per 100,000. The adjusted annual rate of lower-extremity amputation remained stable, at approximately 30 per 100,000. There was a substantial increase in the number of hospital days and in the total charges associated with revascularization procedures. Charges increased from $14.7 million in 1979 (in 1989 dollars) to $30.5 million in 1989.

*Conclusion.*—The use of percutaneous transluminal angioplasty instead of peripheral bypass surgery in selected patients with peripheral vascular disease was expected to substantially reduce costs and the need for amputation. In Maryland, however, numbers of surgical procedures have increased, costs have risen, and the amputation rate remains unchanged. These findings may reflect more frequent diagnosis and an expansion of the indications for angioplasty and bypass surgery.

▶ Isn't it amazing that the prestigious *New England Journal of Medicine* is so uninformed about peripheral arterial disease? Percutaneous transluminal angioplasty (PTLA) is used in the treatment of claudication; rarely is it used in the treatment of end stage limb ischemia. No vascular surgeon is surprised by the published observation that, although the use of PTLA and leg bypass procedures increased over a period of time, the amputation rate remained stable. In fact, the editors were so shocked by this finding that they produced an editorial on the topic in the same issue of the *New England Journal of Medicine.* It is obvious that we vascular surgeons have a large educational chore ahead of us.—J.M. Porter, M.D.

---

**Limitations of Balloon Angioplasty for Vein Graft Stenosis**
Whittemore AD, Donaldson MC, Polak JF, Mannick JA (Brigham and Women's Hosp and Harvard Med School, Boston)
*J Vasc Surg* 14:340–345, 1991                                    11–12

---

*Background.*—A considerable number of autogenous infrainguinal reconstructions fail because of vein graft stenosis—most often developing near anastomoses. Fibrous intimal hyperplasia presumably is the cause. Percutaneous transluminal balloon angioplasty has been proposed as an alternative to surgical revision in the treatment of vein graft stenosis.

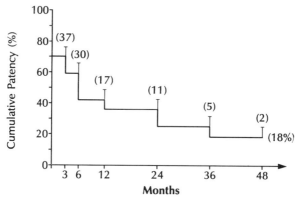

**Fig 11–1.**—The 4-year primary cumulative patency curve associated with balloon angioplasty for vein graft stenoses. (Courtesy of Whittemore AD, Donaldson MC, Polak JF, et al: *J Vasc Surg* 14:340–345, 1991.)

*Series.*—Balloon angioplasty was carried out in 30 patients with 54 stenotic lesions that had developed in autogenous vein grafts after infrainguinal arterial reconstruction.

*Results.*—The primary cumulative 5-year patency rate was 18% (Fig 11–1) and was not related to the length of the stenotic lesion or the need for initial thrombolytic treatment. When a single angioplasty sufficed, 59% of the patients had a patent reconstruction at 3 years, compared with only 6% when repeated dilation was necessary.

*Conclusion.*—Balloon angioplasty is not a consistently effective means of providing long-term secondary patency when vein graft stenosis complicates infrainguinal arterial reconstruction.

▶ This study makes the point that angioplasty is not an effective means for correcting stenosis in vein grafts. The reason that this form of reconstruction performs less well than simple vein patch grafting is unclear (1). However, it should also be noted that angioplasty works less well in the superficial femoral arteries than it does in the higher flow vessels. The observation supports the conclusion that some form of pharmacologic, as opposed to surgical, therapy is needed for the correction of intimal hyperplasia and stenoses in blood vessels.—F.W. LoGerfo, M.D.

*Reference*

1. Whittemore AD, et al: *Ann Surg* 193:35, 1981.

---

**Unsuspected Preexisting Saphenous Vein Disease: An Unrecognized Cause of Vein Bypass Failure**
Panetta TF, Marin ML, Veith FJ, Goldsmith J, Gordon RE, Jones AM, Schwartz ML, Gupta SK, Wengerter KR (Montefiore Med Ctr/Albert Einstein

College of Medicine, New York; Mt Sinai Med Ctr, New York)
*J Vasc Surg* 15:102–112, 1992                                          11–13

*Background.*—Previous experience with unsuspected, preexisting saphenous vein disease prompted a study of 513 infrainguinal arterial bypasses performed with the use of saphenous veins in 1984–1990. Sixty-three diseased saphenous veins were identified. Fifty veins or vein segments with minimal or unsuspected disease were used for the bypasses.

*Results.*—The lesions found in the 63 cases (12%) included thick-walled veins, varicose veins, and postphlebitic sclerotic veins with occlusion or recanalization. Severe changes precluded the use of the vein in 13 cases. Ten of the 50 veins that were used failed at an early stage. At 30 months, the cumulative primary patency rate for these 50 cases was only 32% (Fig 11-2). A review of 21 preoperative duplex ultrasound studies revealed vein abnormalities in 62% of the cases. The histologic findings in diseased veins included intimal and medial thickening, calcification of the vein wall, and luminal recanalization (Fig 11-3).

*Conclusion.*—Unsuspected saphenous vein disease is not infrequent and can cause early or late graft failure. Some cases are detectable by duplex ultrasonography. A thick-walled, calcified, or recanalized vein should not be used if an alternative is available.

▶ Diseased veins unquestionably form very poor bypass conduits. We are readily able to detect a thick-wall, nondistensible segment of vein during hydrostatic dilatation of a reversed vein, which we perform with chilled, autologous heparinized blood. We are in total agreement with the authors that recanalized or thick-walled sclerotic veins give such poor results that they

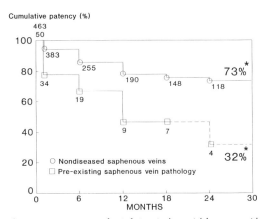

**Fig 11–2.**—Cumulative primary patency for infrainguinal arterial bypasses with autogenous saphenous vein. Vein grafts with preexisting venous disease had significantly decreased patency at all time intervals (* $P \leq$ .001). (Courtesy of Panetta TF, Marin ML, Veith FJ, et al: *J Vasc Surg* 15:102–112, 1992.)

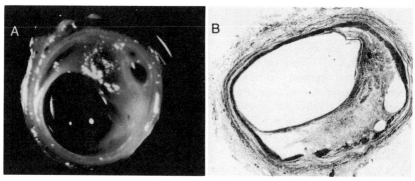

**Fig 11–3.**—Recanalized saphenous vein segment. **A,** this vein would irrigate normally and allow passage of the catherer, thereby allowing recanalized disease to go undetected, although the vein is markedly thickened. **B,** this section clearly demonstrates the thick wall of the vein composed of abundant connective tissue surrounding several recanalized channels. Trichrome stain; original magnification, ×10.) (Courtesy of Panetta TF, Marin ML, Veith FJ, et al: *J Vasc Surg* 15:102–112, 1992.)

should not be used. These veins should be discarded, and alternate autogenous veins should be used for bypass. I do not identify any need for angioscopy to assist in vein evaluation.—J.M. Porter, M.D.

## Unilateral Iliac Artery Occlusive Disease: A Randomized Multicenter Trial Examining Direct Revascularization Versus Crossover Bypass

Ricco J-B (Hospital Jean Bernard, Poitiers, France)
*Ann Vasc Surg* 6:209–219, 1992                                          11–14

*Introduction.*—In a randomized trial patency rates for direct unilateral aortofemoral or iliofemoral prosthetic bypass grafts were compared with those for crossover femorofemoral or iliofemoral bypass grafts in patients with atheromatous occlusive disease of the iliac artery. A total of 143 patients were enrolled in this study.

*Methods.*—Seventy-four patients had crossover procedures and 69 had direct revascularization between May 1986 and March 1991. The groups were comparable with respect to cardiovascular risk factors, symptoms, and atheromatous lesions. Duplex ultrasonography with systolic pressure index estimates was used to follow the patients. Digital subtraction arteriography was done after operation and when hemodynamic abnormalities developed. The mean follow-up was 22 months.

*Results.*—One patient died after direct revascularization. The primary patency rate at 3 years was 90% for patients who had direct revascularization and 79% for those who had crossover bypass. Secondary patency rates at 4 years were 93% and 94%, respectively, which was not a significant difference.

*Conclusion.*—Crossover bypasses may seem to be an attractive approach to unilateral iliac occlusive disease, but direct revascularization is preferred for young patients lacking major surgical risk. The crossover bypass is indicated for patients at risk.

▶ The debate continues as to the optimal repair for the patient with symptomatic unilateral iliac artery occlusive disease. There seems to be no escaping the fact that the femorofemoral bypass is an inferior procedure and simply not comparable to aortofemoral or iliac femoral direct revascularization procedures in terms of patency. Of course, the cross femoral graft is quick and relatively uncomplicated. In the younger patient, however, and especially in the patient with superficial femoral artery occlusion, the femorofemoral bypass appears especially unattractive.—J.M. Porter, M.D.

**Wound Complications of the In Situ Saphenous Vein Bypass Technique**
Reifsnyder T, Bandyk D, Seabrook G, Kinney E, Towne JB (Med College of Wisconsin, Milwaukee)
*J Vasc Surg* 15:843–850, 1992                                                   11–15

*Background.*—Wound complications are frequent after in situ saphenous vein bypass surgery. They may lengthen hospitalization and threaten the viability of the graft.

*Series.*—A total of 126 in situ operations were done in 117 consecutive male patients in 1981–1991. They included 45 femoropopliteal bypasses, 75 femorotibial bypasses, and 6 grafts to the dorsal pedal artery. Sixty-nine procedures were done for ulceration or gangrene, 54 for rest pain, and 3 for claudication. The wound complications were classified as shown in Table 1.

TABLE 1.—Classification of Wound Complications After In Situ Saphenous Vein Bypass

| Class | Wound characteristics | Treatment |
|---|---|---|
| Class 1 | Skin edge necrosis Lymphatic leak | Empiric antibiotics |
| Class 2 | Wound infection or necrosis involving subcutaneous tissue | Culture specific antibiotics |
| | | Wet to dry dressing changes |
| Class 3 | Invasive wound infection to depths of wound about graft | Operative debridement Graft coverage |
| | | Culture specific antibiotics |

(Courtesy of Reifsnyder T, Bandyk D, Seabrook G, et al: *J Vasc Surg* 15:843–850, 1992.)

TABLE 2.—Wound Complications in In Situ Saphenous Vein Bypass Grafts—Degree of Severity, Anatomical Distribution, Type of Treatment, and Time of Onset

| | | Primary location | | | | |
|---|---|---|---|---|---|---|
| Class | No. | Groin | Thigh | Leg | Operative debridement | Mean time to presentation |
| 1 | 19 | 13 | 2 | 4 | 1 | 10.7 days |
| 2 | 12 | 3 | 5 | 4 | 4 | 18.9 days |
| 3 | 13 | 3 | 0 | 10 | 12* | 31.2 days |

Note: Graft coverage: sartorious flap (n = 2), calf muscle apposition (n = 3), slip thickness skin graft (n = 2).
(Courtesy of Reifsnyder T, Bandyk D, Seabrook G, et al: J Vasc Surg 15:843–850, 1992.)

*Results.*—Wound complications developed in 44% of the grafts and included 13 infections that threatened the graft (Table 2). The risk factors for wound infection included lymph leakage and early graft revision for thrombosis, hematoma, retained valve, or arteriovenous fistula. Graft-threatening infections developed a mean of 1 month postoperatively. Most infections were in the distal graft limb. All but 1 of the 13 deep infections required surgical débridement, and 7 required coverage by a flap or split-thickness skin graft. No grafts were lost, and no patient died.

*Conclusion.*—Wound complications have been frequent after in situ saphenous vein bypass surgery, but aggressive management has resulted in the salvage of all grafts.

▶ A disturbing 44% of patients who underwent in situ saphenous vein bypass performed by this very experienced group had significant wound complications develop. Despite successful outcome in the treatment of these patients, their hospitalization was significantly prolonged, and expenses increased. We continue to believe that lower extremity wounds should be closed with a fine subcuticular suture technique; in our experience with reverse vein grafts, this has virtually eliminated skin edge necrosis and localized lymphatic leak.—J.M. Porter, M.D.

---

## Color-Flow Duplex Scanning for the Surveillance and Diagnosis of Acute Deep Venous Thrombosis

Mattos MA, Londrey GL, Leutz DW, Hodgson KJ, Ramsey DE, Barkmeier LD, Stauffer ES, Spadone DP, Sumner DS (Southern Illinois Univ, Springfield)
*J Vasc Surg* 15:366–376, 1992                                            11–16

*Background.*—Color-flow scanning more accurately identifies veins below the knee than conventional duplex imaging does, and it permits

TABLE 1.—Incidence and Location of Deep Venous
Thrombosis by Patients According to Study Group

*No. (%) of patients with DVT
in the specified segment*

| | Diagnostic (N = 75) | Surveillance (N = 99) | p value |
|---|---|---|---|
| Any segment | 40 (53%) | 42 (42%) | NS |
| AK | 32 (43%) | 3 (3%) | $p < 0.001$ |
| BK | 35 (47%) | 41 (41%) | NS |
| CF | 18 (24%) | 1 (1%) | $p < 0.001$ |
| SF | 32 (43%) | 3 (3%) | $p < 0.001$ |
| POP | 27 (36%) | 9 (9%) | $p < 0.001$ |
| TP | 33 (44%) | 39 (39%) | NS |

*Abbreviations: CF*, common femoral; *SF*, superficial femoral; *POP*, popliteal; *TP*, tibioperoneal.
*Percentages* represent the number of patients with thrombi in the specified venous segment (or combination of segments) of either limb divided by the total number of patients in each study group.
(Courtesy of Mattos MA, Londrey GL, Leutz DW, et al: *J Vasc Surg* 15:366–376, 1992.)

TABLE 2.—Incidence and Distribution of Deep Venous
Thrombosis by Limbs According to Study Group

|  | No. (%) of limbs with DVT in the specified segment | | |
|---|---|---|---|
|  | Diagnostic (N = 77) | Surveillance (N = 190) | p value |
| Any segment | 40 (52%) | 44 (23%) | p < 0.001 |
| AK | 32 (42%) | 3 (2%) | p < 0.001 |
| BK | 35 (47%)† | 43 (23%) | p < 0.001 |
| CF | 18 (23%) | 1 (0.5%) | p < 0.001 |
| SF | 32 (42%) | 3 (2%) | p < 0.001 |
| POP | 27 (36%)† | 9 (5%) | p < 0.001 |
| TP | 33 (44%)† | 41 (22%) | p < 0.0003 |

Percentages represent the number of limbs with thrombi in the specified venous segment (or combination of segments) divided by the total number of limbs in each study group.

† Denominator N = 75, 2 limbs not studied below knee.

(Courtesy of Mattos MA, Londrey GL, Leutz DW, et al: *J Vasc Surg* 15:366–376, 1992.)

veins to be surveyed longitudinally. The accuracy of the technique for detecting acute deep venous thrombosis was examined.

*Methods.*—Both color-flow scanning and phlebography were performed prospectively in 77 extremities of 75 patients who were clinically suspected of having venous thrombosis. In addition, 190 limbs of 99 patients who were at high risk of having thrombosis postoperatively were assessed.

*Results.*—Thrombi were about equally frequent above and below the knee in the diagnostic group, but they were far more frequent in below-knee veins in the surveillance group (Tables 1 and 2). The extent of thrombosis is shown in Table 3. Color-flow scanning was 100% sensitive and 98% specific above the knee in symptomatic patients, and it was

TABLE 3.—Extent of Thrombi in Limbs With Deep
Venous Thrombosis

|  | Diagnostic | Surveillance | p value |
|---|---|---|---|
| Occluding | 58% (23/40) | 11% (5/44) | p < 0.00002 |
| Nonoccluding | 42% (17/40) | 89% (39/44) | p < 0.00002 |
| Isolated |  |  |  |
| AK | 9% (3/32) | 33% (1/3) | NS |
| BK | 23% (8/35) | 95% (41/43) | p < 0.001 |
| TP | 15% (5/33) | 83% (34/41) | p < 0.001 |

(Courtesy of Mattos MA, Londrey GL, Leutz DW, et al: *J Vasc Surg* 15:366–376, 1992.)

94% sensitive and 75% specific below the knee. In the surveillance group, the study was only 55% sensitive in detecting thrombi—more than 90% of which were limited to the tibioperoneal veins. The study had negative predictive values of 100% for diagostic extremities and 88% for surveillance extremities. The positive predictive values were 80% for diagnostic extremities and 89% for surveillance extremities.

*Conclusion.*—Color-flow scanning is a highly accurate means of detecting thrombi above and below the knee in patients with symptomatic acute deep venous thrombosis. Below-knee thrombi are not as accurately identified in asymptomatic patients who are at risk of thrombosis, and the role of the study in this group of patients remains uncertain.

▶ Most of us have learned to pay careful attention to the comments of Dr. David Sumner, who is a very careful observer. I am convinced that most experienced vascular labs have achieved an accuracy in venous thrombosis diagnosis, both above and below the knee, that rivals contrast phlebography. However, Dr. Sumner and others point out that if we are doing population surveillance studies rather than deep venous thrombosis symptomatic diagnostic studies, below-knee accuracy decreases considerably. This is important information.—J.M. Porter, M.D.

---

**Lower Extremity Calf Thrombosis: To Treat or Not to Treat?**
Lohr JM, Kerr TM, Lutter KS, Cranley RD, Spirtoff K, Cranley JJ (Good Samaritan Hosp, Cincinnati)
*J Vasc Surg* 14:618–623, 1991                                        11–17

---

*Background.*—Seventy-five patients with isolated calf vein thrombosis diagnosed by duplex ultrasonography were followed prospectively sequential duplex exams at 3-day to 4-day intervals.

*Method.*—A Biosound Phase II device with a 10-mHz phased linear-array probe was used to acquire duplex scans at 3- to 4-day intervals.

*Results.*—Twenty-four patients had propagation of thrombosis, in 11 instances into the popliteal vein or larger veins of the thigh, and in 13 to more proximal calf veins. Forty-nine patients had had surgery, but no particular procedures were significantly associated with propagation of thrombosis. The proximal soleal vein was the most commonly involved single vein segment, whether or not propagation occurred (table). Neither the extent of thrombosis nor the presence of bilateral involvement predicted propagation. In 4 instances, duplex scanning was done because of a highly probable ventilation-perfusion study.

*Conclusion.*—Deep venous thrombosis is not benign, even if it is initially limited to the calf. Long-term sequelae of deep venous insufficiency are as frequent as after more proximal deep venous thrombosis. Based on the likelihood of venous propagation and the high incidence of

Single Vein Segment Involvement

| | Segment involved | Patients |
|---|---|---|
| Propagators | | n = 13 |
| | PSOL | 7 (54%) |
| | DSOL | 4 (31%) |
| | PPTV | 1 (8%) |
| | DPTV | 1 (8%) |
| Nonpropagators | | n = 33 |
| | PSOL | 15 (45%) |
| | DSOL | 4 (15%) |
| | PPTV | 6 (18%) |
| | DPTV | 3 (9%) |
| | PPER | 5 (15%) |

*Abbreviations:* PSOL, proximal soleal vein; DSOL, distal soleal vein; PPTV, proximal posterior tibial vein; DPTV, distal posterior tibial vein; PPER, proximal peroneal vein.
(Courtesy of Lohr JM, Kerr TM, Lutter KS, et al: *J Vasc Surg* 14:618–623, 1991.)

deep venous insufficiency in untreated patients, anticoagulation is recommended on a routine basis for patients with calf vein thrombosis, unless there is a high risk of complications from anticoagulation. Serial duplex scanning is an alternative approach to these patients.

▶ Fifteen percent of the patients with initially isolated calf vein thrombi (serially monitored with duplex scan) propagated thrombi into the popliteal or larger veins. There continues to be no consensus on the optimal treatment of truly isolated calf vein thrombus. Proponents of vigorous treatment cite the 15% to 20% incidence of major proximal vein propagation, as well as the long-term sequelae of valvular insufficiency, which may be reduced by anticoagulation. Opponents cite the relatively infrequent complications of calf deep vein thrombosis and the high cost of routine treatment of all patients. Our current policy is not to treat with anticoagulation and to follow the patients with sequential duplex scans.—J.M. Porter, M.D.

---

**The Reliability of Physical Examination in the Evaluation of Penetrating Extremity Trauma for Vascular Injury: Results at One Year**
Frykberg ER, Dennis JW, Bishop K, Laneve L, Alexander RH (Univ of Florida, Jacksonville)
*J Trauma* 31:502–511, 1991                                          11–18

---

*Background.*—Cases of penetrating extremity injury (PEI) that have any "hard" sign of vascular trauma (i.e., active hemorrhage, distal pulse deficit, distal ischemia, or bruit) are treated by prompt surgical exploration. For penetrating wounds that are in proximity to major extremity arteries that do not manifest any hard signs, exclusion arteriography is the standard method of evaluation. However, some believe that physical examination of occult cases of proximity PEI may be as reliable as arteriography and clearly safer and less costly. The use of physical examination in predicting the presence or absence of significant vascular injury after penetrating extremity injury was evaluated.

*Methods.*—Penetrating wounds between the inguinal ligament and midcalf in the lower extremity, and between the deltopectoral groove and midforearm in the upper extremity were studied. During the 1-year period, 273 male patients and 37 female patients were seen with 366 penetrating wounds to an extremity. Seventy-one percent of the wounds were in a lower extremity. In 78% of the wounds, the PEI was judged to be in proximity to major extremity vessels but produced either no signs or soft signs of vascular injury (a negative physical examination). Fifty-nine wounds (16%) were asymptomatic but were judged not to be in proximity to major extremity vessels, and 21 wounds had at least 1 hard sign of vascular injury (a positive physical examination). Most PEI resulted from gunshot wounds, but stabs and lacerations were most likely to result in major vascular injury to the extremity. Two missed vascular injuries were both in the asymptomatic proximity group.

*Results.*—Eleven arteriograms were performed during the initial evaluation of PEI. Twenty-three extremity vascular injuries required surgical intervention, and 21 produced at least 1 hard sign detectable by physical examination alone. Because all extremity wounds with hard signs had surgically significant vascular trauma, the positive predictive value of physical examination was 100% in this study population.

*Conclusion.*—The overall predictive value of physical examination of PEI for vascular injury approached 100% in this study. The 2 cases of delayed diagnosis in the asymptomatic proximity group were promptly treated and had no morbidity when they became clinically manifest, which suggests that the perceived dangers of delayed diagnosis of vascular injury may be overestimated. In light of costly diagnostic alternatives, physical examination is a reliable and safe method of evaluation for PEI.

▶ These authors conclude that physical examination alone is adequate to detect extremity arterial trauma, and that arteriography is not required for indication of proximity only. These results are interesting, but they are insufficiently persuasive to change my mind. Of course, once my mind is made up, almost no amount of data is sufficient to change it.—J.M. Porter, M.D.

# 12 Plastic, Reconstructive, and Head and Neck Surgery

## Introduction

Plastic and reconstructive surgical advances occurred in many directions during the past year. The articles chosen for review fall into several areas: flap physiology; the Food and Drug Administration (FDA) controversy surrounding silicone gel-filled breast prostheses and the concomitant need to change reconstructive techniques; the definition and treatment of chronic wounds such as pressure sores; the continued search for skin substitutes; and evaluation of newer techniques for treatment of maxillofacial injuries. Advances in head and neck oncology have centered on attempting to find prognosticators of outcome that might aid in therapeutic choices, further attempts at multimodality treatments, and characterization of head and neck tumor responses in children.

Contraindications to pedicled and free flaps have been reported abundantly in the literature. As each contraindication is critically appraised, the data seem to remove the contraindication. For example, age has been removed this year as a contraindication to free flap reconstruction. Smoking seems not to affect anastomotic patency rates. The blood supply to the facial skin was more clearly elucidated so that fear of poor flap design has been lessened. This will also allow design and successful utilization of new flaps such as the facial artery musculomucosal flap described by Pribaz et al. (Abstract 12–5).

Although scientific data do not support the FDA's action of decreasing the availability of gel-filled breast prostheses, the media and patient fears have essentially made procedures using them a nontenable option. One of the best articles showing that there is no increased risk of breast cancer in augmented patients has been included. Because autogenous breast reconstruction remains the only option, articles have been selected that show the efficacy of modification of the transverse rectus abdominis flap.

Chronic wounds have been the subject of many articles in both basic science and clinical journals. The pressure sore is one such wound that lends itself to study. Disa et al. (Abstract 12–6) have reported on the incidence of recidivism of standard operative repairs. This gives a yardstick by which to measure newer nonoperative treatment. The Galveston wound healing research group has reported on the first human trials using growth factors (platelet-derived growth factor-BB and b fibroblast growth factor) for the treatment of pressure sores.

Skin substitutes to use in closure of massive burn wounds are becoming a therapeutic imperative. Cultured epithelial autografts, micrografting techniques, and moisture trapping techniques are all examples of trying to obtain wound closure with other than standard split-thickness skin grafts when donor tissue is at a premium.

Rigid fixation with plates and screws has been replacing wire fixation for maxillofacial fractures recently. Large enough series are being accumulated to allow critical analyses of this technique. Two papers have been included to demonstrate some of the complications of this type of rigid fixation, and one must now weigh the advantages of the methodology against these complications, which can occur with significant incidence.

With the advent of molecular and cell biology, prognosticators of treatment outcome are now being sought for head and neck cancer. These prognosticators can be macroscopic (e.g., size), microscopic (e.g., depth of invasion), or molecular (e.g., cell cytokine receptivity). Each of these has been reviewed this year. Disappointment in single-modality treatment for head and neck cancer continues to lead to trials of multimodality therapy. Two of the best papers, one on induction adjuvant chemotherapy and one on alternating chemotherapy and radiotherapy, are included. Unfortunately, neither of these shows clear advantages over surgical extirpation or radiotherapy alone.

Real advances have been made recently in the treatment of head and neck neoplasms in children. The increased survival of patients with rhabdomyosarcomas in the past 30 years has been remarkable. This is one place in which multimodality therapy has been highly successful.

This has been an excellent year for advances in the field of reconstructive and head and neck surgery. I hope the reader will find the chosen articles as useful as I did in reviewing them.

Martin C. Robson, M.D.

## Plastic and Reconstructive Surgery

**Xanthine Oxidase: Its Role in the No-Reflow Phenomenon**
Punch J, Rees R, Cashmer B, Wilkins E, Smith DJ, Till GO (Univ of Michigan, Ann Arbor)
*Surgery* 111:169–176, 1992                                                                12–1

*Introduction.*—The no-reflow phenomenon is defined as prolonged limb ischemia that becomes irreversible when tissues cannot be reperfused. It has been postulated that production of oxygen radicals may have a major role in reperfusion tissue injury. This hypothesis was further examined in a no-reflow animal model.

*Methods.*—The left femoral vein in Sprague-Dawley rats was exposed and ligated distally. The left femoral artery was occluded for 2, 4, or 6 hours, after which the clamp was released to allow reperfusion. The contralateral limbs were used as controls. Reperfusion was defined as a return of blood flow to 100% of control values for 10 minutes after clamp removal. Venous blood samples and biopsy specimens of skin and muscle were obtained after 2 hours and 4 hours of ischemia to assess the degree of tissue injury. Some animals were pretreated with the xanthine oxidase (XO) inhibitor allopurinol, antioxidant enzymes, or free radical scavengers.

*Findings.*—Laser Doppler studies demonstrated that hind limbs reperfused well after 2 hours or 4 hours of ischemia, but that reperfusion ceased within the first 10 minutes after 6 hours of ischemia. After 4 hours of ischemia, plasma XO levels had increased by threefold when compared with baseline levels. Plasma XO levels peaked 5 minutes after reperfusion and remained elevated throughout the sampling period. Pretreatment with allopurinol reduced XO activity to negligible levels. In all animals pretreated with antioxidant enzymes or free radical scavengers before undergoing 6 hours of ischemia, reperfusion persisted after release of the clamp.

*Conclusions.*—The tissue injury that occurs in long-term ischemia followed by reperfusion is related to oxygen products derived from XO activity. Inhibition of oxygen-derived free radical production with antioxidant enzymes or scavenging the free radicals already produced allows a longer ischemic interval before the no-reflow phenomenon sets in.

▶ Oxygen radicals and arachidonic acid metabolites have been postulated to be important in the development of the no-reflow phenomenon. The source of production of the oxygen radicals has not been adequately demonstrated. The work shows that tissue XO appears to produce the radicals and can be blocked with pretreatment. However, the clinical key will be development of a treatment for the established lack of reperfusion after the episode. Eicosanoid inhibitors, especially those blocking thromboxane production, may prove to be more useful in treating established failure of reperfusion.—M.C. Robson, M.D.

---

**Free Flaps in the Elderly**

Chick LR, Walton RL, Reus W, Colen L, Sasmor M (Univ of Massachusetts, Worcester; Dartmouth-Hitchcock Med Ctr, Hanover, NH)
*Plast Reconstr Surg* 90:87–94, 1992                12–2

---

*Introduction.*—Tissue transfer by microsurgical techniques now allows for reconstruction of acquired defects. Age still poses some problems in microsurgery, however, because the elderly have a higher risk for heart and respiratory problems and infection. A retrospective study assessed the risks of free tissue transfer in an aged population.

*Methods.*—The medical records of all patients who underwent microsurgical free tissue transfer operations were reviewed. Thirty-one of 273 such patients were aged 65 years or older. Data on these elderly patients were compared to those on 90 consecutive patients younger than age 65 years who also underwent the same type of surgery.

*Results.*—The 8 older women and 23 older man had a mean age of 71 years. The mean operative time for a total of 33 free flap microsurgeries was 7.5 hours. The operations were performed under general anesthesia without regional or epidural premedications. The mean hospital stay was 40 days. Twenty patients had at least 1 serious complication within 30 days of the operation. The average age of the 65 male and 25 female patients in the younger group was 37 years, the average operative time was 6.6 hours, and the average hospital stay was 30 days. Chi-sequence analysis showed no significant difference in the rate of wound complications in the 2 groups. The elderly group, however, did have significantly more medical complications than the younger patients.

*Conclusions.*—These results indicate that age alone may not increase morbidity from free tissue transfer operations, which suggests that the elderly can usually expect successful outcomes. Recommendations for older patients undergoing this type of surgery include a thorough medical evaluation, preoperative anesthesia, careful use of medications and antibiotics, close analysis of the technical aspects of the microsurgery, quick performance of the operation, and alertness for problems such as intraoperative hypothermia, pressure sores, and delayed healing.

▶ The authors have successfully demonstrated that age alone is no longer an absolute contraindication to microsurgery. In a series of patients all older than 65 years, no significant increase in operative complications occurred. The medical problems were increased, as expected. Therefore, if free tissue transfer is the best surgical option in an elderly patient, it should not be abandoned simply because of the patient's advanced age.—M.C. Robson, M.D.

---

### Tobacco Smoking and Complications in Elective Microsurgery

Reus WF III, Colen LB, Straker DJ (Dartmouth-Hitchcock Med Ctr, Hanover, NH; Eastern Virginia Med School, Norfolk)
*Plast Reconstr Surg* 89:490–494, 1992                    12–3

---

*Introduction.*—Tobacco smoking has long been considered detrimental to wound healing and surgical outcome after plastic and reconstructive surgery. It is associated with an increased rate of complications in patients undergoing pedicled flap procedures. A retrospective analysis

Recipient-Site Wound Complications in Free-Tissue Transfers

| Complication | Smokers | Nonsmokers |
|---|---|---|
| Anastomotic: | | |
| Patients experiencing flap loss | 5 (5%) | 3 (6%) |
| Number of flaps lost | 5 (5%) | 4 (7%) |
| Flaps successfully salvaged | 9 (9%) | 6 (10%) |
| Delayed healing: | | |
| Responding to local care | 9 (9%) | 7 (12%) |
| Requiring operative intervention | 27 (26%) | 7 (12%) |
| TOTAL | 36 (35%) | 14 (24%) |

(Courtesy of Reus WF III, Colen LB, Straker DJ: *Plast Reconstr Surg* 89:490–494, 1992.)

was done to assess the complication rate in smokers undergoing elective free-tissue transfer.

*Patients.*—Between 1983 and 1990, 93 smokers and 51 nonsmokers (mean age, 45 years) underwent 162 free-tissue transfers. Most smokers discontinued smoking from the time of hospitalization until operation, an average of 7 days. Patients who had quit smoking 2 months to 2 years before operation were excluded from the analysis. Delayed healing at the recipient site was defined as the need for secondary procedures or continued local care to achieve closure after 30 days.

*Results.*—As expected, smokers had a higher incidence of chronic obstructive pulmonary disease. Nonsmokers experienced a slightly higher rate of delayed wound healing at the donor site, but the difference was not statistically significant. Smokers and nonsmokers had similar rates of anastomotic complications, flap loss, return to the operating room for salvage, and uncomplicated flap survival. Yet, 35% of the smokers had delayed wound healing at the recipient site, compared to 24% of the nonsmokers (table). Furthermore, 27% of the smokers required additional procedures to achieve final wound closure, compared to 12% of the nonsmokers. These differences were statistically significant.

*Conclusions.*—Cigarette smokers undergoing elective free-tissue transfer appear to be at increased risk for complications at the flap's interface with the wound or overlying skin graft but not for complications at the site of anastomosis.

▶ Smoking is known to affect wound healing and the microvasculature of flaps. It seemed a logical extension that it might affect anastomotic success of microvessels. This paper shows that this is not the case. Wound problems are increased in smokers but not because of anastomosis patency failure. If wound problems are to be decreased, data are necessary regarding smoking cessation in chronic smokers. No such data are available. Hardesty et al. (1) designed animal experiments for acute smoker cessation, but the results cannot be extrapolated to chronic smokers.—M.C. Robson, M.D.

*Reference*

1. Hardesty R, West S, Schmidt S: Preoperative cessation of cigarette smoking and its relationship to flap survival. Presented at the American Association of Plastic Surgeons Annual Meeting, May 1990, Hot Springs, Va.

---

**The Use of Fasciocutaneous Flaps With Medial Pedicles for Treatment of Burn Contractures in Popliteal Region—A New Approach**
Baş L, Uzunismail A (GATA Haydarpaşa Egitim Hastanesi, Istanbul, Turkey)
*Eur J Plast Surg* 15:124–126, 1992                                        12–4

---

*Introduction.*—Various surgical techniques have been used in the treatment of popliteal burn contractures, including covering the defect with a split-skin graft after contracture release, use of gastrocnemius muscle or musculocutaneous flaps, and use of the saphenous flap as an island. All of these methods, however, have certain drawbacks. A review was made of experience with a medially based fasciocutaneous flap in the treatment of popliteal burn contractures.

*Patients.*—During a 2-year period, 11 men aged 20 to 22 years with chronic popliteal burn contractures stemming from childhood burns underwent operation. None of the patients was able to walk, and 5 had central ulceration in the scarred area. In all cases, the medial side of the distal thigh was intact with sufficient tissue to insure adequate flap elevation. The flaps were designed according to the size of the created defect, but mindful of Hazarika's 5:1 ratio. The follow-up period was 18 to 24 months.

*Methods and Results.*—In the 5 patients with central ulceration, 2 adjacent flaps were transposed to cover the defect after complete excision of the contracture. Of the 10 donor sites, 4 were closed primarily and 6 required skin grafting. Nine donor sites healed uneventfully and partial necrosis developed in 1. In the 6 patients without central ulceration, 2 separated pedicled flaps were used to cover the defects after distal and proximal releasing incisions. Of the 12 donor sites, 3 were closed primarily and 9 required skin grafting. All flaps healed uneventfully with complete survival.

*Conclusions.*—Long-standing burn contractures of the popliteal region can be treated successfully with medially based fasciocutaneous flaps from the distal thigh and proximal calf regions in patients in whom these areas have been preserved.

▶ The techniques in this paper may have specific indications. I disagree that flaps are always necessary for reconstruction of popliteal fossa contractures. Split-thickness skin grafts suffice in the huge majority of cases. However, occasionally a rare neurovascular bundle is skeletonized for a significant distance during contracture release. In these cases, a flap is desirable. It is in these circumstances that I think the authors' flap will prove advantageous.—M.C. Robson, M.D.

## A New Intraoral Flap: Facial Artery Musculomucosal (FAMM) Flap

Pribaz J, Stephens W, Crespo L, Gifford G (Brigham and Women's Hosp, Boston, Mass; Children's Hosp, Boston)
*Plast Reconstr Surg* 90:421–428, 1992                                    12–5

*Introduction.*—Although local cutaneous flaps have been used in facial reconstruction for more than 2,500 years, physicians have only recently combined the principles of using nasolabial and buccal mucosal flaps with an axial musculomucosal flap. The results of using a new axial musculomucosal flap, designated as the facial artery musculomucosal (FAMM) flap, were evaluated.

*Technique.*—The FAMM flap is outlined intraorally by Doppler ultrasound and centered over the facial artery in an oblique orientation. The

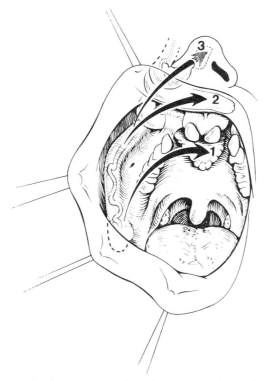

**Fig 12–1.**—Superiorly based FAMM flap may be used to reconstruct defects of hard palate, alveolus, maxillary antrum, nose, upper lip, and orbit. (Courtesy of Pribaz J, Stephens W, Crespo L, et al: *Plast Reconstr Surg* 90:421–428, 1992.)

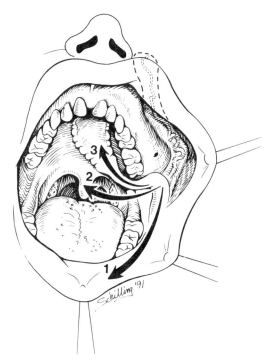

**Fig 12–2.**—Inferiorly based FAMM flap may be used to reconstruct defects of hard and soft palate, tonsillar fossa, alveolus, floor of mouth, and lower lip. (Courtesy of Pribaz J, Stephens W, Crespo L, et al: *Plast Reconstr Surg* 90:421–428, 1992.)

width of the flap usually averages 1.5 to 2 cm, but it may be sized according to the needs of the patient. After the facial artery is ligated and cut, the remainder of the flap is incised and dissection proceeds just deep to the facial vessels. The facial artery must be lifted with the flap to keep the entire flap in an axial orientation. The donor defect is then closed by using a 2-layer approach.

*Results.*—The FAMM flap, when placed superiorly, can be used to close mucosal defects such as those in the anterior hard palate, alveolus, nasal floor, upper lip, and orbit septum (Fig 12–1). When based inferiorly, the FAMM flap can be used to close defects such as those in the posterior hard palate, floor of the mouth, and lower lip (Fig 12–2). Since 1989 this type of operation has been used to correct defects in 15 patients aged 11–82 years, but in 3 other patients the FAMM technique failed.

*Conclusions.*—The FAMM flap has been used successfully to reconstruct a wide variety of difficult oronasal mucosal defects, including defects of the nasal septum, palate, upper and lower lips, and floor of the mouth. Complications can be minimized by insuring that the flap is axial, that the facial artery runs along its total length, and that there are no twists or constraints on the pedicle.

▶ The FAMM flap is versatile and easy to perform. When I have used this flap, it has appeared to fulfill the requirements placed upon it and has been uniformly successful.—M.C. Robson, M.D.

---

**Efficacy of Operative Cure in Pressure Sore Patients**
Disa JJ, Carlton JM, Goldberg NH (Univ of Maryland Hosp, Baltimore)
*Plast Reconstr Surg* 89:272–278, 1992                                    12–6

*Introduction.*—New techniques (e.g., air flotation beds and purified growth factors) have helped to achieve early success in operative closure of pressure sores. This success, along with high recurrence rates and decreasing health resources, suggests that surgical reconstruction of pressure sores is not always necessary. The results in 40 patients who underwent operation for pressure sores were reviewed in an attempt to define those most likely to benefit from surgery.

*Patients.*—During an 8-year period, 66 grade III or IV pressure sores in 40 patients were operated on under the direction of a single surgeon. Patients were divided into 3 groups based on the presence or absence of paraplegia and its cause. There were 21 patients with traumatic paraplegia (mean age, 32 years), 3 with nontraumatic paraplegia (mean age, 22 years), and 16 with nontraumatic, nonparaplegic conditions (mean age, 73 years). The overall mean age was 42 years. Whereas 55 sores were treated by muscle or fasciocutaneous flap, 11 received a cutaneous flap. The mean follow-up was 21 months.

| Comparison of Patients With and Without Recurrence | | |
|---|---|---|
|  | No Recurrence | Recurrence |
| Age (mean) | 43.9 years | 45.7 years |
| Diagnosis: | | |
| TP | 4 (21%) | 15 (79%) |
| NTP | 3 (100%) | 0 (0%) |
| NTNP | 4 (31%) | 9 (69%) |
| Total | 11/35 (31%) | 24/35 (69%) |
| Sores at time of presentation | 14 (1.3/patient) | 44 (1.8/patient) |
| Site: | | |
| Ischial | 33% | 67% |
| Sacral | 26% | 74% |
| Trochanteric | 38% | 62% |
| Complication rate | 38% | 37% |

(Courtesy of Disa JJ, Carlton JM, Goldberg NH: *Plast Reconstr Surg* 89:272–278, 1992.)

*Outcome.*—The operative complication rate was 36%, 21 of 24 complications being flap related. There were no operative deaths. Sores were completely healed at discharge in 80% of the patients. After a mean of 9.3 months, 69% of the patients had recurrent sores, those with traumatic paraplegia being most frequently affected (table).

*Conclusions.*—In the treatment of pressure sores, surgical reconstruction seems ineffective in young patients with traumatic paraplegia and in elderly patients with cerebral compromise. No other considerations could identify patients likely to remain healed after reconstruction.

▶ This may be the most significant paper regarding the treatment of pressure sores to appear in many years. It concerns the recidivism rate after well-performed flap closure of these ulcers. The authors found that 69% of patients had recurrence of the pressure sore within 9.3 months. In the most common subset of traumatic paraplegics, the incidence rose to 79%. Therefore, operative management is not the panacea for pressure sores, and attempts to find other treatment modalities seem indicated.—M.C. Robson, M.D.

### Platelet-Derived Growth Factor BB for the Treatment of Chronic Pressure Ulcers

Robson MC, Phillips LG, Thomason A, Robson LE, Pierce GF (Univ of Texas, Galveston; Amgen Inc, Thousand Oaks, Calif)
*Lancet* 339:23–25, 1992                                                        12–7

*Objective.*—Recombinant human platelet-derived growth factor (rPDGF-BB) greatly accelerates normal soft tissue repair in laboratory animals. A randomized, double-blind, placebo-controlled trial was designed to evaluate the effect of topically applied rPDGF-BB on healing in patients with chronic pressure ulcers.

*Patients.*—Twenty patients aged 21–56 years with pressure ulcers of grades III and IV were randomly assigned to placebo or to rPDGF-BB at doses of 1 μg/mL, 10 μg/mL, or 100 μg/mL, applied topically daily for 28 days. Patients were repositioned every 2 hours throughout the study. Pressure ulcer volumes were measured with alginate molds at baseline and at days 7, 14, 21, and 29. Pressure-relieving devices were used as appropriate.

*Results.*—At the end of the 29-day trial, the mean ulcer volume in patients treated with 1 μg/mL or 10 μg/mL of rPDGF-BB did not differ significantly from that in the placebo-treated patients. All 5 patients treated with 100 μg/mL, however, had a significantly greater reduction in ulcer volume than did placebo-treated patients. None of the patients experienced toxic effects from the treatment. No hypertrophic scarring or keloid formation was observed during the 5-month follow-up. Histologic examination of biopsy samples showed normal active wound healing in all patients. Biopsy samples from ulcers treated with the 100-μg/mL dose tended to have a greater fibroblastic and endothelial cell influx and more provisional extracellular matrix and new vessels.

*Conclusion.*—Topically applied rPDGF-BB at a dose of 100 μg/mL appears to accelerate wound closure in patients with chronic pressure ulcers.

---

**The Safety and Effect of Topically Applied Recombinant Basic Fibroblast Growth Factor on the Healing of Chronic Pressure Sores**

Robson MC, Phillips LG, Lawrence WT, Bishop JB, Youngerman JS, Hayward PG, Broemeling LD, Heggers JP (Univ of Texas, Galveston; Univ of North Carolina, Chapel Hill)

*Ann Surg* 216:401–408, 1992                                    12–8

*Purpose.*—The polypeptide basic fibroblast growth factor (bFGF) has a wide range of biological activities in vitro, including stimulation of cell mitogenesis and chemotaxis. It is a potent mitogen and chemoattractant for capillary endothelial cells that effectively stimulates neovascularization and, ultimately, collagen synthesis in vivo. Results of the first randomized, placebo-controlled trials of bFGF in the treatment of pressure sores in human beings were evaluated.

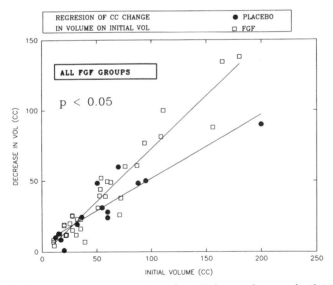

**Fig 12–3.**—Reduction in pressure sore volume after a 30-day period compared with initial volume for all patients treated with bFGF and the placebo. Slopes of the regression curves are statistically different when compared with the F-test ($P < .05$). (Courtesy of Robson MC, Phillips LG, Lawrence WT, et al: *Ann Surg* 216:401–408, 1992.)

*Methods.*—The study included 50 patients at 2 centers with grade III or IV pressure sores extending from the bone to the subcutaneous tissues. Safety was determined at 3 different concentrations of bFGF—1, 5, and 10 $\mu g/cm^2$—at 5 different dosing schedules by assessment of hematologic effects, serum chemistry parameters, urinalysis, absorption, antibody formation, and signs of toxicity. The acute phase of the trial lasted for 30 days. Wound volumes, histologic findings, and photographs were used in evaluation of efficacy.

*Results.*—No patient experienced toxicity or had significant serum absorption or antibody formation. A trend toward treatment efficacy was noted in 6 of the 8 subgroups (Fig 12–3). Treatment with bFGF had a greater healing effect in all subgroups combined, as demonstrated by comparison of the slopes of the regression curves of volume decrease in relation to initial volume. Fibroblasts and capillaries were increased with bFGF. Of 35 patients receiving bFGF, 21 had a 70% reduction in wound volume, as did 4 of 14 patients receiving placebo.

*Conclusions.*—This initial randomized study suggests that topical bFGF treatment may be safe and effective in patients with chronic wounds, in this case, pressure sores. Because of the small number of patients in each subgroup, the lack of significance for the reported trends should not be overinterpreted. The findings of this study are similar to previous studies of contaminated wounds in animals.

▶ Modulation of the processes of wound healing now appears possible. These 2 papers (Abstracts 12–7 and 12–8) represent the first human clinical trials for rPDGF-BB and rbFGF. The model chosen for the study was a chronic pressure ulcer. Based on the previous article by Disa et al. (Abstract 12–6), it is clear that flap reconstruction alone is not the answer in the long-term treatment of these lesions. If the experience reported in these 2 papers can be repeated in larger, multicenter trials, it may be that growth factors will become part of the armamentarium of the surgeon.—M.C. Robson, M.D.

---

**Augmentation Mammaplasty and Breast Cancer: A 5-Year Update of the Los Angeles Study**
Deapen DM, Brody GS (Univ of Southern California, Los Angeles)
*Plast Reconstr Surg* 89:660–665, 1992                    12–9

---

*Objective.*—An estimated 2 million women in the United States have received breast implants. Any increase in the risk of breast cancer is an important public health issue. Outcomes were assessed in 3,112 women followed for a median of 10.5 years after receiving an implant between 1959 and 1980. The follow-up interval ranged from 1 month to about 32 years.

*Findings.*—Twenty-one breast cancers were observed, with nearly 32 expected. The median interval from implant to diagnosis was 8 years (range, 3 to 19 years). None of the patients with cancer had received a polyurethane implant. Among women having implants after age 40 years, 11 cancers were observed, with 14 expected. Cancers were fewer than expected even in women exposed for 10 years or longer. There was no indication that the detection of breast cancer was delayed in women with implants.

*Conclusion.*—The risk of breast cancer was not increased in this large series of women undergoing augmentation mammaplasty.

▶ The controversy about potential complications from silicone implantation has been one of the major subjects of interest in plastic surgery during the past year. Much of the literature has relied on an insufficient database and has reflected more emotion than science. This well-done study of patients with silicone breast implants shows no increased risk of cancer in augmented patients vs. the expected incidence in nonaugmented patients. It is this type of well-performed study that will return this issue from the media to science.—M.C. Robson, M.D.

---

**Double-Pedicle TRAM Flap for Unilateral Breast Reconstruction**
Wagner DS, Michelow BJ, Hartrampf CR Jr (Akron City Hosp, Akron, Ohio; St Joseph's Hosp, Atlanta, Ga)
*Plast Reconstr Surg* 88:987–997, 1991                                    12–10

---

*Indications.*—A double-pedicle transverse rectus abdominis myocutaneous (TRAM) flap offers better flap vascularity and venous outflow as well as midline crossover blood flow. The risk of partial necrosis is less than with a single-pedicle flap. Operating time is prolonged, however, and there is greater abdominal wall morbidity. The double-pedicle flap is indicated when the needed tissue volume exceeds that which can reliably be carried on 1 pedicle or when flap length demands. It also is indicated if the risk of flap necrosis from microvascular dysfunction is increased, or if an abdominal midline scar is a problem.

*Experience.*—A double-pedicle TRAM flap was used in 19% overall of 341 patients having unilateral breast reconstruction, but in 60% of the most recent 50 radical mastectomy reconstructions. Three hernias complicated the single-pedicle procedure and 1 occurred in 66 double-pedicle TRAM reconstructions. Partial flap loss complicated 6% of the single-pedicle reconstructions and 3% of the double-pedicle procedures. Very little abdominal wall morbidity resulted from the double-pedicle procedure, although many patients are unable to do sit-ups.

*Conclusion.*—A single-pedicle TRAM flap is preferred for unilateral breast reconstruction, but a double-pedicle procedure may be indicated to permit a larger, longer, or safer reconstruction. If fascia is harvested conservatively and the abdominal wall is closed directly, abdominal wall complications are infrequent.

### Immediate Breast Reconstruction: Why the Free TRAM Over the Conventional TRAM Flap?

Schusterman MA, Kroll SS, Weldon ME (Univ of Texas MD Anderson Cancer Ctr, Houston)
*Plast Reconstr Surg* 90:255–261, 1992                    12–11

*Introduction.*—There is controversy regarding use of the transverse rectus abdominis myocutaneous (TRAM) flap for immediate breast reconstruction. Partial flap necrosis is a common complication of the TRAM flap that could disrupt the institution of postoperative therapy and evaluation for recurrence. The free TRAM flap based on the inferior deep epigastric vessels has been used in an attempt to decrease this complication. Results with conventional superior-pedicled (cTRAM) and free TRAM (fTRAM) flaps were compared.

*Patients and Methods.*—Of 68 immediate breast reconstructions in 63 patients, 71% were cTRAM and 29% fTRAM flaps. About half of the cTRAM flaps (54%) were unipedicled and the rest bipedicled. In each group, more than 80% were in patients with $T_1$ or $T_2$ lesions. In the group given a cTRAM flap, 29% were node positive, as were 10% of those receiving a fTRAM flap. Overall, 25% of the patients were smokers.

*Results.*—Postoperative chemotherapy was required by 44% of those with a cTRAM flap, but it was delayed in 29% because of flap-related complications. In the group with fTRAM flaps, 35% required chemotherapy, which had to be delayed in 14% because of flap-related complications. There was a 17% rate of partial flap necrosis in the group with cTRAM flaps vs. none in the group with fTRAM flaps. The rate of fat necrosis was 23% in those with cTRAM flaps vs. none of 20 having fTRAM flaps.

*Conclusions.*—Use of the fTRAM flap for immediate breast reconstruction reduces the incidence both of partial flap necrosis and of delays in receiving adjuvant chemotherapy in comparison with the cTRAM flap. The technique is technically simple, and it yields important improvements in blood supply. The fTRAM flap is recommended for selected patients who are being considered for immediate breast reconstruction with autogenous tissue.

▶ With decisions by the Food and Drug Administration decreasing the availability and patient desires for postmastectomy reconstruction with silicone gel-filled prostheses, autologous tissue reconstruction is becoming much more common. The tissue of the abdominal wall transferred as a pedicled flap or divided and reanastomosed in the recipient area as a free flap is the most popular of the autologous tissue reconstructions. As the number of patients increases, dissatisfaction with flaps based on the unilateral rectus muscle is appearing in selected cases. To overcome the complications leading to this dissatisfaction, authors are using modifications such as double pedicles or free tissue transfer. The first of the preceding 2 papers describes indicators and results with double pedicles, and the latter describes a significant experience with free tissue transfer for breast reconstruction.—M.C. Robson, M.D.

---

**The Surgical Applications and Implications of Cultured Human Epidermis: A Comprehensive Review**
Arons JA, Wainwright DJ, Jordon RE (Univ of Texas, Houston)
*Surgery* 111:4–11, 1992                                                                                     12–12

---

*Autologous Grafts.*—Cultured epidermis has been considered an ultimate solution for resurfacing burn wounds. A small biopsy skin specimen can be vastly expanded in 2–3 weeks, but there is a risk that the patient will become more ill during this time, and meticulous laboratory technique is essential. These grafts have not taken consistently. The need for a feeder layer remains controversial.

*Allogeneic Grafts.*—Allogeneic cultures have been used extensively on burn wounds, chronic ulcers, and other types of skin defect. The long-term fate of cultured epidermal allografts remains uncertain, but the grafts can relieve pain and promote rapid epithelialization in chronic wounds. Cultured allografts have been effective in healing chronic ulcers that resist conventional treatment. There is, however, a potential risk of transmitting HIV and other infections. In many respects, skin regenerated from cultured allografts in time resembles normal skin more closely than does that regenerated from conventional split-thickness skin grafts.

▶ It is unusual for us to include review articles in the YEAR BOOK. However, the experience with skin substitutes has resulted in so many articles reported in different ways that a review of the data seems justified. The authors have produced an excellent review that requires careful reading. It gives an unbiased view of the success rates with both autograft and allograft cultured epidermis. The reference list is excellent, and the article should serve as a superior resource.—M.C. Robson, M.D.

---

**Functional Innervation of Cultured Skin Grafts**
English KB, Stayner N, Krueger GG, Tuckett RP (Univ of Utah, Salt Lake City)
*J Invest Dermatol* 99:120–128, 1992                                                                         12–13

---

*Objective.*—In patients with burns, cultured skin grafts lack adnexal structures and probably the highly organized nerve endings around hair follicles as well. With the increasing use of cultured skin grafts, it becomes important to improve methods to maximize graft quality in individual patients. A study was performed in rats to determine whether cultured skin grafts become innervated, and whether their tactile function can be improved by implantation of target tissue.

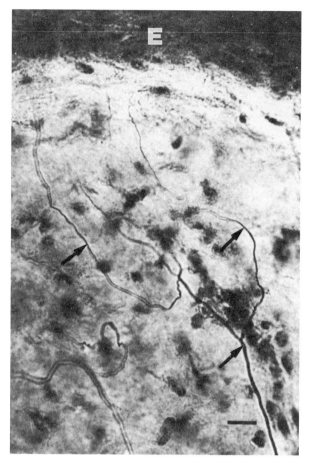

**Fig 12–4.**—Cultured skin 83 days after grafting. Silver-stained nerves (*arrows*) in the dermis of cultured skin outside of a touch dome implant. *Scale bar* = μm. (Courtesy of English KB, Stayner N, Krueger GG, et al: *J Invest Dermatol* 99:120–128, 1992.)

*Methods.*—Thirty-day autologous skin equivalents were cultured for individual adult Sprague-Dawley rats. One group of rats received pure skin equivalent grafts; others had target tissue obtained by 2-mm punch biopsies inserted at the time of grafting. The target tissues consisted of normal skin in 1 group and touch domes, richly innervated areas known to provide tropic or trophic factors for regenerating type I nerves, in another group. Histologic examination was performed at periodic intervals.

*Results.*—Isolated nerve fibers were noted in the cultured skin areas and in implant zones on silver staining of the tissues (Fig 12–4). In both implant and cultured regions, rubbing the grafts with a glass rod or pinching them with a watchmaker forceps evoked a response. Cultured areas showed a decreased afferent response to gentle stroking with a camel-hair brush. Only cutaneous nerves innervating implants that originally had domal tissue showed the characteristic activity of type I neurons innervating touch domes. Return of sensory function was notably better in grafts that took well as opposed to those with episodes of crusting.

*Conclusions.*—Studies in rats indicate that innervation occurs in cultured skin grafts, and that innervation is enhanced by the presence of target tissue. The characteristic type I afferent responses appear to depend on factors other than the nerve alone that are unique to domal tissue. The return of sensory function relies largely on the quality of engraftment.

▶ As patients with larger and larger total body surface area burns survive, skin substitutes will be necessary for wound closure. Innervation of each substitute will be key to long-term function of the new epithelium. This study suggests that innervation of cultured epithelial autografts occurs. It is improved if the donor tissue is specifically selected. This model allows study of neurotropic growth factors to determine whether the innervation can be hastened or made more complete.—M.C. Robson, M.D.

---

**Healing of Partial Thickness Porcine Skin Wounds in a Liquid Environment**
Breuing K, Eriksson E, Liu P, Miller DR (Brigham and Women's Hosp, Boston, Mass)
*J Surg Res* 52:50–58, 1992                                                    12–14

---

*Introduction.*—Maintaining a moist environment in excisional wounds by trapping wound fluid underneath an occlusive dressing prevents deepening of the wound, prevents eschar formation, and accelerates reepithelialization by about 50%. A wound chamber was designed that can be used to expose individual experimental wounds to different physiologic liquids and monitor wound healing.

*Wound Chamber Design and Method.*—The chamber has a flexible transparent vinyl top bonded to an adhesive vinyl base having a central opening of the same size and shape as the wound. The chamber is held in place by a thin layer of medical adhesive. Medium partial-thickness contact burns, 25 × 25 mm, and medium partial-thickness excisional wounds, 25 × 25 mm and 1.2 mm deep, were created under general anesthesia on the backs of Yorkshire pigs. Fluids were added to the chambers with a syringe and a 22-gauge needle. The chambers were replaced every 24 hours.

*Results.*—Burn wounds left uncovered and exposed to air became necrotic (Fig 12–5). Burn wounds covered with empty chambers showed somewhat less necrosis. Partial-thickness burn wounds and excisional wounds left immersed in isotonic saline until healed had much less tissue

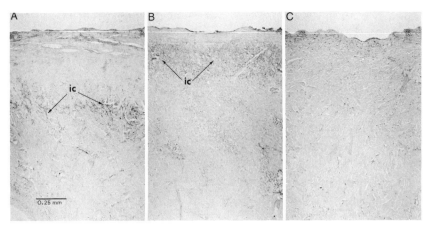

**Fig 12–5.**—Histology of burns at 96 hours. **A,** air-exposed burn with a thick eschar and numerous infiltrating inflammatory cells (*ic*). **B,** burn covered with an empty chamber with a thinner eschar above inflammatory cells. **C,** saline-immersed burn. Eschar is not apparent, and only a few inflammatory cells are seen. Hematoxylin and eosin; original magnification; × 10. (Courtesy of Breuing K, Eriksson E, Liu P, et al: *J Surg Res* 52:50–58, 1992.)

loss than wounds left uncovered. Saline-treated burn wounds formed no eschar and had minimal tissue necrosis. Saline-treated wounds healed without tissue maceration, were less inflamed, and less scar formation resulted compared to air-exposed wounds. As the wounds healed, the daily loss of water, protein, electrolytes, and glucose across the wound surfaces decreased to values found in unwounded skin immersed in saline for 12 days. The addition of hypertonic dextran to the chamber increased fluid loss across the wounds into the chamber compared with that in saline-treated wounds.

*Conclusions.*—The fluid-filled chamber is a useful device for the study of wound healing in a liquid environment.

▶ Moist wound healing has been touted as beneficial since the first observation by Winter (1). However, many of the articles have been anecdotal, and "wound healing" has been used as a generic term. What has been lacking is a sound paper delineating a specific repair process (e.g., epithelization) and demonstrating unequivocal improvement attributable to a liquid environment. This paper does just that. It also shows that the moisture is good for wounds healing by keratinocyte proliferation and migration. These results should not be extrapolated to wounds healing by deposition of extracellular matrix or those healing by contraction.—M.C. Robson, M.D.

*Reference*

1. Winter G: *Nature* 193:243, 1962.

## Microskin Grafting of Rabbits With Pigskin Xenograft Overlay

Lin S-D, Chou C-K, Lai C-S, Yang C-C (Kaohsiung Med College, Kaohsiung, Taiwan)
*Burns* 17:473–477, 1991                    12–15

*Introduction and Methods.*—When meshed grafts are placed, epithelialization of the interstices requires adequate protection with a dressing to prevent drying. The larger the expansion ratio of the graft, the greater the need for an effective dressing. Pigskin xenografts were used to overlay allografts with a 10:1 expansion ratio in rabbits. The overlaid pigskin was removed after 7, 10, or 14 days.

*Observations.*—Eosinophilic changes in epidermal cells and nuclear pyknosis were noted in pigskin after 7 days, but there were areas of newly formed epidermis. On day 14, the pigskin was an eschar or slough. Microskin autografts proliferated actively and expanded beneath the pigskin, and the epidermis showed increasing differentiation. The dermis was well vascularized. Skin texture was nearly normal at 2 weeks when the wound was covered by neoepithelium.

*Conclusion.*—The pigskin xenografts provided favorable conditions for growth of microskin autografts. Further studies of this grafting procedure may be worthwhile.

▶ Microskin grafting, as well as widely spread meshed skin grafts, require protection while the interstitial spaces are closing by epithelialization. Cadaver allografts have provided protection quite well, but suffer from problems of rejection and the ever-present danger of viral transmission. Although porcine xenografts have been used over widely meshed autografts, they have not been demonstrated to be efficient in the micrografting technique. These authors show that xenografts might be useful based on their experimental work. This paper suggests that xenografts may deserve another trial for overgrafting, because the transmission of AIDS and hepatitis is becoming a real risk with the use of allograft skin.—M.C. Robson, M.D.

## Experimental and Clinical Applications of Fibrin Glue

Saltz R, Sierra D, Feldman D, Saltz MB, Dimick A, Vasconez LO (Univ of Alabama, Birmingham; Baptist Med Ctr, Birmingham)
*Plast Reconstr Surg* 88:1005–1017, 1991            12–16

*Background.*—Fibrin glue prepared from human plasma may transmit viral infections. Methods for production of both autologous and single-donor fibrinogen concentrate, however, have been developed. The adhesive strength of fibrin glue was measured, the skin graft take in rats was evaluated, and the results of clinical applications in 73 patients were assessed.

*Methods.*—In vitro mechanical testing was used to measure the shear adhesive strength of glue with fibrinogen concentrations of 20, 40, and 70 mg/mL. Sixteen Sprague-Dawley rats had skin grafts secured with sutures and with single-donor human fibrin glue; donor sites were also treated with fibrin glue and with sutures for controls. The graft take was noted grossly; microscopic analysis assessed the viability of the grafts at 2, 7, 14, and 21 days after operation. A noncontrolled, retrospective review of clinical applications, principally for hand and facial burns and difficult graft sites, also was undertaken.

*Results.*—An increased concentration of fibrinogen was associated with increased shear adhesive strength. Full adhesive strength was attained after a 5-minute incubation in vitro. Histologic evaluation of skin graft healing in rats showed that neovascularization and all phases of healing were the same with glue as with sutures. Donor sites treated with adhesive healed as well as those that were sutured. Histologic examination showed abundant elastic tissue and functional lamellar scar tissue at 14 days, and the amount of anastomotic fibrosis, axonal regeneration, and alignment of fascicles was at least as good with glue as with sutures. Clinical results included minimal blood loss and excellent graft stabilization and requirements for little postoperative care. The single procedure of resurfacing with sheet grafts produced improved esthetic results and complete graft take.

*Conclusions.*—The use of autologous fibrin glue was associated with markedly improved hemostasis, early graft adherence, and excellent graft take. The use of fibrin glue resulted in shorter hospital stays, minimal postoperative care, early return to normal activities, better esthetic results, and increased satisfaction on the part of patients and nurses.

▶ Fibrin glue has not found popularity because previously it required pooled allogenic donors. The risk of viral transmission appeared to be prohibitive. These authors discuss techniques to make single-donor autologous fibrin glue and demonstrate its efficacy in a series of patients. A multi-center trial now seems indicated to learn whether this experience can be duplicated.—M.C. Robson, M.D.

---

**External Rhinoplasties: Indications for Use**
Teichgraeber JF, Riley WB, Russo RC (Univ of Texas, Houston; The Carle Clinic, Urbana, Ill)
*Br J Plast Surg* 45:47–54, 1992                                                    12–17

---

*Background.*—The external approach to rhinoplasty is increasing in popularity among otolaryngologists, but there are few reports of its use in the plastic surgery literature. The technique and indications for external rhinoplasty and its role in nasal surgery were examined.

*Patients.*—The external rhinoplasty technique was used in 563 patients during a 5-year period. Of these, 452 were female patients, and 111 were male patients; the mean age was 29.5 years. Sixty-three operations were secondary rhinoplasties. The most common indications were a severely twisted nose and augmentation rhinoplasty, followed by major revision surgery, congenital deformity, septoplasty, and septal perforation. Several graft types were used, including shield tip grafts from the septum or ear; cartilaginous columellar struts, using septum cartilage or homograft irradiated cartilage; and dorsal onlay grafts. Cranial bone was usually used when bone was needed, and dorsal cartilage from the septum or ear was used when cartilage was needed. Ten percent of patients had "spreader" grafts. All patients were followed for at least 18 months.

*Results.*—Compared to a previous series of endonasal rhinoplasties, the external exposure allowed for more predictable results. The Rethi incision helped to maintain and augment tip support, and augmentation of the nasal dorsum and spine was more accurate. Incidence of dislocation and shifting was decreased. No complications were attributable to the external approach, although 1 patient had dehiscence of the columellar scar that healed by secondary intention. Supratip edema and anesthesia were more common than with the endonasal approach, sometimes persisting for 6–9 months and probably resulting from disruption of the venous, lymphatic, and nervous connections of the tip. Operative time was increased only in primary cosmetic operations with minimal tip and dorsal work. Patients were unconcerned about the transcolumellar scar. Septal perforations were closed successfully in 19 of 22 cases.

*Conclusions.*—External rhinoplasty is a useful procedure, especially for patients with a severely twisted nose, or a need for secondary or augmentation rhinoplasty, or correction of congenital deformities or septal perforation. It is also helpful in the teaching and learning of rhinoplasty. There are no complications from this approach.

▶ This large series of patients in whom external rhinoplasties were performed demonstrates the procedure's utility. The paper carefully outlines the operative technique, shows the indications to be considered, and discusses possible pitfalls. External rhinoplasty is becoming commonplace, and this article will benefit the surgeon unfamiliar with its intricacies.—M.C. Robson, M.D.

---

**The Fate of Plates and Screws After Facial Fracture Reconstruction**
Francel TJ, Birely BC, Ringelman PR, Manson PN (Maryland Inst for Emergency Med Services System, Baltimore; Johns Hopkins Univ, Baltimore)
*Plast Reconstr Surg* 90:568–573, 1992                    12–18

---

*Background.*—Rigid plate and screw fixation is widely used in the management of complex facial fractures. Rigid fixation facilitates bone healing and preserves the facial dimensions. Although complications associated with the use of the rigid plate and screw fixation have been reported, the fate of reconstructive hardware in facial reconstruction has not been examined. A retrospective review was made of the complications associated with facial plate and screw fixation.

*Patients.*—During a 5-year period, 507 patients underwent open reduction with plate and screw fixation for 1,112 facial fractures. The patients ranged in age from 17 to 74 years, and 72% were male trauma victims. Of the 507 patients, 157 (31%) had open fractures and 350 (69%) had closed fractures. The fate of the hardware was assessed at least 18 months after operation.

*Results.*—During the follow-up period, reconstructive hardware had to be removed in 61 patients (12%), and 21 of them (34.4%) required removal of multiple plates. The maxillary buttress region and the mandible were the most common sites from which hardware was removed. Thirty-seven patients required removal because of infection and 24 because of other symptoms, including exposure (15%), prominent hardware (13%), or pain (11.5%). Symptoms prompting hardware removal varied by anatomical divisions. The average time to removal was 3.7 months for infection and 38 months for pain. Hardware removal rates were not influenced by the type of metallic plating system used at the initial reconstruction.

*Recommendations.*—Infection and exposure rates associated with the use of reconstructive hardware in complex facial fractures can be minimized with antiseptic irrigations, by avoiding mucosal damage, by paying attention to proper mucosal closure, and by correct placement of the plates.

▶ These authors pioneered in the wide use of plates and screws for internal fixation of facial fractures. Their patients included all comers with severe maxillofacial injuries and were not highly selected from a small group of "ideal" cases. Therefore, they have been able to collect 1,112 fractures in 507 patients. They have now helped all reconstructive surgeons by carefully evaluating the fate of the implanted hardware. Certainly, the plates and screws were sometimes problems, with 12% of patients requiring removal. The authors suggest techniques to decrease the incidence of complications in these patients.—M.C. Robson, M.D.

---

## Experience With Rigid Fixation of Mandibular Fractures and Immediate Function

Anderson T, Alpert B (Univ of Louisville, Louisville, Ky)
*J Oral Maxillofac Surg* 50:555–560, 1992                     12–19

---

*Objective.*—The results of using rigid fixation in selected mandibular fractures were examined in 52 patients with 75 fractures. The technique essentially was limited to injuries that ordinarily would have been treated by open reduction and internal fixation and to patients in whom maxillomandibular fixation had to be avoided.

*Patients.*—All of the fractures resulted from blunt trauma. No patient was grossly infected before reduction. The fractures were rigidly fixed after placement of maxillomandibular fixation, which then was promptly released or removed. Most fractures were fixed with plates and bicortical screws. The majority of procedures were performed transorally.

*Results.*—Twelve of the 52 patients had complications, e.g., infection, scarring, and facial nerve paresis. Twelve of the 75 fractures became infected, and 3 of the infected patients had unsightly, bound-down scars as a result. Seven infections necessitated tooth and appliance removal or débridement. All infections involved teeth in the line of fracture. Extraoral surgery appeared to dispose to infection. Three of the 14 comminuted fractures became infected.

*Conclusion.*—Rigid fixation of mandibular fractures with limited postoperative function seems to be a valid means of avoiding prolonged maxillomandibular fixation in selected patients despite a risk of infection.

▶ Conceptually, rigid internal fixation eliminating the need for maxillomandibular immobilization would be a real advance in the treatment of mandibular fractures. Unfortunately, as demonstrated by this article, this has not proved to be the case. Complications are high, as shown by a high infection rate, bound-down scars, and facial nerve injury. There are patients in whom maxillomandibular immobilization is truly contraindicated. In these cases, possibly acceptance of the higher complication rate is justified.—M.C. Robson, M.D.

---

**Preliminary Observations on Isotretinoin-Induced Ear Malformations and Pattern Formation of the External Ear**
Lammer E (California Birth Defects Monitoring Program, Emeryville)
*J Craniofac Genet Dev Biol* 11:292–295, 1991                12–20

---

*Background.*—Retinoic acid is a morphogenic substance that can induce a variety of extremity malformations, including duplications and reduction type defects, in chick embryos. Its role in controlling the pattern formation of other structures is not clear. Since 1984, several fetuses and infants whose mothers used isotretinoin, (13-*cis* retinoic acid) during the first trimester of pregnancy have been followed up longitudinally. The unusual craniofacial malformations in these fetuses and infants were examined.

*Data Analysis.*—Isotretinoin induced a characteristic pattern of craniofacial malformations, especially of the external ear. A consistent pattern was reduction of external ear structures derived from tissue of the second branchial arch, with relative sparing of structures derived from the first branchial arch. The specific types of auricular malformations included partial duplications and tissue reductions and displacements. The tragus was frequently elongated along its superior-inferior axis, with a vertically oriented crus helicis. The shape and location of the external ear canal were always linked to the size of the tragus, so that a canal was never present when the tragus was absent.

*Discussion.*—The similarities in isotretinoin-induced external ear malformations and the types of extremity malformations induced by retinoic acid suggest that retinoic acid can also alter the pattern formation of developing craniofacial structures. It appears that the isotretinoin-induced external ear malformation results from an altered pattern formation along the dorsal-ventral axis of the first and second branchial arches.

▶ Plastic surgeons and dermatologists beware. Retinoic acid is being used more and more frequently on women's facial skin. This article addresses potential birth defects of the craniofacial area in fetuses of mothers exposed to retinoic acid. Previously, limb development was shown to be affected by retinoic acid.—M.C. Robson, M.D.

## Head and Neck Surgery

### Prognostic Factors in the Recurrence of Stage I and II Squamous Cell Cancer of the Oral Cavity

Jones KR, Lodge-Rigal RD, Reddick RL, Tudor GE, Shockley WW (Univ of North Carolina, Chapel Hill)
*Arch Otolaryngol Head Neck Surg* 118:483–485, 1992          12–21

*Introduction.*—Few physicians have recommended elective neck dissection or radiotherapy for all stage I/II oral cancers despite a high risk of occult neck disease. A retrospective study identified patients at increased risk of recurrence after excision of stage I/II oral cavity cancer.

*Series.*—Forty-nine of 71 patients seen in 1981–1988 with oral cavity cancers were available for follow up after at least 2 years. The 33 men and 18 women had a median age of 64 years. Eighteen patients had $T_1$, $N_0$ tumors, whereas 31 had $T_2$, $N_0$ tumors.

*Findings.*—Twenty of the 49 patients (41%) had recurrences, 9 locally, 8 in the neck, and 3 at both sites. Recurrences appeared a median of 6 months after excision. Eleven patients were salvaged by surgery and/or radiotherapy. Margin status and depth of invasion were the most significant factors predicting recurrence. Perineural invasion also was a factor. A positive surgical margin and a tumor depth exceeding 5 mm each increased the risk of recurrence by nearly threefold, and these risks were multiplicative.

*Discussion.*—Unfortunately, neither margin involvement nor tumor depth is a useful preoperative predictor of recurrence. Nevertheless, positive margins should be immediately reexcised if feasible.

▶ Positive margins in small ($T_1$ and $T_2$) lesions in the oral cavity and a tumor depth exceeding 5 mm predict tumor recurrence. These data should be useful in determining the need for reoperation or larger resection. Unfortunately, only the tumor depth can help preoperatively, and then only if the biopsy is done in the opportune locality with the greatest depth. Further prognostic papers will be useful for the head and neck surgeon.—M.C. Robson, M.D.

---

**Interleukin 2 Receptors on Squamous Cell Carcinomas of the Head and Neck: Characterization and Functional Role**
Cortesina G, Sacchi M, Galeazzi E, Johnson JT, Whiteside TL (Univ of Torino, Italy; Univ of Pittsburgh, Pa)
*Acta Otolaryngol* 112:370–375, 1992                                    12–22

---

*Introduction.*—Recombinant interleukin-2 (IL-2) has been used to stimulate natural killer cells to become lymphokine-activated killer cells that can destroy a wide range of human tumor cells. Such cells are helpful in the adoptive immunotherapy of certain types of cancer. Interleukin-2 receptors on squamous cell carcinomas in the head and neck region were quantified.

*Methods.*—Expression of binding sites for IL-2 was demonstrated by radiobinding studies on squamous cell carcinoma lines in vitro. Cytocentrifuged tumor cells were examined by immunoperoxidase staining using monoclonal antibody to the p70 subunit of IL-2 receptors.

*Findings.*—High-affinity binding sites for IL-2 were demonstrated on the tumor cells, and positive immunostaining was reproducibly observed. Studies in a nude mouse model suggested a functional role for these receptors. Low doses of IL-2 inhibited growth of 11 of the 16 tumor cell lines tested.

*Implication.*—Interleukin-2 in low dosage might have a direct effect on squamous cell head and neck tumors, which express high-affinity IL-2 receptors.

▶ Molecular and cell biologists will make the next great advance in the treatment of head and neck cancer. Demonstration of IL-2 receptors in some tumors suggests possible treatment of these with exogenous rIL-2. If the treatment of human tumors explanted to "nude" mice is predictive, then this technique might be a real advance. I eagerly await results of a clinical trial.—M.C. Robson, M.D.

### Induction Chemotherapy in Head and Neck Cancer: Results of a Phase III Trial

Mazeron J-J, Martin M, Brun B, Grimard L, Lelièvre G, Vergnes L, Haddad E, Feuilhade F, Piedbois P, Strunski W, Peynègre R, Pierquin B, Le Bourgeois J-P (Hôp Henri Mondor, Créteil, France; Hôp Intercommunal de Créteil)

*Head Neck* 14:85–91, 1992        12–23

*Background.*—When the diagnosis is made at an advanced stage, patients with squamous cell carcinoma of the head and neck (SCCHN) have a poor prognosis. Although chemotherapeutic debulking in these patients leads to a high response rate, induction chemotherapy has yet to produce improvement in locoregional control and cause-specific and overall survival. A phase III trial compared induction therapy followed by radical local treatment with radical local treatment alone in patients with stages II–IV SCCHN.

*Methods.*—The study sample comprised 131 patients with biopsy-proven stage II, III, or IV squamous cell carcinoma of the oropharynx or mouth seen at 1 of 2 French medical centers. Patients were stratified by site, tumor size, and nodal status before randomization. One group received induction chemotherapy consisting of bleomycin, 10 mg/m²/day in continuous infusion from day 1 to day 5; methotrexate, 120 mg/m² on day 2; 5-fluorouracil, 600 mg/m² on day 2; and cisplatin, 120 mg/m² on day 4, every 4 weeks for 3 cycles, followed by definitive locoregional treatment. The other group received locoregional treatment only. The selection of radiotherapy and/or surgery as definitive treatment was made before randomization.

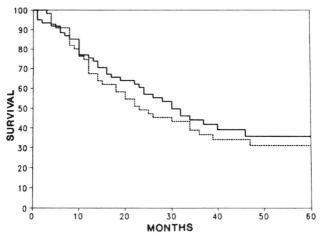

**Fig 12–6.**—Survival (percentage of patients) in months for both the experimental (*dotted line*) and control group (*solid line*). Log-rank test, P = .49. (Courtesy of Mazeron J-J, Martin M, Brun B, et al: *Head Neck* 14:85–91, 1992.)

*Results.*—There were 116 evaluable patients. Induction therapy yielded a complete response rate of 7% and a partial response rate of 42%. After locoregional therapy, complete response was achieved in 76% of the group given chemotherapy and in 89% of the control group. There were no differences between the groups with regard to survival, cause-specific survival, or pattern of relapse, with median survivals of 22 months in the group given chemotherapy and 29 months in controls (Fig 12-6). Most of the few toxic complications of chemotherapy were related to cisplatin, the dose of which was reduced to 100 mg/m² for 35 patients.

*Conclusions.*—The induction chemotherapy regimen examined here does not improve locoregional control or survival in patients with advanced SCCHN compared with locoregional treatment alone. These patients should receive induction or adjuvant chemotherapy only in prospective, randomized trials of new drugs or combinations.

---

### Treatment of Advanced Squamous-Cell Carcinoma of the Head and Neck With Alternating Chemotherapy and Radiotherapy

Merlano M, Vitale V, Rosso R, Benasso M, Corvò R, Cavallari M, Sanguineti G, Bacigalupo A, Badellino F, Margarino G, Brema F, Pastorino G, Marziano C, Grimaldi A, Scasso F, Sperati G, Pallestrini E, Garaventa G, Accomando E, Cordone G, Comella G, Daponte A, Rubagotti A, Bruzzi P, Santi L (Natl Inst for Cancer Research, Genoa, Italy; S. Paolo Hosp, Savona, Italy; Galliera Hosp, Genoa; Celesia Hosp, Genoa; S. Martina Hosp, Genoa; et al)
*N Engl J Med* 327:1115–1121, 1992                                    12–24

---

*Background.*—Radiotherapy is the conventional treatment in patients with advanced, unresectable head and neck squamous cell carcinoma. Survival outcomes are poor, however. Whether rotational chemotherapy/radiotherapy treatment would improve survival rates in such patients was investigated.

*Methods.*—The series included 157 patients who were randomly assigned to receive either combined chemotherapy and radiotherapy or radiotherapy alone. Eighty patients were given 4 cycles of cisplatin (20 mg/m²) and fluorouracil (200 mg/m²) intravenously daily for 5 days alternating with three 2-week courses of radiotherapy (20 Gy per course). Those assigned to radiotherapy alone (77 patients) received up to 70 Gy, 2 Gy daily, 5 days a week. Patient groups were similar in terms of age, gender, performance status, disease stage, and primary tumor sites.

*Results.*—Complete responses were significantly different in each group. In the group given combined treatment, 34 patients had complete responses compared with 17 receiving only radiotherapy. The overall response rates were similar between the 2 groups. Local relapses occurred in 12 of the 34 patients with complete response who received combined treatment and in 10 of the 17 patients with complete re-

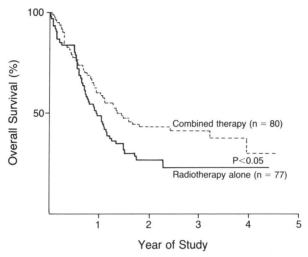

**Fig 12–7.**—Overall survival in the treatment groups. (Courtesy of Merlano M, Vitale V, Rosso R, et al: N Engl J Med 327:1115–1121, 1992.)

sponse who received radiotherapy. There was a significant difference in survival rates that favored the combined therapy arm (Fig 12–7). Median survival was 16.5 months in the group given combined treatment as opposed to 11.7 months in the group given radiotherapy alone.

*Implications.*—Alternating chemotherapy and radiotherapy increases median survival and in this series doubled the survival probability for 3 years as compared with radiotherapy alone. Local disease, however, cannot be controlled in more than half of the patients who receive combined therapy. Therefore, improved methods of management are needed.

▶ Multiple modality treatment of head and neck cancer remains theoretically sound. However, when put to the statistical trial, it has been difficult to show advantages over single treatment alone such as surgical extirpation or radiotherapy. In the first paper (Abstract 12–23), adjunctive induction chemotherapy plus operative extirpation was no better than extirpation alone. In the second paper (Abstract 12–24), alternating chemotherapy and radiotherapy increased the median survival and doubled the 3-year survival rate. However, local recurrences were not improved with the combination treatment. Both of these studies were well done with adequate numbers to show differences, if indeed differences existed.—M.C. Robson, M.D.

## Cigarette Smoking, Alcohol, and Nasopharyngeal Carcinoma: A Case-Control Study Among U.S. Whites

Nam J, McLaughlin JK, Blot WJ (Natl Cancer Inst, Bethesda, Md)
*J Natl Cancer Inst* 84:619–622, 1992                                    12–25

*Background.*—Nasopharyngeal carcinoma (NPC) is extremely common among certain Chinese populations, but it is relatively rare among white persons in the United States. Epidemiologic studies of NPC conducted in Asia have implicated several environmental factors. In the United States, some studies have implicated several environmental factors. In the United States, some studies have implicated cigarette smoking as a risk factor for NPC, but others could not confirm such an association. A case-control analysis was conducted to investigate the role of cigarette smoking and alcohol consumption as risk factors for NPC in the United States.

*Methods.*—The cases were 204 white American men and women who had died of NPC, and the controls were 408 white American men and women who had died of causes unrelated to cigarette smoking or alcohol use. Information on smoking habits and alcohol intake was obtained mainly from surviving spouses.

*Results.*—The risk of NPC increased with increasing pack-years of cigarette smoking. The odds ratio (OR) for NPC among cigarette smokers with 60 or more pack-years of smoking compared with that for lifelong nonsmokers exceeded 3 for both men and women. The risk for NPC also increased with alcohol consumption. Cigarette smoking and alcohol consumption were independent risk factors, with cigarette smoking having a stronger effect than alcohol (table).

Odds Ratios (ORs) for NPC Associated With Smoking and Drinking

| Cigarette smoking, pack-years | Alcoholic beverage intake, drinks/wk | | | Total * | |
|---|---|---|---|---|---|
| | 0-3 | 4-23 | 24+ | OR | 95% CI |
| ≤30 (light use) | 1.0 | 0.6 | 1.4 | 1.0 | — |
| 31-59 (medium use) | 1.5 | 2.3† | 2.6§ | 2.2 | 3.3-3.5 |
| ≥60 (heavy use) | 2.2† | 2.3† | 5.2§ | 3.1 | 1.9-5.4 |
| Total ‖ | | | | | |
| OR | 1.0 | 0.9 | 1.8 | — | |
| 95% CI | — | 0.5-1.4 | 1.1-3.1 | | |

Note: All odds ratios were adjusted for sex.
* Risks of smoking were adjusted for alcohol intake.
†P <.05.
‡P <.01.
§ Risks of alcohol intake were adjusted for smoking.
(Courtesy of Nam J, McLaughlin JK, Blot WJ: *J Natl Cancer Inst* 84:619–622, 1992.)

*Conclusion.*—Cigarette smoking and, to a lesser extent, alcohol intake are risk factors for NPC in the white American population.

▶ Data from this case-control study of the National Mortality Followback Survey document the strong association of cigarette smoking with the increased risk of NPC. Alcohol consumption was also an independent risk factor, but had a lesser impact than that of cigarette smoking. The results of this study are somewhat unusual because other epidemiologic studies have documented diet, Epstein-Barr infection, and other environmental factors in the causation of NPC.

As with any large epidemiologic study of questionnaires when medical records are unavailable, inaccuracies may exist that would influence the conclusions. However, cigarette smoking, and perhaps alcohol consumption, may partially explain the occurrence of NPC in the otherwise low-risk white American population.—T.J. Eberlein, M.D.

### The Indications for Elective Treatment of the Neck in Cancer of the Major Salivary Glands

Armstrong JG, Harrison LB, Thaler HT, Friedlander-Klar H, Fass DE, Zelefsky MJ, Shah JP, Strong EW, Spiro RH (Mem Sloan-Kettering Cancer Ctr, New York City)
*Cancer* 69:615–619, 1992                                                          12–26

*Purpose.*—The selection criteria for elective treatment of the neck in patients with locally confined major salivary gland cancers are not well defined. To define selection criteria for elective neck dissection (END) in these patients, a retrospective record review was performed.

*Patients and Treatment.*—Between 1939 and 1982, 474 patients with newly diagnosed, locally confined, major salivary gland cancers and no evidence of distant metastatic disease underwent tumor resection as indicated by tumor extent. Sixty-seven patients (14%) with clinically evident lymph node spread underwent therapeutic neck dissections. Sixteen of them (24%) received postoperative neck irradiation at a median dose of 4,500 cGy. Of 474 patients, 90 (19%) underwent END. Although no strict selection criteria were used, END was performed mostly in patients with high-grade and more advanced tumors.

*Results.*—Lymph node involvement was confirmed pathologically in all 67 patients who underwent therapeutic neck dissection. Of 90 patients with clinically negative necks who underwent END, 34 (38%) had occult pathologically positive nodes. In addition, occult node metastases were found in the intraparotid or periparotid nodes of 10 patients and in the submandibular specimens of 3. In all, 47 of the 407 patients with clinically negative necks had pathologically positive nodes. Multivariate analysis identified size and grade as significant risk factors for occult metastases. Tumors 4 cm or greater in diameter were associated with a 20%

risk of occult disease compared with a 4% risk for smaller tumors. The risk of occult disease was 49% for high-grade tumors, regardless of histologic type, compared with a 7% risk for intermediate- or low-grade tumors.

*Conclusions.*—Routine END in patients with salivary gland tumors and no clinical evidence of neck involvement is not warranted, but END should be considered in those with high-grade or large tumors.

▶ The findings that salivary tumors at least 4 cm in diameter or high grade histologically tend to metastasize are shown in a series large enough to be believed. Because both of the prognosticators can be determined by a careful physical examination and fine-needle biopsy before definitive resection, they should be useful in assessing the role of END. A follow-up series after these prognosticators are used to determine therapy would be helpful to know if they can be relied upon.—M.C. Robson, M.D.

---

**Salivary Gland Neoplasms in Children**
Callender DL, Frankenthaler RA, Luna MA, Lee SS, Goepfert H (Univ of Texas MD Anderson Cancer Ctr, Houston)
*Arch Otolaryngol Head Neck Surg* 118:472–476, 1992          12–27

---

*Introduction.*—Less than 5% of all salivary gland tumors occur in children and young adults, and these neoplasms account for less than 10% of all head and neck tumors in pediatric patients. The records of 29 patients aged 3–16 years, seen between 1944 and 1987 with nonvasoformative salivary gland neoplasms were reviewed.

*Pleomorphic Adenoma.*—Eight patients had pleomorphic adenoma, the only benign neoplasm encountered. Most patients were seen initially with a slowly enlarging mass. The parotid gland was involved in 6 lesions. All of the adenomas were resected, and no recurrences developed during a mean follow-up of 16 years.

*Malignancies.*—Most patients with malignant salivary gland neoplasms had an enlarging parotid or submandibular mass. Mucoepidermoid carcinoma was the most common malignancy and usually involved the parotid gland. Seventeen of the 21 patients with malignant tumors remained free of disease for a mean of 13.6 years. Two others were alive with disease, and 2 died of disease. The absolute 5-year survival rate was 90%. Two of 5 surgical salvage procedures succeeded. Four patients required resection of the main facial nerve trunk, and 6 others had resection of 1–3 facial nerve branches.

*Conclusions.*—Benign parotid tumors in children may be controlled by parotidectomy. It often is not necessary to sacrifice the facial nerve. Postoperative radiotherapy may be indicated when a high-grade lesion, soft tissue extension, or perineural invasion is present. Salvage surgery has given disappointing results.

▶ At first, this article is deceiving. It suggests that the most common salivary gland tumors in children are malignant. Careful reading explains that this is a quirk of the M.D. Anderson Hospital, and that indeed most salivary gland tumors and most parotid tumors are benign. Hemangiomas, arteriovenous malformations, and pleomorphic adenomas make up the majority of parotid tumors. Pediatric tumors present most frequently as a mass and not with pain or a nerve defect. The good news in this article is that even patients with malignant tumors do well after excision.—M.C. Robson, M.D.

---

**Pediatric Head and Neck Rhabdomyosarcoma**
MacArthur CJ, McGill TJI, Healy GB (Children's Hosp, Boston, Mass)
*Clin Pediatr* 31:66–70, 1992                                    12–28

---

*Introduction.*—Although rhabdomyosarcoma (RMS) in children is a rare occurrence, it is the most common malignant soft tissue tumor in the pediatric population. Rhabdomyosarcoma most often occurs in the head and neck region, accounting for 40% of all RMS cases. The current approach to the diagnosis and treatment of pediatric head and neck RMS was examined.

*Diagnosis.*—A thorough physical examination in young children may require general anesthesia. Computed tomography with contrast is the most useful radiographic modality for determining tumor size and extent, and evaluating bone or skull-base involvement. Magnetic resonance imaging is most useful for evaluating vascular invasion and obtaining finer soft tissue details. Incisional biopsy is usually performed if the lesion is recognized early. Excisional biopsy may also be possible. After tissue confirmation, chest CT and bone scanning should be performed to exclude distant metastatic involvement.

*Treatment.*—Rhabdomyosarcoma must be treated aggressively, both locally and immediately, because the tumor has a proclivity for local invasion and tends to metastasize at the high rate. Local tumor is controlled with surgery and radiation therapy. The risk of distant metastases is controlled with chemotherapy. In children with group II or higher grade tumors, radiation therapy is used in conjunction with chemotherapy or surgery to control local disease or nodal drainage.

*Survival.*—Before 1960, RMS was uniformly fatal. Since the introduction of multimodality treatment regimens, however, survival in children with RMS has improved significantly. Current survival rates are more than 60% for those who do not have metastases when RMS is first diagnosed. Five-year survival rates as high as 83% have been reported in children whose tumor is completely resected and who are treated systemically to reduce the risk of distant metastases. Five-year survival rates decline to 52%, however, when residual tumor is left behind because of inaccessibility or CNS invasion. Survival after relapse remains poor, with 32% surviving for 1 year and 17% surviving for 2 years. The prognosis in children with distant metastases at the time of diagnosis remains poor.

*Conclusions.*—It is hoped that, through the continued combined efforts of medical oncologists, radiotherapists, and surgeons, the improvements in survival achieved during the past 20 years in children with RMS in the neck and head region will continue.

▶ This article describes the success story of multimodality treatment for RMS. If multimodality treatment allows for total resection, 83% survival is now possible. When total resection is limited by CNS invasion or distant metastases, the survival rate drops to 52%. Considering that the tumor was almost uniformly fatal 30 years ago, this is a great improvement.—M.C. Robson, M.D.

---

**Types and Causes of Pain in Cancer of the Head and Neck**
Vecht CJ, Hoff AM, Kansen PJ, de Boer MF, Bosch DA (Dr Daniel den Hoed Cancer Ctr, Rotterdam, The Netherlands; Academic Med Ctr, Amsterdam, The Netherlands)
*Cancer* 70:178–184, 1992                                                12–29

---

*Introduction.*—Types of pain and their causes were examined in a series of patients with head and neck cancer. The 14 men and 11 women had an average age of 57 years. A numerical rating scale was used to score pain.

*Findings.*—Nineteen of the 25 patients had nociceptive pain — pain of new onset that was linked with active tissue damage by recurrent tumor, tumor-related inflammation, ischemia, trauma, or infection. Nine of these patients had actual nociceptive pain, 8 had nociceptive nerve pain, and 2 had referred pain. Nociceptive pain was caused by a recurrent tumor in many of the cases, but in 3 instances, it was secondary to benign inflammation. Six patients had neuropathic pain secondary to the sequelae of neck dissection.

*Treatment and Response.*—If oral medication failed, nerve blocks were used in patients with nociceptive pain. Stellate and trigeminal blocks and stereotactic mesencephalotomy all were used. Nine patients received antitumor therapy for recurrent tumor causing pain. Non-nociceptive pain usually was managed with amitriptyline or carbamazepine. Seventy-two percent of the patients were relieved after as many as 4 attempts to alleviate pain. Antitumor treatment succeeded in only 3 patients.

*Conclusion.*—Assessing the type and cause of pain in patients with head and neck cancer is helpful in defining appropriate treatment.

Nearly three fourths of the study patients, who had severe pain, were relieved, chiefly by symptomatic measures.

▶ The authors conclude that the type and cause of pain in patients with cancer of the head and neck can be determined. This can lead to the administration of proper symptomatic treatment directed at the underlying cause. In most cases, several attempts to treat the pain were required before relief was achieved. This is a good start toward trying to analyze pain in these patients and developing a rational approach to therapy.—M.C. Robson, M.D.

**Arterial Anatomy of the Face: An Analysis of Vascular Territories and Perforating Cutaneous Vessels**
Whetzel TP, Mathes SJ (Univ of California, San Francisco)
*Plast Reconstr Surg* 89:591–603, 1992                    12–30

*Introduction.*—Physicians have known about the 14 individual arteries that form the cutaneous arterial circulation of the face and scalp for

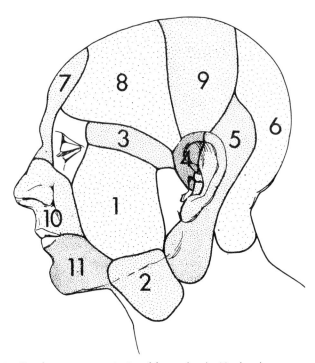

**Fig 12–8.**—Vascular cutaneous territories of face and scalp. Numbered areas represent individual cutaneous vascular territories of face supplied by following arteries: *1,* transverse facial; *2,* submental; *3,* zygomatico-orbital; *4,* anterior auricular; *5,* posterior auricular; *6,* occipital; *7,* supratrochlear; *8,* frontal branch of superficial temporal; *9,* parietal branch of superficial temporal, *10,* superior labial, and *11,* inferior labial. (Courtesy of Whetzel TP, Mathes SJ: *Plast Reconstr Surg* 89:591–603, 1992.)

more than a century, but the precise locations of the arteries' perforation sites have not been determined. Various methods were used to define the extent and location of certain arteries and their relationship with various facial muscles and fascia.

*Methods.*—Twenty-one fresh cadavers aged 23–89 years at the time of death provided specimens for studying the following vessels: the transverse facial, anterior auricular, occipital, submental, frontal, and parietal branches of the superficial temporal, zygomatico-orbital, posterior auricular, supratrochlear, and superior and inferior labial arteries. Three methods were used to define the vessels: selective ink injections, subdermal dissection after blue latex injection, and selective lead oxide injection. Three steps determined the site of perforating arteries and measured the predictability of their location relative to bone and surface landmarks: dissection and measurement of perforator sites, thermographic localization of these sites in vivo, and statistical analysis of perforation site measurements. The relationship of the perforating arteries to the facial fascia, muscles of facial expression, and deeper structures of the face was studied by deep dissection and tranverse section dissection and by transverse section radiographs.

*Results.*—The 90 selective ink injections in 14 facial arteries defined 11 cutaneous vascular territories (Fig 12-8). This technique demonstrated that all areas adjacent to the midline extended into the contralateral areas. Overall, these mapping techniques found 3 distinct patterns of arterial vascularization: small, densely populated musculocutaneous perforating vessels that supply the anterio face, large and sparsely distributed fasciocutaneous perforators, that supply the lateral region of the face, and small, densely packed fasciocutaneous perforators that supply the scalp.

*Conclusions.*—These findings outline and further define the anatomy of the cutaneous vessels of the face and scalp. They provide the anatomical framework to potentially revise or improve current procedures in reconstructive or esthetic surgeries on the face.

▶ This meticulous description of arterial supply to the face should be read and kept as a ready reference by surgeons operating in the head and neck area. By combining this paper with Corso's work (1), the reader will have an excellent basis for designing incisions and flaps on the face.—M.C. Robson, M.D.

*Reference*

1. Corso P: *Plast Reconstr Surg* 27:160, 1961.

### Laryngotracheal Resection and Reconstruction for Subglottic Stenosis

Grillo HC, Mathisen DJ, Wain JC (Massachusetts Gen Hosp, Boston; Harvard Med School, Boston)
*Ann Thorac Surg* 53:54–63, 1992                          12–31

*Introduction.*—A single-stage resection and reconstruction was used to treat inflammatory stenosis of the subglottic larynx and upper trachea in 80 consecutive patients, excluding those with neoplastic disease.

*Patients.*—Fifty patients had lesions secondary to intubation for ventilatory support; 7 had stenosis of traumatic origin; 19 patients had idiopathic laryngotracheal stenosis. Many patients had systemic disorders. Most of the postintubation patients and many others had been treated previously. Forty-two patients had a tracheostomy in place.

*Management.*—Surgery was delayed in 9 patients. In most patients, a cervical collar incision was used. Most resections extended for 2–4.5 cm. The anterolateral cricoid arch was resected in all patients; in addition, posterior larygneal stenosis was removed when present. The posterior cricoid plate was salvaged. In 31 patients a posterior membranous tracheal wall flap was used to resurface the exposed cricoid cartilage.

*Results.*—One postoperative death occurred, caused by myocardial infarction. The long-term outcome was excellent in 18 patients, good in 48, and satisfactory in 8. Two operations were considered failures. Three patients had good initial results but were lost to follow-up.

*Conclusion.*—Laryngotracheal resection and reconstruction in 1 stage can avoid complex multistage surgery in many patients with subglottic stenosis, but careful timing of surgery and exacting operative technique are essential.

▶ This is an excellent series of difficult cases treated by the master of tracheal reconstruction. The paper should be read in full and the excellent diagrams studied. No other group has attacked this problem with the same fervor as Grillo and his colleagues.—M.C. Robson, M.D.

# 13 Noncardiac Thoracic Surgery

## Introduction

This chapter, noncardiac Thoracic Surgery, comprises principally the treatment of thoracic malignancies. Specifically, lung cancer has become the number one killer of men and women in the United States (1). The care of patients with primary pulmonary or other thoracic malignancies in previous years has followed a sequential course leading from the thoracic surgeon for primary therapy to the oncologist or radiotherapist for the treatment of recurrent disease. Long-term survival has been essentially unchanged in the past two decades. Approximately 50% of patients successfully treated surgically die of their disease (2), and, unfortunately, it is still a minority of patients who present with operable lesions (2). The morbidity of traditional surgical approaches remains high, with traditional thoracotomy a major source of morbidity and mortality. Indeed, elective lobectomy and pneumonectomy carry the highest mortality for an elective procedure when compared to other operative resections of malignancy (3).

This current situation has stimulated the search for additional prognostic factors that would allow more specific identification for prognostic subgroups of patients with primary resectable lung cancer. Molecular markers, as expressed by a tumor's genetic make-up, surface antigens, and secreted serum markers, are currently under study. In addition, traditional prognostic factors, including evidence of vascular or lymphatic invasion, as well as specific light microscopic findings are also being re-reviewed for clues leading to more specific prognostication for patients with stage I and stage II lung cancer. These prognostic factors, as they become established, will need to be understood by the thoracic surgeon in terms of their significance in selecting patients for specific treatment strategies. This fact is especially important because the thoracic surgeon is often the first individual to encounter the patient with a potentially resectable lung nodule. A firm understanding of the patient's prognosis will allow for selection of patients for specific adjuvant therapies and clinical trials as thoracic surgeons seek to make a further impact on the survival in this disease.

Multimodality therapy as primary treatment for thoracic malignancies has become more common in recent years. These primary treatment strategies using multimodality approaches have necessitated closer working relationships between medical oncologists, thoracic surgeons, and radiotherapists, as well as a better understanding of each others' methods as they are combined in primary treatment.

The multimodality approach to non–small-cell lung cancer (NSCLC) has been most prominent in the treatment of locally advanced NSCLC, specifically in patients who have etiologically documented stage IIIA disease. The efficacy of traditional operative approaches and approaches including neoadjuvant chemotherapy and/or radiotherapy is important to determine. The appropriate sequencing of the multimodality approach to stage IIIA lung cancer depends on the resultant operative morbidity and mortality, as well as the ability of each of these strategies to demonstrate practicality and universality.

The use of adjuvant surgery in the performance of pulmonary metastectomy has been a traditionally confusing area, with reported series difficult to interpret and indications for surgical resection hard to define. The need for appropriate surgical intervention in patients with pulmonary metastasis is clear. This section addresses this very important, clinical situation with the review of five articles that address the outcome of pulmonary metastectomy in the treatment of metastatic carcinoma, as well as metastatic sarcoma.

Specific problems in thoracic oncology are then examined. Updates on the appropriate diagnosis and therapy of malignant thymoma are reviewed, as are specific problems related to the AIDS population of patients. The surgeon's role in the treatment of myasthenia gravis is again considered, given the important nature and often confusion state of the literature concerning this disease.

Thoracoscopy has been used for more than 50 years in the diagnosis and management of intrathoracic disease. However, with the advent of small miniaturized video cameras that allow for excellent intrathoracic visualization via minimally invasive techniques, the role of thoracoscopy has expanded from the purely diagnostic into the therapeutic realm. This has led to a resurgence of surgeons devising new operative techniques in the treatment of surgical disease, as has been reflected in the thoracic surgical literature in the past year. It is extremely important for thoracic surgeons to constantly synthesize new surgical techniques as they are described, and compare and contrast them with standard operative techniques. Indeed, the origin of many standard operative procedures is rooted in a mixture of an understanding of the biology of the pathology being treated, as well as the anatomy of the organ to be resected. It is possible, and in many instances probable, that minimally invasive thoracic surgical techniques will be centered more specifically on the anatomical surgical resection of the lesion with some disregard for its biological activity.

It would appear important at this time for surgeons not to quickly adopt new techniques as they are reported, but to continue to retain a healthy skepticism of each report, recognizing that current standard operative procedures are the result of many years of clinical investigation and trial. Thoracoscopic surgery will undoubtedly continue to change, and this change will be stimulated by the surgeon's enhanced understanding of the clinical behavior of malignant disease, as well as the development of new operative technology that will provide safer and less morbid means of operative intervention.

The equation that seeks to relate operative morbidity and mortality to either palliative or curative outcome is the one surgeons use to determine indications for operative intervention. Thoracoscopic surgery has the potential to radically alter this equation. As the morbidity and mortality of operative intervention decrease, indications for surgical intervention may change. These facts require an enhanced understanding and participation of thoracic surgeons in the management of patients with thoracic disease.

Video-assisted thoracic surgery may some day entirely replace the conventional operative approaches to the chest. However, if it is to do so in an orderly fashion by which the patient's benefit is maximized, thoracic surgeons must carefully evaluate each new report in light of his or her own practice and surgical training. We have carefully selected articles that represent the most concise, substantive reports in thoracoscopic surgery. In many instances we have reviewed several articles on the same procedure because the authors differ in technique and resultant morbidity and mortality.

We have reviewed the application of thoracoscopic surgery from reports around the world concerning the diagnosis and therapy of pleural disease, parenchymal disease, mediastinal disease, and diseases of the chest wall. It is clear that advances in thoracoscopic technique are the products of surgeons worldwide whose ingenuity and surgical expertise are once again devising new approaches to thoracic disease.

David J. Sugarbaker, M.D.

*References*

1. Boring CC, et al: CA 42:19, 1992.
2. Mountain CF: *Semin Oncol* 15:236, 1988.
3. Ginsberg RJ, et al: *J Thorac Cardiovasc Surg* 86:654, 1983.

## Thoracic Surgical Oncology

New Prognostic Factors in Non–Small-Cell Lung Cancer

### Detection of Large Cell Component in Small Cell Lung Carcinoma by Combined Cytologic and Histologic Examinations and Its Clinical Implication

Fushimi H, Kikui M, Morino H, Hosono Y, Fukuoka M, Kusunoki Y, Aozasa K, Matsumoto K (Osaka Univ, Suita, Japan; Osaka Prefectural Habikino Hosp, Habikino, Japan; Nara Med College, Kashirhara, Japan)
*Cancer* 70:599–605, 1992                                          13–1

*Background.*—The International Association for the Study of Lung Cancer (IASLC) pathology panel has proposed a classification of 3 subtypes of small cell lung carcinoma (SCLC): pure SCLC, mixed small cell/large cell carcinoma (mixed SC/LC), and combined SCLC. Previous studies evaluating the usefulness of the modified IASLC classification for SCLC usually examined only histologic specimens. A combination of cytologic and histologic specimens was used to evaluate the classification of SCLC according to the modified IASLC system.

*Method.*—Histologic specimens, cytologic specimens obtained by brushing or fine-needle aspiration, and sputum cytologic specimens from 430 patients with SCLC were examined.

*Findings.*—The frequency of SCLC was approximately 15% in patients whose diagnosis was made with any diagnostic procedure. As in other studies, the prognosis of SCLC was unfavorable, with a median survival in this series of 256 days. Patients with mixed SC/LC had a poorer response to treatment and worse prognosis than those with pure SCLC. When classified with biopsy specimens, the median survival for mixed SC/LC was 144 days vs. 285 days for pure SCLC. Classification with cytologic specimens obtained by brushing or fine-needle aspiration showed a median survival of 160 days for mixed SC/LC vs. 275 days for pure SCLC. Classification by sputum cytologic specimens showed a median survival of 47 days for mixed SC/LC and 259 days for pure SCLC.

*Conclusion.*—The patients with mixed SC/LC had a poorer response to treatment and significantly shorter survival when compared to patients with pure SCLC diagnosed by any procedure. Mixed SC/LC should be distinguished from pure SCLC. Brushing and/or aspiration are useful and sensitive procedures for obtaining cytologic specimens. Cytologic and biopsy specimens used together confirmed the utility of the IASLC classification when defining a treatment schedule and predicting patient survival.

▶ The authors point out an important fact: Patients who have a mixed SC/LC pathology have a worse prognosis than patients with pure SCLC tumors. Indeed, this conclusion is supported by other data that demonstrate approximately 15% to 20% of small cells do not respond to chemotherapy

(1–3). This is important in assessing the prognosis in this group of patients. In addition, these patients who have no pathologic evidence of mediastinal node involvement may be considered for operative resection followed by chemotherapy (4). The rationale for surgery in patients with mixed cell type is that surgery remains the best therapy for non–small-cell tumors followed by chemotherapy for the small cell component. The existence clinically of these mixed tumors supports more recent hypotheses suggesting a common neuroendocrine origin for all lung cancers.—D.J. Sugarbaker, M.D.

*References*

1. Mentzer SJ, et al: *Chest* 103(suppl):S349, 1993.
2. Lynch TJ: *Chest* 103(suppl):S349, 1993.
3. Elias A: *Chest* 103(suppl):S349, 1993.
4. Shields TW, et al: *J Thorac Cardiovasc Surg* 84:481, 1982.

---

**Vascular Invasion in Non–Small-Cell Lung Carcinoma**

Roberts TE, Hasleton PS, Musgrove C, Swindell R, Lawson RAM (Univ Hosp of South Manchester, Manchester, England; Wythenshawe Hosp, Manchester; North Staffordshire Hosp Ctr, Stoke on Trent, England; Christie Hosp, Manchester)
*J Clin Pathol* 45:591–593, 1992
        13–2

---

*Background.*—Vascular invasion allows metastasis of several types of malignant neoplasms, including breast, cervical, and endometrial carcinoma. Whether there is a correlation between vascular invasion and prognosis in non–small-cell carcinoma of the lung was investigated in a specific search for invasion of vascular channels by tumor cells.

*Method.*—Eighty-seven patients who had resections for 64 squamous cell carcinomas and 23 adenocarcinomas of the lung were followed for 5 years. Histologic sections were studied for evidence of vascular invasion using a van Gieson stain. Invasion was classified as vascular if the tumor was seen within pulmonary arteries or veins, and lymphatic if tumor cells were seen without areas that had a definite and clearly identifiable endothelial lining. Survival data were analyzed using the log rank test.

*Findings.*—The 5-year survival rate in the 87 patients was 32%. Vascular invasion was found in 77% and lymphatic invasion in 44%. The patients with lymphatic permeation had recurrence and died earlier than those without lymphatic permeation. Prognosis was not related to the presence or absence or proportion of blood vessels having vascular invasion, intimal fibrosis, or tumor necrosis.

*Conclusion.*—Unlike findings in other common solid tumors, there was no correlation between the presence of vascular invasion and survival in patients with squamous and adenocarcinoma of the lung. Lymphatic permeation was associated with a poor prognosis, with recurrence and shorter survival.

▶ The importance of blood vessel invasion (BVI) and lymphatic vessel invasion (LVI) as prognostic factors have been in dispute. Takise analyzed prognostic factors in 75 patients with resected stage I non–small-cell lung carcinoma (NSCLC). In his study, the presence of BVI in the tumor was highly significant as a poor prognostic sign (absent, 84% 5-year survival; present, 49%; P = .02) (1).

Shields, reporting from the Veterans Administration Adjuvant Treatment Group, evaluated the importance of LVI and BVI in 685 men with resected lung cancer of all histologic subtypes. In node-negative patients, LVI did predict for poorer outcome (LVI present, 42% 3-year survival; LVI absent, 63%; P < .05) (2). In this study the presence of BVI did not add significantly to the prognostication of survival.

The study by Roberts et al. would support LVI as an important prognostic factor that should be considered in the development of adjuvant treatment strategies in resected stage I and stage II NSCLC.—D.J. Sugarbaker, M.D.

*References*

1. Takise A, et al: *Cancer* 61:2083, 1988.
2. Shields TW: *Surg Gynecol Obstet* 157:185, 1983.

---

## Relation of Neovascularisation to Metastasis of Non–Small-Cell Lung Cancer

Macchiarini P, Fontanini G, Hardin MJ, Squartini F, Angeletti CA (Univ of Pisa, Pisa, Italy; Univ of Alabama, Birmingham)
*Lancet* 340:145–146, 1992                    13–3

---

*Introduction.*—Some experimental studies have shown that angiogenesis spurs tumor growth and also permits tumor cells to enter the general circulation. The mechanism of this neovascularization is currently unknown. Whether the intensity of angiogenesis correlates with metastasis of non–small-cell lung cancer (NSCLC) was investigated in tumor specimens from 87 patients with $T_1N_0M_0$ NSCLC were studied. The 84 male and 3 female patients had a mean age of 60 years.

*Findings.*—Twenty-two patients had postoperative metastases. The microvessel count (Fig 13–1) and density were higher in these patients then in those with no evidence of metastases. There were significant differences between the 2 groups regarding tumor size and proliferation. On stepwise multivariate logistic regression analysis, only microvessel density was significantly related to metastasis.

*Conclusions.*—Metastasis is probably dependent on the intensity of angiogenesis. This finding may assist in the identification of patients who may need systemic treatment after radical surgery.

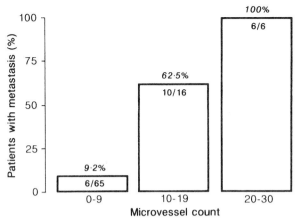

**Fig 13–1.**—Relationship between frequency of postoperative metastasis and microvessel counts. Microvessel counts are per ×200 field. (Courtesy of Macchiarini P, Fontanini G, Hardin MJ, et al: *Lancet* 340:145–146, 1992.)

▶ The clinical relevance of angiogenesis factor was not apparent until recently. This factor, produced by tumors, induces the neovascularization of tumors to allow continued growth. The factor has been isolated by Folkman et al. (1, 2), but its usefulness in clinical trials remains unclear. Further understanding of the mechanisms of neovascularization may allow for development of therapeutic strategies that seek to interrupt this process.

The report from Macchiarini et al. needs to be validated in larger, better-controlled studies. However, its importance in suggesting the significance of tumor vascularization in predicting prognosis in NSCLC should not be overlooked. Weidner et al's report of this fact in breast cancer may lead to new adjuvant strategies in this disease (3).

Thus the importance of this prognostic factor may imply the use of conventional therapies and represent the basis for new approaches to tumor therapy.—D.J. Sugarbaker, M.D.

*References*

1. Folkman J, et al: *Nature* 288:551, 1989.
2. Folkman J, Haudenschild C: *Nature* 288:551, 1980.
3. Weidner N, et al: *N Engl J Med* 324:1, 1991.

### Correlation of L-*myc* RFLP With Metastasis, Prognosis and Multiple Cancer in Lung-Cancer Patients

Kawashima K, Nomura S, Hirai H, Fukushi S, Karube T, Takeuchi K, Naruke T, Nishimura S (Natl Cancer Ctr Research Inst, Tokyo, Japan; Natl Cancer Ctr Hosp, Tokyo)

*Int J Cancer* 50:557–561, 1992                                                      13–4

*Introduction.*—A close correlation has been reported between restrictions-fragment-length polymorphism (RFLP) of L-*myc* and the extent of lung cancer metastasis. This finding was examined in a larger group of lung cancer patients.

*Methods.*—Tumors and portions of normal resected lung tissue were obtained from 252 randomly selected Japanese patients with lung cancer. Histopathologic diagnoses of these tissues were made and DNA was isolated. Southern blot hybridization was used to monitor L-*myc* RFLP. Bands were identified as long (L) or short (S).

*Results.*—Twenty-six of 64 patients with L-L bands (41%) and 140 of 188 patients with L-S or S-S bands (75%) had lymph node metastases. Metastases to distant organs occurred in 3 of 64 patients with the L-L type (5%) and in 45 of 188 patients with L-S or S-S bands (24%). The overall prognosis was also poorer for patients with S-S or S-L bands.

*Conclusions.*—Good correlation was found between L-*myc* RFLP and lung cancer metastasis. Polymorphism was also correlated with a poor prognosis and the incidence of multiple cancers.

▶ The importance of this study lies in its clear demonstration that the genetic code of a particular lung cancer can accurately predict survival and the development of metastasis. In this study it was the presence of RFLP of L-*myc* that was closely correlated with the presence of lymph node metastasis and survival.

Very soon, the genetic make-up of early stages I and II non–small-cell lung cancer will influence the use of conventional adjuvant therapy. In addition, methods of genetic manipulation may allow for genetic biological therapies in the near future.—D.J. Sugarbaker, M.D.

### *ras* Gene Mutations as a Prognostic Marker in Adenocarcinoma of the Human Lung Without Lymph Node Metastasis

Sugio K, Ishida T, Yokoyama H, Inoue T, Sugimachi K, Sasazuki T (Kyushu Univ, Fukuoka, Japan)

*Cancer Res* 52:2903–2906, 1992                                                      13–5

*Background.*—Mutations in the *ras* gene family often transform the *ras* gene into an oncogene. Previous studies have shown that K-*ras* mutations in adenocarcinoma of the lung are associated with a poor progno-

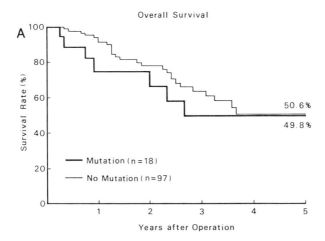

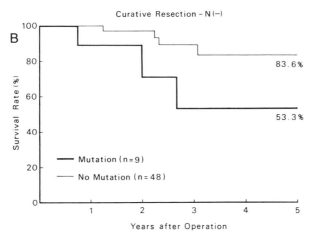

**Fig 13–2.**—Kaplan-Meier survival curves after surgery for adenocarcinoma of lung, with respect to presence or absence of *ras* gene mutation. **A,** overall survival ($P = .1513$ by generalized Wilcoxon test). **B,** cases of curative resection without lymph node metastasis ($P = .0212$ by generalized Wilcoxon test). Numbers of patients with stage I and stage III-A disease were 44 and 4 in *ras*-negative group and 8 and 1 in *ras*-positive group, respectively. (Courtesy of Sugio K, Ishida T, Yokoyama H, et al: *Cancer Res* 52:2903–2906, 1992.)

sis. The relationship between mutations at codons 12, 13, and 61 in the entire *ras* gene family and the clinical prognosis were examined.

*Methods.*—High-molecular-weight DNA was isolated from tissue samples of 115 Japanese patients who had undergone surgical resection for lung adenocarcinomas. Selective amplification of codons 12, 13, and 61 was performed in K-*ras*, H-*ras*, and N-*ras* genes by the polymerase chain reaction (PCR). The PCR products were spotted and hybridized with labeled oligonucleotide probes to determine codon point mutations.

*Results.*—Mutated codons were detected in 18 tissue samples (15.7%). Seventeen mutations occurred in K-*ras*: 15 at codon 12 and 2 at codon 13. A single mutation was also found at codon 61 of N-*ras.* Mutations were significantly more likely to occur in men (16 mutations in 69 men) than in women (2 mutations in 46 women). The mutation rate was significantly higher among smokers (20.8%) than among nonsmokers (7%). There was no correlation between heavy and light smoking and mutations, nor was a significant difference noted in mutation rates between male smokers and nonsmokers. The overall 5-year survival rate was similar for patients with (49.8%) and without (50.6%) codon mutations (Fig 13–2). For patients undergoing complete (curative) resectioning, however, the 5-year survival rate was significantly better among those with a normal *ras* gene (83.6%) than in those with point mutations (53.3%).

*Conclusion.*—The presence of *ras* gene mutations may be a negative prognostic factor, especially in early-stage adenocarcinoma of the lung.

▶ The *ras* protein family is thought to mediate the signal transduction that controls the growth of cells (1). *ras* Genes are expressed in almost all mammalian cells, and *ras* proteins are essential for normal cell growth and physiology (2). Malignant transformation may be attributable to mutated *ras* genes that send continual growth signals leading to unregulated cell growth. The *ras* proteins receive transforming potential as a result of point mutation of the encoding gene. The presence of K-*ras* mutations is known to be common in non–small-cell lung cancer (3). The K-*ras* region produces p21 proteins that are detectable with immune histochemical techniques.

This study is important because it validates the significance of K-*ras* mutations as a negative prognostic variable in surgically resected patients with adenocarcinoma. In addition, the fact that smoking in female patients was associated with a higher incidence of K-*ras* mutation suggests the inductability of genetic aberrations by cigarette smoking. Of interest was the fact that there was no correlation between the amount of smoking and the mutation rate in females.

The presence of K-*ras* mutations in resected tumors may become an indication for conventional adjuvant therapy.—D.J. Sugarbaker, M.D.

*References*

1. Carbone D, Minna J: Molecular biology of lung cancer, in Broder, S (ed): *Molecular Foundations of Oncology.* Baltimore, Williams and Wilkins, 1991, pp 339–366.
2. Rodenhuis S, Slebos RJ: *Cancer Res* S2:52665, 1992.

**Prognostic Value of Nuclear DNA Content and Expression of the *ras* Oncogene Product in Lung Cancer**

Miyamoto H, Harada M, Isobe H, Akita HD, Haneda H, Yamaguchi E,

Kuzumaki N, Kawakami Y (Hokkaido Univ, Sapporo, Japan)
Cancer Res 51:6346–6350, 1991
13–6

*Objectives.*—The growth characteristics of tumors, particularly DNA content, are important in assessing prognosis. Study was made of the prognostic value of nuclear DNA content, estimated by flow cytometry, as well as *ras* oncogene expression in tumor sections taken surgically from 112 non–small-cell lung cancer (NSCLCs). Monoclonal antibody rp-35 was used to detect the p21 protein product of *ras* in paraffin-embedded sections.

*Findings.*—Of the 84 tumors examined by flow cytometry, 77% had DNA aneuploid patterns. Positive reactions for *ras* protein were obtained in 56% of squamous cell cancers and 68% of adenocarcinomas. Patients with DNA diploid tumors had a better 5-year survival rate than those with aneuploid tumors. Those with p21-negative tumors survived significantly longer than those with p21-positive tumors, especially strongly positive tumors. The degree of *ras* protein expression did not correlate with the nuclear DNA content.

*Conclusion.*—Prognostic assessment of patients with NSCLC may be aided by estimating nuclear DNA content and expression of the *ras* oncogene in addition to the stage of disease.

▶ Flow cytometry is a useful technique that can rapidly provide a reproducible, quantitative analysis of cellular characteristics. This technique is automated and can examine tumor samples of $10^5$ cells in a few minutes (1). The analysis can be performed on fresh tissue or on archival, paraffin samples.

Flow cytometry measures 2 cellular characteristics having biological relevance to prognosis. First, it measures the DNA content of tumor cells, or ploidy. Aneuploid tumor cells have an abnormal amount, whereas diploid cells have a normal amount. Ploidy has been related to the clinical and biological aggressiveness of tumors. The second characteristic is the fraction of cells in different phases of the cell cycle, in particular, the percentage of cells in the S phase, or synthetic phase. The index of cells in the S phase is a indication of the tumor's proliferative activity.

The study by Miyamoto et al. is important because it demonstrates the ability of flow cytometry to predict survival on the basis of ploidy in NSCLC. It is also of note that K-*ras* was also a predictor of poor outcome but was independent of the ploidy status. Thus, in the same population of patients, 2 independent variables were identified.—D.J. Sugarbaker, M.D.

*Reference*

1. Merkel DE, et al: *J Clin Oncol* 5:1690, 1987.

### Tumor-Associated Antigen 43-9F Is of Prognostic Value in Squamous Cell Carcinoma of the Lung: A Retrospective Immunohistochemical Study

Battifora H, Sorensen HR, Mehta P, Ahn C, Niland J, Hage E, Pettijohn DE, Olsson L (City of Hope Natl Med Ctr, Duarte, Calif; State Univ Hosp, Copenhagen, Denmark; Univ of Colorado, Denver; Receptron, Inc, Concord, Calif)
*Cancer* 70:1867–1872, 1992                                                     13–7

*Background.*—The only criterion of current prognostic value in squamous cell lung carcinoma (SLC) is node staging. The monoclonal antibody 43-9F is associated with an SLC-related antigen and is not reactive with small cell lung carcinomas.

*Objective.*—An immunohistochemical study was carried out to examine primary tumor specimens from 231 patients with lung cancer. Squamous cell lung carcinoma was present in 130 patients, adenocarcinoma in 64, small cell carcinoma in 10, large cell carcinoma in 16, and adenosquamous carcinoma in 11. Formalin-fixed, paraffin-embedded tissue specimens were examined for immunoreactivity with 43-9F antibody.

*Findings.*—Patients whose tumors were negative for 43-9F had a significantly poorer outlook than those whose tumors contained 43-9F epitope-positive cells. This was the case for squamous cell lung tumors but not for adenocarcinoma. In SLC, the 43-9F staining pattern was the most significant single prognostic factor. Reactivity with 43-9F did not correlate with the degree of keratinization or with other prognostic factors in patients with SLC or adenocarcinoma.

*Conclusion.*—Expression of 43-9F is a useful prognostic marker in SLC that can be determined before treatment.

▶ This report is of interest because it is one of the few that describes a positive prognostic factor. The presence of the antigen 43-9F on squamous tumors was associated with improved survival. It is of additional interest in that it is one of the few predictors for squamous cancers, because no association between this antigen and survival was noted in the group with adenocarcinoma in this study.—D.J. Sugarbaker, M.D.

### Correlation of Expression of H/Le$^y$/Le$^b$ Antigens With Survival in Patients With Carcinoma of the Lung

Miyake M, Taki T, Hitomi S, Hakomori S (Kitano Hosp, Osaka, Japan; Kyoto Univ, Kyoto, Japan; Univ of Washington, Seattle)
*N Engl J Med* 327:14–18, 1992                                                   13–8

*Background.*—Patients with various histologic types of lung cancer have a high level of H/Le$^y$/Le$^b$ antigen expression. This phenomenon may be associated with deletion of A and B blood group antigens. The

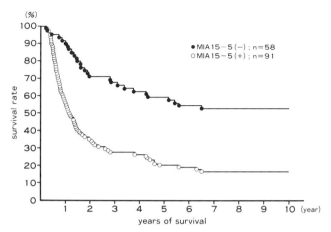

**Fig 13-3.**—Survival in 149 patients with lung cancer, according to expression of MIA antigen in tumor. The *P* value was determined with the log-rank test. (Courtesy of Miyake M, Taki T, Hitomi S, et al: N *Engl J Med* 327:14–18, 1992.)

possibility was examined that expression of this antigen, defined by the monoclonal antibody MIA-15-5, may be of prognostic value.

*Methods.*—The antibody was used to stain tissue sections from 149 patients with primary lung cancer. The survival curves of patients with positively staining tumors were compared with those of patients with negatively staining tumors.

*Findings.*—Whereas 91 patients had MIA-positive tumors, 58 had MIA-negative tumors. The 5-year survival rate in the first group was significantly lower than survival in the second group, rates being 21% and 59%, respectively. The survival rates also differed significantly among the 67 patients with squamous cell carcinoma, proportions being 10.5% of those with MIA-positive findings and 62% of those with MIA-negative findings. Survival differences between patients with MIA-positive and MIA-negative tumors also were significant among patients with blood groups A and AB, but not among those with B or O types. According to multivariate analysis, positivity best correlated with 5-year mortality, followed by lymph node status and tumor size. Sex, age, and blood group did not correlate with mortality (Fig 13-3).

*Conclusions.*—Because MIA positivity, or immunohistologic staining by MIA-15-5, is correlated inversely with survival among patients with primary lung cancer, this finding may be of prognostic value.

▶ The prognostic importance of blood group antigen A expression in patients with resected non–small-cell lung cancer (NSCLC) was reported by Lee et al. (1). The ABH blood group antigens are known to be on the surface of many different epithelial cells, along with erythrocytes. The presence of expressed ABH blood group antigens on the surface of cancer cells has been linked in studies to cellular differentiation and maturation.

The H/Le$^y$/Le$^b$ antigen is a carbohydrate antigen related to blood group antigen H (2). The expression of this antigen on the surface of tumor cells is high, and this includes cases of NSCLC. The blood group A and B antigens are thought to be the precursor antigens to the H/Le$^y$/Le$^b$ on the surface of tumor cells. The expression of the latter antigen is thought to be related to deletion of blood group A and B antigens. Previous studies in other tumors have shown that the presence of this deletion is associated with a greater potential for invasion.

Miyake et al. used the antibody MIA-15-5 to detect H/Le$^y$/Le$^b$ on the surface of resected cancer cells. This study is of great importance, given the very significant level of association of survival with antigen expression. Thus this report was selected based on the probability that detection of this antigen will soon be in clinical use as a staging adjunct. Because tumors that express H/Le$^y$/Le$^b$ on their cell surfaces are the same ones that don't express A and B antigens, this report appears to confirm the conclusions of Lee et al. regarding the importance of the expression of blood group A antigen.—D.J. Sugarbaker, M.D.

*References*

1. Lee JS, et al: N Engl J Med 324:1084, 1991.
2. Lee JS, Hong WK: N Engl J Med 327:47, 1992.

---

### Postoperative Increase in Soluble Interleukin-2 Receptor Serum Levels as Predictor for Early Recurrence in Non–Small-Cell Lung Carcinoma

Tisi E, Lissoni P, Angeli M, Arrigoni C, Corno E, Cassina E, Ballabio D, Benenti C, Barni S, Tancini G (San Gerardo Hosp, Milan, Italy)
*Cancer* 69:2458–2462, 1992
13–9

---

*Background.*—Major surgery leads to immunosuppression, and in cancer patients this could promote the growth of existing micrometastases. Interleukin-2 (IL-2) is an important cytokine in the regulation of immune responsiveness, and activated T lymphocytes can release a soluble form of IL-2 receptor (SIL-2R) into the circulation. An increased risk of relapse might be expected in patients with non–small-cell lung cancer who have a rise in the SIL-2R content postoperatively.

*Study Design.*—Sixty consecutive patients with epidermoid lung carcinoma or adenocarcinoma participated in the study. Twenty-one had node involvement. The median follow-up was 10 months. Levels of SIL-2R were estimated by enzyme immunoassay.

*Findings.*—Forty patients (67%) had elevated levels of SIL-2R preoperatively, and the mean level significantly exceeded control values. Whereas 32 patients had a decline in the serum level of SIL-2R postoperatively, 28 did not. Relapse occurred in 19 patients and was more frequent in those with adenocarcinoma than in those with epidermoid cancer. Relapse also was more common in patients with involved nodes and those with higher SIL-2R values a month postoperatively. Preoperative levels of SIL-2R did not differ significantly between patients who relapsed and those who remained free of disease.

*Conclusion.*—Postoperative determination of the serum level of SIL-2R may help to predict the risk of early relapse in patients with operable non–small-cell lung cancer.

▶ Interleukin-2 is a cytokine known to be involved in the host antitumor response. It is produced by activated T helper lymphocytes and produces its activity by binding to surface receptors of IL-2. In addition, activated T lymphocytes may release SIL-2R into the bloodstream, where it competes with IL-2 surface receptors for the available IL-2 in the blood. Thus the available IL-2 is decreased. In this way, high levels of SIL-2R may indicate an immunosuppressed state (1).—D.J. Sugarbaker, M.D.

*Reference*

1. O'Garra A: *Lancet* 1:942, 1989.

NEW SURGICAL APPROACHES TO THERAPY OF NON–SMALL-CELL LUNG CANCER

**Survival After Resection of Stage II Non–Small-Cell Lung Cancer**
Martini N, Burt ME, Bains MS, McCormack PM, Rusch VW, Ginsberg RJ (Mem Sloan-Kettering Cancer Ctr, New York City; Cornell Univ Med College, New York City)
*Ann Thorac Surg* 54:460–466, 1992                                    13–10

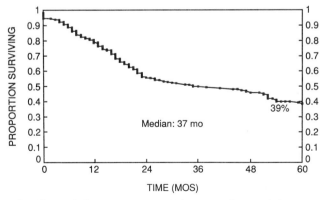

**Fig 13–4**—Overall survival after resection in stage II lung cancer (n = 214). (Courtesy of Martini N, Burt ME, Bains MS, et al: *Ann Thorac Surg* 54:460-466, 1992.)

*Introduction.*—Resection is the preferred approach to patients with early invasive lung carcinoma involving only the hilar or pulmonary nodes, but recurrences are frequent and overall survival is not encouraging. No adjuvant measures have proved to be helpful.

*Series.*—A total of 214 patients with stage II non–small-cell lung cancer (NSCLC) underwent resection with complete mediastinal node dissection. Adenocarcinoma was present in 116 patients, and squamous cancer in 98. There were 35 $T_1N_1$ and 179 $T_2N_1$ tumors in the series. Half of the patients had only a single involved $N_1$ node.

*Treatment.*—Most patients (68%) had lobectomy, 31% had pneumonectomy, and 1% underwent wedge resection or segmentectomy. Lobectomy was adequate for all but 1 of the patients with $T_1N_1$ disease. Only 22% of the patients received external radiotherapy postoperatively. Eleven patients were given chemotherapy.

*Results.*—The postoperative mortality rate was 3.3%; all deaths occurred in patients with $T_2$ lesions. The overall 5-year survival rate was 39% for patients with $N_1$ disease (Fig 13–4). Patients with tumors 3 cm or less in diameter had the best outlook. Involvement of multiple lymph nodes significantly worsened the prognosis. Postoperative irradiation appeared to reduce local and regional recurrences only in patients with squamous cancer. Sixteen new cancers developed, 7 of them primary lung cancers.

*Conclusions.*—Complete resection is the best approach to stage II NSCLC. Postoperative radiotherapy may limit recurrences in patients with squamous cancer but has not improved survival. The fact that most recurrences are distant metastases indicates the need for effective systemic measures once nodal disease is present.

▶ The standard therapy of patients with stages I and II NSCLC remains surgical resection. This report emphasizes the inadequacy of surgery in the majority of patients who have nodal metastasis. This is consistent with the findings of the National Surgical Adjuvant Breast and Bowel Project in breast cancer (1). That group demonstrated that a single nodal metastasis is an indicator of systemic disease, thus the extent of surgical resection, i.e., local control, will not affect survival. In addition, it appears that the number of involved nodes is not of importance to survival in patients with breast cancer, which is where the analogy with NSCLC appears to break down. In the study by Martini et al., patients with 1 node positive did significantly better than patients with multiple nodes. Thus NSCLC has some halstedian character to it in that resection of regional lymph nodes appears to be of therapeutic value, at least in the case of a single node.

These differences from breast cancer may reflect differences in the anatomy of lymphatic drainage of the lung versus the breast, or other immune factors. The important message in this study for thoracic surgeons is that the adequacy of anatomical surgical resection appears to be more important in NSCLC. This must be kept in mind, particularly as we evaluate new thoracoscopic techniques in which local excision is often the primary goal.—D.J. Sugarbaker, M.D.

*References*

1. Fisher B, et al: *Surg Gynecol Obstet* 140:528, 1975.

## Surgery and the Management of Peripheral Lung Tumors Adherent to the Parietal Pleura

Albertucci M, DeMeester TR, Rothberg M, Hagen JA, Santoscoy R, Smyrk TC (Creighton Univ, Omaha, Neb; Univ of Southern California, Los Angeles)
*J Thorac Cardiovasc Surg* 103:8–13, 1992          13–11

*Introduction.*—Proper treatment of tumors that adhere to the parietal pleura remains uncertain. No strong evidence supports extrapleural or en bloc resection. Data were reviewed concerning 37 patients with lung cancer, seen between 1976 and 1988, who had peripheral $T_3$ lesions. Twenty-eight tumors were considered $T_3$ lesions based on the clinical and imaging findings, whereas 9 others thought to be $T_2$ lesions were found at exploration to adhere to the parietal pleura.

*Management.*—Radiotherapy was given preoperatively to 28 patients and postoperatively to 7. Twenty-one patients had en bloc removal of the tumor and chest wall, which included part of the vertebral body in 9 of them. Sixteen patients had extrapleural resection around the primary tumor. Pneumonectomy was performed in 20 instances.

*Results.*—Thirty patients in all had tumor extending through the visceral pleura and into the parietal pleura. Six of the 16 patients who had extrapleural resection had local recurrences, as did only 2 of the 21 undergoing en bloc resection. Actuarial survival rates were 30% at 5 years and 22% at 10 years. Survival was significantly better for patients having en bloc chest wall resection when only those lacking node involvement were analyzed.

*Conclusions.*—Some lung cancers invading the parietal pleura go undetected on preoperative evaluation. Pleural adherence almost always signifies extension through the parietal pleura. A tumor adherent to the pleura overlying the chest wall should be resected en bloc in patients with $N_0$ and $N_1$ disease.

▶ The adequacy of surgical resection is again highlighted in this study. The standard teaching in many thoracic surgical texts and training centers is that tumors fixed to the chest wall should be resected en bloc with the chest wall and undergo preoperative irradiation. Furthermore, it is standard teaching that tumors adherent to the parietal pleura, but "moveable," can be resected in the extrapleural plane.

This report demonstrates that extrapleural dissection in these cases constitutes inadequate surgical therapy and suggests that these tumors be resected en bloc with the chest wall when possible. Moreover, we can infer that postoperative radiotherapy should be given when parietal pleural invasion is noted on pathologic examination of the specimen if a chest wall resection was not performed. The question remains as to whether postoperative radiation is indicated if a chest wall resection was carried out and the margins are clean. Previous reports suggest that, "when in doubt radiate." This is because of the limited morbidity of postoperative radiotherapy to the chest wall and the high mortality of local tumor recurrence.—D.J. Sugarbaker, M.D.

▶↓ The next 2 reports (Abstracts 13–12 and 13–13) concern the treatment of stage IIIA non–small-cell lung carcinoma (NSCLC) with neoadjuvant chemotherapy followed by surgery. The treatment of ipsilateral mediastinal node-positive NSCLC with surgery alone has been disappointing. Five-year survival rates of 5% to 8% are reported when the entire cohort of patients is considered (1). This fact has led to multimodality therapy of the disease with the neoadjuvant (preoperative) use of platinum-based chemotherapy regimens. Neoadjuvant chemotherapy may be of superior benefit for several reasons: (1) The patient is treated earlier in the course of the disease than if the treatment were given after postoperative recovery; (2) tumor clones with higher mitotic indexes would be expected to metastasize to lymph nodes, and these cells should be more sensitive to chemotherapeutic agents; (3) the tumor blood supply is intact before surgery, therefore maximal drug delivery could be expected; (4) hypoxia is a well-described mechanism of both chemo- and radioresistance. Incompletely resected cells may be the result of surgery, and these cells may be hypoxic because of disruption of their blood supply.

The important question to be addressed by these studies is what the combination and sequence of therapy should be. The morbidity and mortality of the treatment strategy must be weighed against the survival benefit.—D.J. Sugarbaker, M.D.

*Reference*

1. Strauss GM et al: *J Clin Oncol* 10:829, 1992.

---

**Preoperative Chemotherapy and Radiation Therapy for Stage IIIa Carcinoma of the Lung**
Yashar J, Weitberg AB, Glicksman AS, Posner MR, Feng W, Wanebo HJ
(Roger Williams Cancer Ctr, Providence, RI; Brown Univ, Providence)
*Ann Thorac Surg* 53:445–448, 1992          13–12

---

*Introduction.*—A pilot study was begun in 1985 to administer chemotherapy and radiotherapy concomitantly to 36 patients who had stage

IIIa non–small-cell lung carcinoma (NSCLC) with positive mediastinal nodes. Nineteen patients had large cell carcinoma, 10 had squamous cell carcinoma, and 7 had adenocarcinoma.

*Treatment.*—Two cycles of induction chemotherapy including *cis*-platinum and etoposide were administered. At the same time, patients received irradiation to the tumor and mediastinum in a total dose of 55 Gy, with an additional 540 cGy to the tumor alone. Resection was scheduled 4 to 6 weeks after the end of treatment, and chemotherapy was repeated postoperatively; 2 cycles of adjuvant therapy were given at 28-day intervals.

*Results.*—Thirty-one patients (86%) underwent resection. Five patients had no definite gross tumor at the time of thoracotomy and in 6 others shrinkage of the tumor occurred. Radical penumonectomy was necessary in 27 cases. Sterilization of the primary site and mediastinal nodes was proved histologically in 28% and 47% of patients, respectively. Operative mortality was 5.6%. Six patients had radiologic findings of acute respiratory distress, and 3 others had bronchopleural fistulas. Twelve patients followed for a median of 27 months had a 3-year survival rate of 62%. Eight of 10 patients with no microscopic disease were alive without disease 5 months to 5 years postoperatively, and local control had been achieved in 9 of the 10.

*Conclusion.*—Preoperative chemotherapy including *cis*-platinum and concomitant radiotherapy is well tolerated by patients with stage IIIa NSCLC. It promotes tumor resectability and improves survival.

---

**Induction Chemotherapy With Mitomycin, Vindesine, and Cisplatin for Stage III Unresectable Non–Small-Cell Lung Cancer: Results of the Toronto Phase II Trial**

Burkes RL, Ginsberg RJ, Shepherd FA, Blackstein ME, Goldberg ME, Waters PF, Patterson GA, Todd T, Pearson FG, Cooper JD, Jones D, Lockwood G (Mt Sinai Hosp, Toronto, Ont, Canada; Toronto Hosp; Ontario Cancer Inst, Toronto)
*J Clin Oncol* 10:580–586, 1992                    13–13

---

*Introduction.*—The primary curative therapy for non–small-cell lung cancer (NSCLC) is surgery, yet few patients have operable disease when first seen. Chemotherapy regimens have also been of limited usefulness in NSCLC. Mitomycin, vindesine, and cisplatin (MVP) induction chemotherapy, previously reported to be effective in patients with stage IIIA unresectable $N_2$ NSCLC, was evaluated.

*Methods.*—The study group of 39 patients included 32 men and 7 women whose median age was 60 years. Fourteen had adenocarcinoma/ large cell tumors and 25 had squamous cell carcinoma. Two cycles of MVP were administered. Responders underwent thoracotomy for resection and 2 further courses of MVP.

*Results.*—Four patients died of chemotherapy-induced sepsis. Of the remaining 35 patients evaluated for clinical response, 22 were also assessed for surgical response. The overall clinical response rate was 64%: 8% complete response (CR) and 56% partial response (PR). All 3 patients achieving CR had squamous cell carcinoma. Three pathologic CRs occurred, all in the group with squamous cell carcinoma (2 were clinical PRs and 1 was a clinical CR). The major surgical complication was bronchopleural fistula, which caused 2 deaths. Two patients experienced mitomycin pulmonary toxicity. Recurrence developed in 8 of 18 completely resected patients; the median time to recurrence was 20.6 months. Overall, 28 patients died and 20 had recurrent or progressive disease. The median survival and 3-year survival were greater for patients who had complete resection than for the group was a whole (29.7 months and 40% vs. 18.6 months and 26%, respectively).

*Conclusion.*—In patients with limited NSCLC, MVP is an effective, although toxic, regimen. Complete resection, which can be accomplished in most responders, offers prolonged survival.

▶ The report by Yashar et al. (Abstract 13–12) demonstrates the ability of neoadjuvant therapy to downstage patients. The fact that 5 patients had no viable tumor in the resected specimen and 6 patients had "shrinkage of tumor" is an important finding. The overall resection rate of 86% is slightly higher than previously reported. The postoperative mortality rate of 5.6% is high, as is the fact that 9 of 31 patients had significant postoperative morbidity. Specifically, the development of bronchopleural fistula in 3 of 31 patients is distressing. This unacceptable level of morbidity and mortality is most likely the result of preoperative concomitant radiotherapy. Previous reports have suggested that preoperative radiotherapy when given above 40 cGy is accompanied by unacceptable postoperative complications. Survival data on 12 patients followed for 3 years in this phase II retrospective study provide no basis for conclusions regarding survival.

The study by Burke et al. (Abstract 13–13) is also enlightening, given the high mortality from the preoperative MVP regimen. Four deaths in 39 patients would prohibit this regimen from being generic therapy. Mitomycin appears to be the agent most likely to be responsible for toxicity. The high operative morbidity and mortality is undoubtedly linked to preoperative therapy. The important finding in this study would appear to be that NSCLC will show a clinical and pathologic response in the neoadjuvant setting. The regimen described is prohibitive in its toxicity. Regimens relying on platinum as a base may be of equal efficacy with reduced toxicity.—D.J. Sugarbaker, M.D.

PULMONARY METASTECTOMY: OPERATIVE INDICATIONS AND OUTCOME

▶↓ The indications for pulmonary metastectomy have remained unchanged in recent years. The efficacy of this approach has been difficult to establish because of the inability to run phase II randomized trials in which one arm receives no operative therapy. Generally, the indications remain as follows:

(1) The primary site must be completely controlled as assessed radiographically; (2) there must be no other sites of metastatic disease; (3) the patient must have sufficient pulmonary reserve for resection; (4) the disease must be completely resectable as assessed by the surgical team (1).

The efficacy of pulmonary metastectomy in prolonging survival has been linked to several factors in the literature. The number of lesions is important, as is the cell type of the primary lesion and, in some reports, the disease-free interval.—D.J. Sugarbaker, M.D.

*Reference*

1. Todd TR: *Chest* 103 (suppl): S401, 1993.

---

**Colorectal Lung Metastases: Results of Surgical Excision**
McAfee MK, Allen MS, Trastek VF, Ilstrup DM, Deschamps C, Pairolero PC
(Mayo Clinic and Found, Rochester, Minn)
*Ann Thorac Surg* 53:780–786, 1992                    13–14

---

*Introduction.*—Pulmonary resection for metastatic colorectal carcinoma remains a controversial issue. The factors affecting long-term prognosis are not well understood.

*Methods.*—Pulmonary resection was carried out in 139 consecutive patients during a 28-year period. The patients, 73 men and 66 women, had a median age of 64 years. All had a solitary adenocarcinoma as the primary colorectal neoplasm. In 86% the pulmonary metastases were asymptomatic, and 71% had a solitary metastasis. The operation consisted of wedge excision in 68 patients, lobectomy in 53, lobectomy and wedge excision in 9, pneumonectomy in 5, and bilobectomy in 4. Twenty patients also underwent resection of localized extrapulmonary colorectal cancer. The patients were followed for a median of 7 years.

*Outcomes.*—The operative mortality rate was 1.4%. The 5-year survival was 31%, and the 20-year survival, 16%. For patients with solitary metastases, however, the 5-year survival improved to 37%, compared with 19% for those with 2 metastases and 8% for those with more than 2. The 5-year survival was 47% in patients with a normal level of carcinoembryonic antigen (CEA) and 16% in those with an increased CEA level. Patients with and without resected extrapulmonary disease both had 5-year survivals of about 30%. In 19 patients who had repeat thoracotomy for recurrent metastases, survival 5 years after the second operation was 30%.

*Conclusions.*—Surgical resection of colorectal lung metastases appears to be a safe and effective procedure that can be done even in patients with resectable extrapulmonary disease. Patients must be followed carefully; if metastases recur, thoracotomy can be repeated with fairly good long-term survival.

▶ This study is important because it suggests that the CEA level at the time of metastectomy is an important prognostic factor. Given that most of the lesions were solitary, it is not surprising that a large number of anatomical resections were carried out. It should be stressed that a new primary non–small-cell lung carcinoma (NSCLC) can develop in the patient with a history of previous colorectal cancer; in this case, it was adenocarcinoma.

Metastases do not spread to lymph nodes as a rule, thus wedge resection is adequate surgery in this instance. However, because the nature of these solitary tumors could not be determined on frozen section, they were treated as primary lung carcinoma with adequate standard regional resections. Therefore, anatomical resection should be done as if a primary NSCLC were being removed (1).—D.J. Sugarbaker, M.D.

*Reference*

1. Todd TR: *Chest* 103 (suppl): S401, 1993.

---

**Pulmonary Resection for Metastatic Breast Cancer**
Staren ED, Salerno C, Rongione A, Witt TR, Faber LP (Rush-Presbyterian-St Luke's Med Ctr, Chicago)
*Arch Surg* 127:1282–1284, 1992                                              13–15

---

*Introduction.*—Surgical resection of pulmonary metastases has not been widely practiced despite some reports of its therapeutic potential. In 3 series from the late 1970s, the 5-year survival rates were 14% to 33% after resection of metastatic carcinoma from the breast. The outcome after surgical resection of pulmonary metastases from breast cancer was compared with that after systemic chemotherapy and/or hormonal therapy.

*Methods.*—From a cancer registry at the study institution, 63 patients with breast cancer and metastatic disease confined to the lung were identified. Whereas 33 underwent surgical excision of the pulmonary metastases, 30 were treated medically. Data examined included initial cancer stage, type of breast surgery, and characteristics of pulmonary nodules.

*Results.*—The surgically treated and medically treated groups were comparable in age, initial stage of breast cancer, and interval from breast cancer surgery to presentation with lung metastases (48 months and 44 months, respectively). Nine patients treated surgically received adjuvant systemic therapy and 4 had adjuvant radiation therapy; 8 treated medically also underwent local radiation therapy. The mean survival in the surgically treated group was 55 months, significantly longer than in the medically treated group (33 months). The overall 5-year survival rate after lung recurrence was also significantly greater after surgical than after medical treatment (36% vs. 11%). There was no correlation between survival and the location or number of lung metastases.

*Conclusion.*—Selected patients with breast cancer and pulmonary metastases may gain a survival benefit from surgical resection. Candidates include those able to undergo thoracotomy, those with surgically resectable disease, and those whose workup indicates no extrapulmonary disease.

▶ This is an interesting report of pulmonary metastectomy in patients with breast carcinoma because metastatic breast cancer has not been an indication for metastectomy in the past. Although the study was retrospective and not randomized, the survival benefit in the surgical group, as well as the 5-year survival, are impressive. The key to selection of these patients for operative therapy is the absence of metastatic disease at other sites. This criterion will exclude most patients presenting with pulmonary metastatic disease. The outcome is not unexpected, because previous reports of conventional therapy have noted the more refractory nature of visceral metastatic breast disease compared to bony metastatic disease (1).—D.J. Sugarbaker, M.D.

*Reference*

1. Henderson IC: Chemotherapy for advanced disease, in Bonadonna G (ed): *Breast Cancer: Diagnosis and Management.* New York, John Wiley & Sons, 1984, pp 274–280.

---

### Surgical Treatment of Pulmonary Metastases From Uterine Cervical Cancer: Operation Method by Lung Tumor Size

Seki M, Nakagawa K, Tsuchiya S, Matsubara T, Kinoshita I, Weng S-Y, Tsuchiya E (Cancer Inst, Tokyo, Japan)
*J Thorac Cardiovasc Surg* 104:876–881, 1992                     13–16

---

*Background.*—With proper patient selection, surgical resection of metastatic pulmonary tumor can improve long-term survival over other methods of treatment. Different modes of resection are needed for metastases from different types of tumor. A retrospective study sought to determine the extent of surgery needed for individual patients with pulmonary metastases of primary squamous cell carcinoma of the uterine cervix.

*Patients.*—Pulmonary resection for metastatic tumors of the uterine cervix was performed in 32 patients, most of the primary tumors were squamous cell carcinomas. The average age was 59 years. Most patients (26) underwent lobectomy, 3 had pneumonectomy, 2 had segmentectomy, and 1 had wedge resection. The resection was macroscopically radical in 25 cases and palliative in 7. Some 42% of the patients had positive lymph nodes, and 34% had microscopic satellite lesions around the

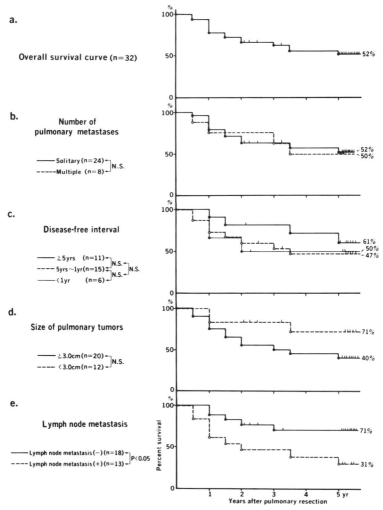

**Fig 13–5.**—Survival curve after pulmonary resection. Comparison of survival by 4 factors. (Courtesy of Seki M, Nakagawa K, Tsuchiya S, et al: *J Thorac Cardiovasc Surg* 104:876-881, 1992.)

main metastasis. The mode of pulmonary resection was correlated with the pathologic findings of the metastases.

*Findings.*—Of the 20 patients with pulmonary metastases at least 3 cm in diameter, 65% had secondary lymph node involvement; in the same group, 50% had microscopic satellite lesions. Of 12 patients with metastases smaller than 3 cm, none had accompanying lymph node involvement and only 1 had microscopic satellite lesions. The overall 5-year survival was 52%, with a trend toward improved survival in those with metastases less than 3 cm (Fig 13–5).

*Conclusions.*—These findings suggest that different approaches to re-section are need for individual patients with pulmonary metastases from the uterine cervix. Those with pulmonary lesions measuring at least 3 cm in diameter should have lobectomy with lymph node dissection. For those whose lesions measure less than 3 cm, wedge resection with a dis-ease-free margin of 2 cm or more may be sufficient.

▶ The incidence of metastatic cervical cancer is low in the United States. This study is important to the thoracic surgeon because it demonstrates that as metastatic lesions increase in size, they have the ability to metastasize to regional lymph nodes. Therefore, an anatomical resection should be carried out for metastatic lesions of significant size. In the current study the measure of 3 cm was used. The size at which lesions gain metastatic potential could be expected to differ with differing cell types and tumor grades. The rela-tively high incidence of satellite lesions in this study would also support the consideration of larger resections during pulmonary metastectomy.—D.J. Sugarbaker, M.D.

## Five-Year Survival After Pulmonary Metastasectomy for Adult Soft Tissue Sarcoma

Casson AG, Putnam JB, Natarajan G, Johnston DA, Mountain C, McMurtrey M, Roth JA (Univ of Texas MD Anderson Cancer Ctr, Houston)
*Cancer* 69:662–668, 1992                                    13–17

*Introduction.*—In adults with soft tissue sarcomas, complete resection of isolated pulmonary metastases is associated with improved survival. Evaluation was made of the prognostic factors associated with survival for longer than 5-years after complete resection of pulmonary metasta-ses in adults with soft tissue sarcoma.

*Patients and Treatment.*—During a 5-year period, 68 patients under-went at least 1 thoracotomy for histologically proven pulmonary metas-tases of adult soft tissue sarcoma. Of these, 58 who had complete resec-tion were followed for at least 5 years or until death. Thirty patients underwent repeat exploration for second recurrences. In all, 139 thora-cotomies were done to remove 385 proven metastases.

*Results.*—The median survival was 25 months, and the absolute 5-year survival rate was 26% of patients. Six patients with unresectable metasta-ses had a median survival of 6 months; they were not included in the analysis. At a median follow-up of 76 months, 11 patients were disease free. Improved survival was associated with the independent prognostic factors of doubling time of 40 days or more (37 vs. 15 months), unilat-eral disease observed on preoperative radiographs, (33 vs. 15 months), 3 or fewer nodules on preoperative CT, (40 vs. 14 months), 2 or fewer nodules resected (40 vs. 17 months), and the histologic finding of malig-nant fibrous histiocytoma rather than other tumors (33 vs. 17 months).

On multivariate analysis, the number of nodules detected on preoperative CT was a significant prognostic factor.

*Conclusions.*—The described criteria are useful in predicting the survival of patients undergoing pulmonary metastasectomy for adult soft tissue sarcomas. The number of nodules detected on preoperative CT should be used routinely. No patient with potentially resectable disease should be denied surgery on the basis of a single prognostic factor, however.

▶ This study was of interest because it suggested that, along with other criteria for resection of metastatic disease, tumor doubling time was of significance in this population. This is because of the occasional aggressive nature of metastatic soft tissue sarcoma, which can display doubling times less than the 40-day cutoff used in this study. The population of patients with soft tissue sarcoma is often made up of young persons, and aggressive surgical intervention is often hard to avoid. This report provides solid criteria for decision making in this often difficult clinical situation.—D.J. Sugarbaker, M.D.

### Resection of Pulmonary Metastases From Uterine Sarcomas
Levenback C, Rubin SC, McCormack PM, Hoskins WJ, Atkinson EN, Lewis JL Jr (Mem Sloan-Kettering Cancer Ctr, New York City; Univ of Texas MD Anderson Cancer Ctr, Houston)
*Gynecol Oncol* 45:202–205, 1992                    13–18

*Background.*—Information regarding resections for pulmonary metastases in gynecologic patients with primary tumors is limited. Data were reviewed on patients with uterine sarcomas who had undergone resec-

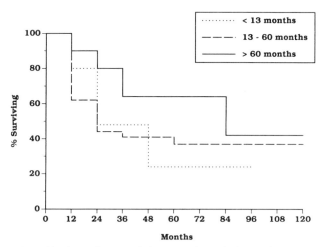

**Fig 13–6.**—Survival by disease-free interval. (Courtesy of Levenback C, Rubin SC, McCormack PM, et al: *Gynecol Oncol* 45:202–205, 1992.)

tions of pulmonary metastases, with particular attention being given to long-term survival and analyses of prognostic variables.

*Patients.*—Forty-five eligible patients met inclusion requirements, including hysterectomy for uterine sarcoma, no extrathoracic tumor at time of metastases, known thoracic disease evaluated as operable, histology consistent with uterine sarcoma, and no medical contraindications to thoracotomy. The mean age at diagnosis of metastases was 50 years.

*Results.*—Unilateral lesions were present in 32 patients, 1 nodule was seen in 23 patients, and 31 patients had nodules larger than 2 cm. At completion of thoracotomy 16 patients had residual disease. The actuarial 5-year and 10-year survival rates after hysterectomy for uterine sarcoma were 65% and 50%, respectively, with a mean follow-up of 89 months. The rates of 5-year and 10-year survival after resection of pulmonary metastases were 43% and 35%, respectively, with a mean follow-up 25 months. The mean survival for those with unilateral disease was 39 months and for those with nodules 2 cm or larger, 30 months. Based on the interval between hysterectomy and initial pulmonary resection, patients were divided into 3 groups. Metastatic disease was diagnosed within 1 year of hysterectomy in 12 patients, between 1 and 5 years in 23, and after 5 years in 10. The mean survival for postthoracotomy patients in each group was 32 months, 31 months, and 64 months, respectively. No significant statistical differences were noted among these groups (Fig 13–6). The size and number of metastases, disease-free intervals, and patient age were not significant.

*Conclusion.*—Long-term survival was achieved in a substantial proportion of patients in this study. No single risk factor was accurate enough to exclude individual patients from consideration for thoracotomy.

▶ This report, based on clinical data from 2 of the biggest cancer centers in the United States, reviews a large series of patients with uterine cancer metastatic to the lung. The series again suffers from lack of a non-surgical control, but the data do demonstrate that metastectomy can be performed in this cell type with comparable survival statistics. None of the traditional prognostic factors for predicting improved survival in pulmonary metastectomy was of importance in this study (1).—D.J. Sugarbaker, M.D.

*Reference*

1. Mentzer SJ, et al: *J Surg Oncol,* 1993: In press.

## Challenging Problems for the Thoracic Surgeon

### Primary Bony and Cartilaginous Sarcomas of Chest Wall: Results of Therapy

Burt M, Fulton M, Wessner-Dunlap S, Karpeh M, Huvos AG, Bains MS, Martini N, McCormack PM, Rusch VW, Ginsberg RJ (Mem Sloan-Kettering Cancer Ctr, New York City)
*Ann Thorac Surg* 54:226–232, 1992                                    13–19

*Introduction.*—Primary osteogenic sarcomas and chondrosarcomas of the chest wall are uncommon, with few studies on their treatment and outcome having been reported. The treatment of these tumors during a 40-year period was reviewed.

*Patients and Therapy.*—Between 1949 and 1989, chondrosarcoma was diagnosed in 96 patients and osteosarcoma arising in the chest wall in 41. Complete data were available for 88 patients aged 5–86 years with chondrosarcoma and 38 patients aged 11–78 years, with osteosarcoma. Primary treatment for cartilaginous sarcoma of the chest wall consisted of resection in 84 patients, radiation therapy in 3, and chemotherapy in 1. Of the 38 patients with osteosarcoma of the chest wall, 13 underwent resection alone, 3 had resection with radiation therapy, 15 had resection with chemotherapy, 3 had radiation therapy alone, 2 had radiation therapy and chemotherapy, 1 had chemotherapy alone, and 1 was not treated.

*Results.*—The median follow-up for the 88 patients with chondrosarcoma of the chest wall was 56 months; the overall 5-year survival was 64%, and overall median survival, 148 months. Metastases at presentation, metastases at any time during the course of disease, age beyond 50 years, incomplete or no resection, and local recurrence were highly predictive of poor survival. Sex, tumor grade, and tumor size had no significant impact on survival. The median follow-up for the 38 patients with osteosarcoma of the chest wall was 12 months; the overall 5-year survival was 15%, and overall median survival, 12 months. The presence of synchronous metastases and metastases at any time during the course of disease was significantly associated with poor survival, whereas age, sex, tumor size, local recurrence, and extent of resection had no impact on survival.

*Conclusions.*—The 5-year survival for patients with a primary chest wall osteosarcoma is significantly poorer than that in patients with a primary chest wall chondrosarcoma. Complete chest wall resection significantly improves survival in patients with primary chondrosarcomas, but not in those with primary osteogenic sarcomas.

▶ The current report is of interest because it provides a strong contrast of the efficacy of surgical resection in 2 sarcomas of the chest wall. Chondrosarcomas, as noted in this study, are well controlled by surgical resection when adequately resected. In contrast, the efficacy of surgical resection could not be established for osteosarcoma.

The conclusion is clear that tumor biology, and not primary therapy, determines prognosis. This realization is important because new treatment strategies are based more on tumor biology and less on the anatomical extent of the primary lesion.—D.J. Sugarbaker, M.D.

▶↓The treatment of thymic neoplasms has been surgical resection. Selection of patients for postoperative radiotherapy and/or chemotherapy has been based on pathologic stage at the time of resection. Reported here are the results of this traditional approach at a major cancer center, following a report in which the usefulness of flow cytometry is assessed in predicting the need for primary multimodality therapy in this disease.—D.J. Sugarbaker, M.D.

---

**Thymoma: The Prognostic Significance of Flow Cytometric DNA Analysis**
Pollack A, El-Naggar AK, Cox JD, Ro JY, Sahin A, Komaki R (Univ of Texas MD Anderson Cancer Ctr, Houston)
*Cancer* 69:1702–1709, 1992                                         13–20

---

*Introduction.*—Some patients with thymoma and favorable prognostic factors nevertheless experience recurrence and aggressive tumor behavior. Whether flow cytometric (FCM) analysis of nuclear DNA content holds prognostic value was studied in 25 patients with thymoma who were followed for a mean of over 5 years.

*Treatment.*—Seventeen patients had gross total tumor resection and 8 underwent subtotal resection. Definitive megavoltage radiotherapy was then given to 17 cases. Nine patients received chemotherapy within 6 months after diagnosis.

*Results.*—The mean FCM-determined percent of cells in S phase was 5.6; this parameter was unrelated to the outcome. Sixteen patients with diploid tumors had a 5-year disease-free survival rate of 85%, compared with 33% for 9 having aneuploid tumors. The respective figures were 89% and 50% in patients having total tumor resection.

*Conclusion.*—Flow cytometric analysis of nuclear DNA is a useful means of predicting relapses of thymoma, but further study is needed to determine whether the DNA index is a prognostic factor independent of stage of disease and extent of surgery.

### Thymoma: Treatment and Prognosis

Pollack A, Komaki R, Cox JD, Ro JY, Oswald MJ, Shin DM, Putnam JB Jr
(Univ of Texas MD Anderson Cancer Ctr, Houston)
*Int J Radiat Oncol Biol Phys* 23:1037–1043, 1992               13–21

*Introduction.*—Research continues to outline the clinical pathology of thymomas—slow-growing, malignant-type, epithelial neoplasms. Patients with noninvasive thymomas usually undergo surgery to remove the lesion, with 80% having a 5-year survival rate. Treatment of the invasive disease is still controversial. The results of a retrospective study of 36 patients treated for thymoma at the University of Texas M.D. Anderson Cancer Center were examined.

*Methods.*—Of the 83 individuals with a diagnosis of a thymic neoplasm, 36 had most of their treatment at the present cancer center and had an average follow-up of 66 months. After diagnosis and staging, 21 patients had total resection, 5 had subtotal resection, and 10 had biopsy only. Twenty-two individuals received radiation therapy and 12 had chemotherapy.

*Results.*—All 11 patients with stage I and the 8 with stage II disease had total resections, but only 1 patient with stage III and 1 with stage IVA had this type of surgery. All patients undergoing subtotal resection had stage III disease. The disease-free survival (DFS) for stages I–IVA were 74%, 71%, 50%, and 29%, respectively, which demonstrated a significant difference for survival by stage. The DFS differed significantly for the type of surgery, with the group having total resection having a 74% 5-year DFS; the group undergoing subtotal surgery group had a 60% DFS, and the biopsied group, a 20% DFS. Patients with invasive thymomas who received radiation therapy had a significantly longer length of survival than those who did not. The 5-year DFS tumor histology showed that 68%, 77%, and 40% had lymphocyte predominant, epithelial predominant, and mixed type cells, respectively.

*Conclusions.*—The Center's preferred method of staging and treatment for thymomas now includes total tumor resection when possible, radiation after surgery at about 50 Gy for the total, noninvasive resections and for invasive thymomas, and mixed therapy (radiation treatment and chemotherapy) for those tumors that cannot be resected.

▶ Flow cytometry appears to hold some promise in predicting poor clinical outcomes in patients with malignant thymoma. This is of particular importance in thymic tumors, because light microscopic findings often are not useful, and therapy is frequently based only on gross findings of invasion at surgery.

The postoperative treatment of all resected thymic tumors with radiotherapy is the thrust of the recommendation made in this report. The addition of chemotherapy to the incompletely resected group remains suspect because this systemic treatment is applied to localized, albeit unresectable disease.

Chemotherapy used in this fashion has failed to show consistent efficacy in other neoplasms (1–3).—D.J. Sugarbaker, M.D.

*References*

1. Cooper JD: *Chest* 103 (suppl):S334, 1993.
2. Macchiarini P, et al: *Cancer* 68:706, 1991.
3. Maggi G, et al: *Ann Thorac Surg* 51:152, 1991.

---

**Management of Myasthenia Gravis by Extended Thymectomy With Anterior Mediastinal Dissection**
Nussbaum MS, Rosenthal GJ, Samaha FJ, Grinvalsky HT, Quinlan JG, Schmerler M, Fischer JE (Univ of Cincinnati Med Ctr, Cincinnati, Ohio; Jewish Hosp of Cincinnati)
*Surgery* 112:681–688, 1992                                                13–22

*Introduction.*—Thymectomy is effective in limiting the progress of myasthenia gravis when done early enough, but many neurologists are hesitant to refer patients with early or mild disease. The surgical results were studied in 48 patients with myasthenia gravis who, between 1979 and 1991, underwent extended transsternal thymectomy.

*Patients.*—The mean age at surgery was 39 years. Forty patients had generalized myasthenia gravis, and 8 had ocular myasthenia only. Most patients had no other associated medical disorders. The mean duration of illness at the time of surgery was about 4 years.

*Operative Findings.*—Six patients had a thymoma and 10 others had some degree of thymic hyperplasia. Seventeen patients, most of whom were taking prednisone, had an involuted thymus. Fifteen patients had normal thymic histology.

*Outcome.*—There were no operative deaths, but 21% of the patients had surgical morbidity. One patient had a sternal dehiscence requiring reoperation, and 1 required reintubation for respiratory arrest. All but 3 patients had symptomatic improvement, and 46% experienced a drug-free remission. Three of 6 patients with thymoma and 4 of 10 with thymic hyperplasia were able to discontinue drug therapy. Two patients with thymoma died of progressive disease.

*Conclusion.*—Extended transsternal thymectomy offers an excellent chance of drug-free remission, or at least symptomatic improvement, to patients with myasthenia gravis.

▶ The role of thymectomy in the treatment of myasthenia gravis has only recently been accepted by the neurologic community. This well-prepared report reaffirms the efficacy of thymectomy. The debate continues, however, as to the appropriate approach to thymectomy. The transsternal approach remains the most widely used procedure, although transcervical resection in certain centers has attained similar results (1). The principle remains, however, that all thymic tissue must be removed by either approach. Newer thoracoscopic techniques as they are developed are certain to revive this controversy.—D.J. Sugarbaker, M.D.

*Reference*

1. Cooper JD, et al: *Ann Thorac Surg* 45:242, 1988.

### Treatment of AIDS-Related Bronchopleural Fistula by Pleurectomy

Crawford BK, Galloway AC, Boyd AD, Spencer FC (New York Univ, New York City)
*Ann Thorac Surg* 54:212–215, 1992                                              13–23

*Background.*—The number of patients with AIDS and spontaneous pneumothorax associated with *Pneumocystis carinii* infection has increased yearly. Because of the diffuse nature of the parenchymal disease in patients with AIDS who have spontaneous pneumothorax, standard intercostal tube drainage often fails to close the bronchopleural fistula. The effectiveness of aggressive surgical therapy in patients with AIDS who had persistent bronchopleural fistulas was assessed.

*Patients.*—Between March 1989 and September 1991, 44 patients with AIDS and spontaneous pneumothorax were treated with intercostal tube drainage. In 28 patients (64%), the fistula closed and the chest tubes could be removed. Two patients (4.6%) died of unrelated progressive disease with the chest tubes in place. The remaining 14 patients (32%) had persistent air leaks for more than 10 days and underwent 15 thoracotomies and 1 sternotomy. Two patients had contralateral thoracotomoies on subsequent admissions. The bronchopulmonary fistula was closed directly with suture or staples in 15 operations and resected by lobectomy in 1 case. Adjuvant parietal pleurectomy was also performed in all 14 patients. A lung tissue biopsy specimen was obtained from the area of air leakage. Each patient received perioperative prophylactic cephalosporin intravenously.

*Results.*—One patient (7%) died of uncontrolled sepsis. The 13 survivors were discharged home within 7–28 days after operation. Examination of lung tissue obtained during operation demonstrated *P. carinii* in 13 patients (93%), tuberculosis in 2 (14%), and pathologic changes characteristic of cytomegalovirus in 2. Six patients (43%) had evidence of subpleural necrosis. At the time of this report, 6 patients were still alive, 4 had died, and 3 were lost to follow-up.

*Conclusions.*—For selected patients with AIDS who have spontaneous pneumothorax and no response to conventional tube thoracostomy, surgical closure of the bronchopulmonary fistula combined with pleurectomy may be an effective option.

▶ The combination of AIDS and a spontaneous pneumothorax can be one of the most difficult clinical problems facing the thoracic surgeon. This report is included because it gives some rationale of a graded approach to therapy in this patient group. Initial therapy with a chest tube for drainage is usually successful. This would appear to be the standard approach in most centers at present. It is the use of surgical closure and pleurectomy as reported in this series that is of value because it confirms that pleurectomy does provide a high likelihood of success, both in terms of control of the bronchopulmonary fistula and successful discharge from the hospital.

Also of note is the fact that active infection with *P. carinii* was found at the site of the air leak in most patients (93%), despite presumed adequate medical therapy. Thus it would seem logical to continue anti-*Pneumocystis* therapy in all patients with AIDS and an active bronchopulmonary fistula regardless of the known status of the *Pneumocystis* infection.—D.J. Sugarbaker, M.D.

Thoracoscopy

*Pleural*

▶↓ Advances in thoracoscopic surgery have been the result of advances in intrathoracic visualization. The surgeon's eyesight has been extended into the chest. The range of procedures that can be performed safely with only enhanced visualization is limited, however, and further advances will depend on new technology that extends the surgeon's sense of palpation into the chest. Nevertheless, we need to understand that this limitation of current techniques is to be expected if we are to avoid pushing the limit of the technology beyond safe boundaries.

The technique of thoracoscopic surgery is old and well known. The current use of mediastinoscopes or specially made thoracoscopes has allowed surgeons to visualize the thoracic cavity in a limited fashion. It is appropriate to begin our review of the advances in thoracoscopic surgical techniques with a recent report of a conventional scope used to diagnose unknown pleural disease in a group of patients under general anesthesia.—D.J. Sugarbaker, M.D.

---

**Pleural Effusions: Is Thoracoscopy a Reliable Investigation? A Retrospective Review**
Kendall SWH, Bryan AJ, Large SR, Wells FC (Papworth Hosp, Cambridgeshire, England)
*Respir Med* 86:437–440, 1992                                          13–24

---

*Introduction.*—Fiberoptic thoracoscopy is being used increasingly to diagnose pleural disease under local anesthesia. Of 620 patients referred from 1985 to 1989 with a pleural effusion of unknown origin, 48 had no diagnosis after cytologic study of pleural fluid and blind pleural biopsy. These patients then underwent surgical thoracoscopic assessment.

*Findings.*—Malignant disease, most frequently mesothelioma, was diagnosed in 24 patients and benign disease in 16. In 8 patients no diagnosis was made; 2 of these patients recovered, but 6 had persistent symptoms and were later found to have malignant disease. Thoracoscopy was 83% sensitive for a malignant or benign diagnosis and 100% specific. The predictive value of a negative result was 25%. Two patients died after thoracoscopy, and 2 had prolonged air leaks. The average hospital stay after the procedure was 2 days.

*Conclusions.*—Surgical thoracoscopy can be helpful in diagnosing pleural effusion when standard procedures have failed, but the cost implications of wider use of this measure are uncertain.

▶ The importance of this study is that it establishes the fact that a surgeon can adequately assess pathology in the chest to the point of determining an accurate diagnosis using small trocar sites and direct vision via a fiberoptic thoracoscope. This is done when blind or radiologically directed procedures have failed, which is important because the older literature has suggested that open thoracotomy is required when "noninvasive" measures fail (1–3). Although this may seem obvious, this report is included because it makes the historical transition between open thoracotomy and video-assisted procedures currently in development. When a diagnosis of pleural disease is the indication of surgery, simple thoracoscopy can be performed with simpler equipment at lower cost.—D.J. Sugarbaker, M.D.

*References*

1. Miller J: *Ann Thorac Surg* 52:1036, 1991.
2. Hucker J, et al: *Ann Thorac Surg* 52:1145, 1991.
3. Rusch VW, Mountain C: *Am J Surg* 154:274, 1987.

## *Pulmonary Resection for Diagnosis and Therapy of Benign Disease*

▶↓ Thoracoscopic lung resections have been made possible by the development of the endostapler. Previous staplers required large incisions with their resultant morbidity and mortality. With the aid of the video thoracoscope, closed lung biopsy has become one of the principal indications for the use of thoracoscopy. Note the slightly different techniques used in the following reports. The indications for lung biopsy remain essentially unchanged, although the presumed lower morbidity of the procedure may move the obtaining of a pathologic diagnosis to an earlier place in the natural history of medical lung disease.—D.J. Sugarbaker, M.D.

## Videothoracoscopic Wedge Excision of the Lung

Miller DL, Allen MS, Trastek VF, Deschamps C, Pairolero PC (Mayo Clinic

and Found, Rochester, Minn)
*Ann Thorac Surg* 54:410–414, 1992                                    13–25

*Introduction.*—The routine use of thoracoscopy had to wait for the development of minature video cameras that attach to the flexible thoracoscope to observe this procedure by a televised screen. By combining this technology with percutaneous stapling instruments, the percutaneous pulmonary wedge excision has become possible for all lung areas. The results of using videothoracoscopy to perform percutaneous wedge excision procedures were studied in a consecutive series of patients.

*Methods.*—Seven women and 3 men (median age, 60 years) had 14 pulmonary wedge excisions using the videothoracoscopic method. Five patients had preoperative spirometry studies, and all 10 underwent coagulation studies before surgery.

*Technique.*—All thoracoscopic wedge excisions of the lung are performed under general anesthesia. After a 2-cm incision is made along the midaxillary line in the seventh intercostal space and single-lung ventilation is completed, an open-ended cylindric plastic tube is inserted and the solitary pulmonary nodule, located and a specimen removed for analysis. The videothoracoscope is then reinserted into the expanded lung for inspection. Once the air leak is found, an endostapler completes the percutaneous wedge excision, followed by dry gauze abrasive pleurodesis.

*Results.*—All 10 patients had a tissue diagnosis without thoracotomy; 3 patients were found to have metastatic cancer and 1 had a caseating granuloma. Three other patients had benign lung disease, 1 had a bronchoalveolar carcinoma, and 2 had percutaneous apical bleb excision. No intraoperative complications or deaths occurred during the 90-minute (median) procedure. Specimens ranged in size from 3 to 8 cm with the 4 solitary pulmonary nodules being less than 1 cm. The patients required parenteral narcotic agents or nonsteroidal anti-inflammatory drugs for pain after surgery. After 6 months of follow-up, the 3 patients with metastatic cancer and the 1 with granuloma had no recurrence of symptoms. All of the other patients improved except for the 1 with diffuse bilateral bronchoalveolar cell cancer who had no response to chemotherapy.

*Conclusions.*—The videothoracoscopic wedge lung excision has excellent diagnostic accuracy without increasing morbidity or mortality.

---

**Thoracoscopic Lung Biopsy**
McKeown PP, Conant P, Hubbell DS (Univ of South Florida, Tampa)
*Ann Thorac Surg* 54:490–492, 1992                                    13–26

*Background.*—Traditional thoracoscopy was limited by restricted access and the inadequacy of available light sources and instruments. The technology of laparoscopic video endoscopy was integrated with unique endoscopic instruments to perform thoracoscopic lung biopsies in patients with diffuse lung pathology.

*Technique.*—The procedure is done under general anesthesia. Endoscopic instruments for obtaining a thoracoscopic lung biopsy sample include a camera and standard straight laparoscopes with diameters of 5, 7, and 10 mm, trochars, an endoscopic stapler for obtaining biopsy specimens, endoscopic forceps, and endoscopic scissors. The lung may be deflated with a double-lumen endotracheal tube with contralateral ventilation. In smaller patients or in those with marginal pulmonary function, decreased tidal volume double-lung manual ventilation with a single-lumen tube may be used, although this approach limits visualization of the thoracic cavity. The procedure requires 3 incisions, two 10–mm incisions to accommodate the thoracoscope and the instruments, and one 12–mm port to accommodate the endoscopic stapler. The ports are placed far enough apart to avoid obstruction of vision. Experience in endoscopy is required to become proficient with remote hand-eye coordination.

*Experience.*—Thoracoscopic pulmonary wedge excisions using the new technology were performed successfully in 3 adults and 1 child. Video monitors simultaneously displayed and recorded the operative images. In all patients a chest tube was inserted through 1 of the port sites at the end of the procedure. The number of patients undergoing thoracoscopic procedures at the present hospital has increased since this preliminary experience, and many other centers are now using the new technology.

*Conclusion.*—Video thoracoscopic lung biopsy using innovative instruments is an effective, rapidly evolving technique that has a wide range of other potential applications.

---

**Imaged Thoracoscopic Lung Biopsy**
Lewis RJ, Caccavale RJ, Sisler GE (Robert Wood Johnson Univ, New Brunswick, NJ)
*Chest* 102:60–62, 1992                                                    13–27

---

*Introduction.*—Lung biopsy requiring a thoractomy can result in significant morbidity in patients with progressive pulmonary disorders. A new technique, imaged thorascopic surgery, can obtain adequate lung tissue without performing a thoractomy.

*Patients.*—Eleven patients ranging in age from 27 to 77 years underwent the procedure. Indications for biopsy included diffuse interstitial pulmonary infiltrates, massive bullous disease, and suspected metastatic breast cancer.

*Technique.*—The patient is administered general anesthesia and placed in the lateral position. Three incisions are made for insertion of a diagnostic telescope and instruments. The intrathoracic organs are projected onto a monitor, allowing the entire operating room team to have a full view. Specimens can be taken from appropriate areas of the lung without making a formal thoracotomy incision.

*Results.*—All 11 procedures obtained adequate tissue for pathologic and microbiological examination. Each patient was extubated in the recovery room. Postoperative pain was significantly reduced relative to thoractomy, because there was no need for placement of a retractor with rib distraction. Within 1 week of discharge from the hospital, the patients were able to resume their normal activities.

*Conclusion.*—Imaged thoracoscopic surgery can be a useful method of obtaining lung biopsy specimens, particularly from patients in a weakened condition. The procedure is more complex and tedious, however, than a traditional thoracotomy.

▶ Because of the lack of reports from large multi-institutional trials, we have included these 3 reports (Abstracts 13–25, 13–26, and 13–27) on closed lung biopsy.

The operative technique is different in the 3 reports. The first 2 use 3 ports for the procedure. The report by Lewis et al. (Abstract 13–27) utilizes 2 incisions, 1 for the camera and a larger incision for placement of a conventional stapler and dissection. Indeed, in this approach an incision is made that is close to the size used in the conventional approach. The use of the smaller endostapler would appear to be preferred because it can be introduced via a 12-mm port.

Several points deserve further emphasis. The first port is for introduction of the thoracoscope, which permits thorough inspection of the thorax and placement of the subsequent working ports. The exact locations of these ports are dependent on the location of the visualized pathology. The ports should use 12-mm trocars so that the stapler can easily be placed from both sides. The surgeon should always work where he or she can see the monitor looking over the patient (1).

Multiple lobes may be biopsied to improve the accuracy of the procedure, although this is not always necessary (2, 3). Further, after successful lung biopsy, ports need to be inspected for evidence of bleeding from a lacerated intercostal vessel. Marcaine 0.25% is injected in and around trocar sites to improve postoperative pain control. We use small chest tubes that are removed in the recovery room if the chest x-ray study shows full lung expansion and there is no evidence of an air leak. The chest tube is always left in place if the patient is to continue to receive positive pressure ventilation.—D.J. Sugarbaker, M.D.

*References*

1. Landreneau RJ, et al: *Ann Thorac Surg* 54:800, 1992.
2. Newman SL, et al: *Am Rev Respir Dis* 132:1084, 1985.
3. Boutin C, et al: *Chest* 82:44, 1982.

### Surgical Thoracoscopy: Indications and Technique: Early Results in Spontaneous Pneumothorax

Inderbitzi R, Furrer M, Striffeler H (Inselspital Bern, Switzerland)
*Chirurg* 63:334–341, 1992                                           13–28

*Background.*—The severe postoperative pain occurring after early thoracoscopic procedures was a major drawback because patients were afraid to breathe and cough, leading to shallow breathing and its sequelae, along with accumulation of bronchial secretions. Modern thoracic endoscopies have very small diameters and dramatically improved optics. New video technology allows the guided manipulation of surgical instruments that have been redesigned for this specific application. Consequently, endoscopic thoracic surgery is now minimally invasive.

*Patients.*—In 1990 and 1991, 221 patients underwent video-thoracoscopic surgery for a variety of indications, including spontaneous pneumothorax, chylothorax, empyema, sympathectomy, tumor resection, diagnostic lung biopsy, h  othorax, and chronic pleural effusion. The average operating tim. was 4 minutes. Only immunosuppressed patients were given perioperative antibiotic prophylaxis.

*Results.*—No infections of the incision sites or openings in the thoracic cavity developed. None of the patients died as a result of the procedure, but 8 died within 30 days of operation, 7 of pleurodesis secondary to malignant disease and 1 of acute aortic dissection. Autopsy did not identify any aortic or pleural injury casued by the thoracoscopic instruments. Most of the other complications occurred in early use and were avoided with increasing experience. Since January 1990, 65 patients have undergone endoscopic treatment for spontaneous pneumothorax. In the first 16 patients the thoracoscopic procedure was limited to obtaining an overview and pleurodesis with fibrin or talc. Since March 1990, 49 patients with spontaneous pneumothorax have been treated according to a 4-step diagnostic algorithm. Forty-three patients had persistent or recurrent spontaneous pneumothorax and 6 had an acute first event. The approach was from the back and under local anesthesia in patients with idiopathic or primary spontaneous pneumothorax, and from the side under general anesthesia inpatients with spontaneous pneumothorax secondary to chronic lung disease or with a history of previous episodes. To date, 3 of the 49 patients with spontaneous pneumothorax (6%) have had an early recurrence after thoracoscopic treatment.

*Conclusions.*—Thoracoscopic surgery is minimally invasive and avoids the functional burden of thoracotomy. Its long-term efficacy for a variety of indications, however, remains to be determined.

▶ This report from Switzerland is one of the first to describe the use of minimally invasive techniques in the treatment of spontaneous pneumothorax. This is important because our own experience suggests that is an ideal application of this technique. We differ from this approach in that we use a 3-cannula technique, placing the camera port in the midaxillary line between the fifth interspace and the 2 working ports in the anterior position third interspace and posterior to the scapula in the third or fourth space. Apical bullectomy is easily accomplished, as is manual pleurodesis.

We again remove the chest drain in the recovery room as described above. The indications for repair of spontaneous pneumothorax remain unchanged at present, although as this procedure becomes refined, the ability to avoid prolonged hospitalization by prompt closure of the fistula becomes attractive as first-line therapy.—D.J. Sugarbaker, M.D.

## Pulmonary Resection for Diagnosis and Therapy of Malignant Disease

▶ The next 3 articles that are reviewed represent the largest series to date that summarize a large experience from several institutions. It is important to realize that these are initial reports, and that the stated rates of morbidity and mortality can be expected to decline as the experience of the surgical team increases and instrumentation and technology improve.

It is interesting to note the differences in technique and management. The new intraoperative approaches appear to call for reappraisal of traditional postoperative management as well. What we appear to be witnessing is a total change, in many instances and diseases, in the way we treat patients intraoperatively and manage them postoperatively. The big winner of this change would appear to be the patient who may experience less morbidity and mortality than with traditional approaches.—D.J. Sugarbaker, M.D.

---

### Present Role of Thoracoscopy in the Diagnosis and Treatment of Diseases of the Chest

Mack MJ, Aronoff RJ, Acuff TE, Douthit MB, Bowman RT, Ryan WH (Humana Hosp Med City Dallas, Dallas, Tex)
*Ann Thorac Surg* 54:403–409, 1992                                  13–29

---

*Introduction.*—The use of thoracoscopy has been limited to the diagnosis of pleural disease. Recent advances in endoscopic equipment and refinement in surgical techniques, however, have expanded its application. Video thorascopic procedures have recently been used in 70 patients with various intrathoracic disease that would previously be treated by "open" techniques.

*Procedures.*—All procedures were performed under general endotracheal anesthesia. A rigid telescope and camera attached to a video monitor was inserted through the seventh intercostal space. Twenty-one patients underwent wedge resection of pulmonary nodules using an endoscopic mechnical stapling device. Twenty patients underwent thoracoscopy for the diagnosis and treatment of pleural disease, including 11 patients with indeterminate diagnoses after thoracentesis. Other procedures included excision of the pericardium and drainage of pericardial

space in 6 patients, dorsal thoracic sympathectomy in 6, apical blebec-
tomy and pleurodesis in 6, and lung biopsies for the diagnosis of diffuse
lung disease in 5. Additional procedures performed included biopsy of
hilar masses, biopsy of esophageal mass, excision of a mediastinal cyst,
and drainage of a spinal abscess.

*Outcome.*—There was no mortality associated with thoracoscopy. Except for patients who were chronically ill or had limited pulmonary reserve preoperatively, none of the patients required routine postoperative
care in the intensive care unit. The hospital stay averaged 3.4 days and
was often as short as 1 day.

*Summary.*—Because of its less invasive nature and decreased morbidity, the role of thoracoscopy has been markedly expanded in the diagnosis and treatment of thoracic disease.

▶ The authors applied thoracoscopic techniques to a wide range of thoracic
disease. Of interest is the use of $CO_2$ insufflation to improve on the degree of
atelectasis. We have found that with adequate split-lung anesthesia, this is
not required. In some situations, the use of $CO_2$ insufflation can cause serious problems. These situations are primarily hemodynamic in nature and result from the tamponade effect of positive pressure in the chest. It appears
that pressure above 5 cm of water leads to this type of difficulty. We do not
use $CO_2$ on a routine basis for these reasons.

It is also of note that wedge resection for diagnosis of a pulmonary lesion
does not usually constitute adequate therapy. The surgeon needs to be ready
to perform a more definitive procedure either at the time of thoracoscopy if
frozen section diagnosis is adequate, or subsequently, based on the permanent pathologic examination. This represents a change in approach for most
thoracic surgeons and thus needs to be emphasized.—D.J. Sugarbaker, M.D.

### Thoracoscopic Resection of 85 Pulmonary Lesions

Landreneau RJ, Hazelrigg SR, Ferson PF, Johnson JA, Nawarawong W, Boley
TM, Curtis JJ, Bowers CM, Herlan DB, Dowling RD (Univ of Pittsburgh, Pitts-
burgh, Pa; St Luke's Med Ctr, Milwaukee, Wis)
*Ann Thorac Surg* 54:415–420, 1992                                    13–30

*Background.*—Video-assisted thoracic surgery (VATS) is used as an
adjunct to traditional diagnostic thoracoscopy. Because of advances in
endoscopic surgical equipment and laser technology, closed, surgical,
pulmonary resection via thoracoscopy is now possible. Recent experience with this procedure was reviewed.

*Patients and Procedures.*—Sixty-one consecutive patients with lesions
of less than 3 cm in the outer third of the lung underwent 85 thoracoscopic wedge resections. Most of the 31 women and 30 men had un-
diagnosed pulmonary parenchymal lesions. All tumors (mean diameter,
1.3 cm) were removed intact either by withdrawal through a trocar or by

Histologic Evaluation of 85 Lesions Resected in
61 Patients

46 benign lesions in 28 patients

| | |
|---|---|
| Interstitial fibrosis/pneumonia | 29 |
| Nocardia | 1 |
| Rheumatoid | 2 |
| Hamartoma | 3 |
| Anthroscilicosis | 1 |
| Pulmonary infarct/scar | 4 |
| Granulomata | 2 |
| Sclerosing hemangioma | 1 |
| Sarcoid nodules | 2 |
| Cytomegalovirus pneumonitis | 1 |

39 malignant lesions in 33 patients

13 primary lung cancers in 13 patients

| | |
|---|---|
| Adeno/large cell | 6*;† |
| Bronchioalveolar | 3† |
| Squamous | 2† |
| Carcinoid | 1 |
| Small Cell | 1 |

26 metastatic cancers in 20 patients

| | |
|---|---|
| Sarcoma | 2 |
| Lymphoma | 4 |
| Colon | 3 |
| Breast | 3 |
| Renal | 3 |
| Hepatocellular | 10 |
| Melanoma | 1 |

*Subsequent lobectomy was performed in 2 patients.
†Subsequent formal segmentectomy was performed in 3 patients (1 with bronchioalveolar, 1 with squamous, and 1 with adenocarcinoma).
(Courtesy of Landreneau RJ, Hazelrigg SR, Ferson PF, et al: *Ann Thorac Surg* 54:415–420, 1992.)

enclosure within a sterile glove, thus avoiding possible tumor spillage within the thoracic cavity.

*Results.*—The histologic evaluation of the 83 lesions is shown in the table. Forty-six of the resected lesions (28 patients) were benign, whereas 29 represented interstitial fibrosis-pneumonia, 4 were pulmonary infarct-scars, and 3 were hamartomas. Thirty-three patients had 39 malignant lesions, 13 of which were primary lung tumors. Twenty patients had 26 metastatic cancers. Five of the 61 patients were found to have bronchogenic cancer, and they underwent either segmentectomy

(3) or lobectomy (2). Surgical complications were minimal, and only 1 patient died.

*Conclusions.*—A shortened hospital stay (a mean of 5.7 days compared with 7–10 days for open resection) and reduced morbidity may result from using VATS. This minimally invasive approach may also reduce postoperative pain. Selected patients may benefit significantly if the VATS approach continues to be successful.

---

### Thoracoscopic Neodymium: Yttrium Aluminum Garnet Laser Resection of a Pulmonary Metastasis

Dowling RD, Wachs ME, Ferson PF, Landreneau RJ (Univ of Pittsburgh, Pittsburgh, Pa)
*Cancer* 70:1873–1875, 1992                                                                 13–31

---

*Introduction.*—Thoracotomy with wedge resection is the standard surgical approach to new lung lesions in patients who have a history of malignant disease. Substantial morbidity results from the thoracotomy incision.

*Case Report.*—Man, 59, had a 2-cm nodule in the right upper lung field 2 years after radical removal of a $T_3N_0M_0$ renal cell carcinoma. There were no related symptoms, and examination findings were unremarkable. Lung function was normal, as were CT studies of the head and abdomen. After induction of general anesthesia, a thoracoscope was introduced using a double-lumen endotracheal tube. A single discrete 2-cm lesion was noted subpleurally in the right upper lobe. A 28-F chest tube then was placed through a trocar site. A neodymium:yttrium/aluminum/garnet laser fiber was passed via the operating thoracoscope and used to excise the lesion with a margin of normal tissue. The tumor bed was treated to minimize air leakage. A clear cell carcinoma was found with negative resection margins. Minimal air leakage resolved on the second postoperative day. The patient was discharged on day 4 when a chest radiograph showed complete expansion of the lung.

*Conclusion.*—Thoracoscopic resection using a laser may be an ideal surgical approach to selected patients having peripheral pulmonary nodules that may be metastases.

▶ These are 2 important reports (Abstracts 13–30 and 13–31) because they demonstrate the practicality of laser lung resection through the thoracoscope. The laser represents an alternative method to electrocautery of delivering thermal energy. It can be used in the contact or noncontact mode. For parenchymal lung resections, the noncontact mode is preferable. The neodymium:yttrium/aluminum/garnet laser is the one best suited for lung resections in our experience. The fact that dark colors attract the thermal energy and light colors reflect it is cleverly used by Landreneau and colleagues. Dissection through the lung parenchyma is slowed when either a branch of the pulmonary artery or bronchus is encountered. This then allows the surgeon to apply clips, divide the structure, and proceed with the parenchymal resection.

An additional note is that many of the patients in this series would be considered high risk for conventional resection but did undergo potential curative resection via the video-assisted technique. This will be an additional benefit of the technique, because more elderly and high-risk patients will be candidates for resection. In addition, the eschar that the laser produces appears to effectively control air leaks, a persistent problem in the performance of nonanatomical lung resections.—D.J. Sugarbaker, M.D.

---

**One Hundred Consecutive Patients Undergoing Video-Assisted Thoracic Operations**

Lewis RJ, Caccavale RJ, Sisler GE, Mackenzie JW (Univ of Medicine and Dentistry of New Jersey, New Brunswick)

*Ann Thorac Surg* 54:421–426, 1992                    13–32

---

*Introduction.*—The limited access visualization of thoracoscopy has recently been overcome by using solid-state systems and micro cameras to produce a video-assisted thoracic surgical procedure. This new technique allows complex intrathoracic operations and eliminates the thoracotomy incision and its accompanying clinical problems. The use of video-assisted thoracic surgery in 100 patients was reviewed. The 51 female and 49 male patients had an average age of 61 years and underwent 113 procedures.

*Technique.*—All patients had one-lung ventilation during the surgery. The diagnostic telescope of the video monitor is placed perpendicular to the monitor. Most of the operations require 3 incisions, 1 in the sixth or seventh intercostal space and 2 others for inserting and manipulating the instruments. At no time is pressure applied to the ribs. After thoracic exploration, the flexible bronchoscope is inserted and the necessary procedures are performed with conventional instruments.

*Results.*—Nineteen of the 22 patients with primary lung maligancies had cervical mediastinoscopy. Sixteen of the 19 had nodes negative for malignancy. In the patients who had wedge resection by video-assisted thoracic surgery, each node biopsied was negative for cancer. Wedge resection was a curative procedure in 12 patients who had a variety of cancers. Video-assisted thoracic surgery found 14 patients to have benign lesions after resection. Other conditions identified by the video procedure included metastatic lesions, diffuse pulmonary disease, recurrent pneumothorax, pleural effusions, bullous disease, and problems of the pericardium and esophagus. No patients died, but 10 experienced complications from the procedure, including 6 who had air leaks for 7–10 days after the operation.

*Conclusions.*—These early results suggest that the video-assisted thoracic operation offers a way to avoid thoracotomy and its associated discomfort and complications.

▶ This report is of interest because the technique described does not require special endostaplers but uses conventional technology. The dissection is done through a smaller than usual thoracotomy, with the assistance of the video camera. Video-assisted thoracic surgery, or so-called VATS, has practical applications, particularly in the performance of larger resections via limited incisions.

Further, 19 patients who had resections for lung cancer had cervical mediastinoscopy. By performing cervical mediastinoscopy, the authors reduce the chance of performing futile surgery in this high-risk group. We would endorse the use of cervical mediastinoscopy in patients who are at risk for conventional surgery, but are candidates for VATS resection.

The final point is that cervical mediastinoscopy will not, in all likelihood, be replaced by thoracoscopic node biopsy in the majority of cases. This is because of the ability, afforded by mediastinoscopy and not by thoracoscopic biopsy, to palpate the mediastinum to digitally and biopsy the contralateral nodes.—D.J. Sugarbaker, M.D.

*Reference*

1. Sugarbaker DJ, Strauss GM: *Semin Oncol* 1993. In press.

## Endoscopy Assisted Microthoracotomy: Initial Experience

Donnelly RJ, Page RD, Cowen ME (The Cardiothoracic Ctr, Liverpool, England)
*Thorax* 47:490–493, 1992                                        13–33

*Background.*—Thoracic surgeons have used thoracoscopy for diagnostic purposes and minor therapeutic procedures for more than 70 years, but there are only sporadic reports of its use for major surgical procedures within the thorax. Endoscopic-guided intrathoracic surgery is now being performed for indications that traditionally required formal thoracotomy.

*Procedure.*—After the lung is collapsed, a laparoscope with a camera attached is introduced into the pleural cavity via a stab incision through the sixth intercostal space. One or 2 additional stab incisions are made as needed for introduction of surgical instruments into the chest. Instruments specifically designed for endoscopic surgery include endoscopic scissors and an endoscopic cutting stapler that cuts between 2 parallel rows of staples. All instruments are inserted through trocars. With an assistant holding the laparoscope, the surgeon manipulates the instruments within the chest while watching the video monior.

*Patients.*—Twenty-one patients aged 17–75 years underwent endoscopic-guided intrathoracic procedures under general anesthesia with a double-lumen endotracheal tube. Patients were positioned and draped as for conventional posterolateral thoracotomy. In 8 patients lung tissue was removed for examination and 8 underwent removal of a solid pulmonary mass. Five patients were investigated for recurrent or persistent pneumothraces. Patients were extubated immediately after the operation and given intramuscular opiate analgesia for the first 24 hours, followed by oral acetaminophen.

*Results.*—Wedge excision for removal of a solid pulmonary mass was complete in all 8 patients. There were no perioperative complications or deaths, and patients were discharged home after a mean hospital stay of 3.4 days. One patient in whom a second pneumothorax developed 7 days after endoscopic pleurectomy required pleurodesis.

*Conclusion.*—Endoscopic surgery within the thorax is expected to become a routine procedure within the near future, but this technique should be attempted only by thoracic surgeons experienced in both thoracoscopy and general thoracic surgery.

▶ This report from England confirms many of the principles of the previous reports. One important point alluded to in the discussion is that thoracoscopy for the treatment of metastatic disease would appear inadequate if the goal of complete cytoreduction is maintained. Although the temptation to resect 1 or 2 nodules via thoracoscopy is real, the inability to carefully palpate the atelectatic lung bimanually will prevent complete cytoreduction in many cases. Complete cytoreduction is a critical factor in extending the survival of patients having pulmonary metastectomy (1–3).—D.J. Sugarbaker, M.D.

*References*

1. Freidman B, et al: *Thorac Cardiovasc Surg* 34:120, 1986.
2. Swoboda L, Tomes H: *J Thorac Cardiovasc Surg* 34:149, 1986.
3. Todd TR: *Chest* 103 (suppl):S401, 1993.

**Percutaneous Localization of Pulmonary Nodules for Thoracoscopic Lung Resection**

Mack MJ, Gordon MJ, Postma TW, Berger MS, Aronoff RJ, Acuff TE, Ryan WH (Humana Hosp Med City, Dallas, Tex)

*Ann Thorac Surg* 53:1123–1124, 1992                    13–34

*Introduction.*—The inability to locate lesions deep within the lung can limit the ability to remove pulmonary nodules by videothoracoscopic techniques. The use of percutaneous localization for such nodules was investigated.

*Technique.*—After the patient is accepted as a candidate for removal of a pulmonary nodule by thoracoscopy, the likelihood of locating it endoscopically is assessed. If the clinicians believe a lesion is unlikely to be identified, it is located fluoroscopically or by CT. A needle from the localizer system is placed through the chest wall and into the nodule, its placement verified from multiple angles. A hook wire is then put through the needle into the lesion, and the needle is withdrawn. In the operating room, a 10-mm endoscope is placed through a trocar, and the site of entry of the wire into the lung is identified. A laser is used to make a circumferential score on the visceral pleura around the wire, a core of lung tissue is developed, and the nodule with the hook wire embedded in it is withdrawn.

*Results.*—Nine lesions were identified and removed from 6 patients. Surgical margins were adequate. The technique is easy and has not led to any unexpected morbid effects.

▶ This report addresses an important problem during thoracoscopic nodulectomy. It points up the fact that lesions deeper than in the outer third of the lung are very difficult to remove (1).

The use of wire placement is a technique that deserves further study. In most instances, the second thoracoport should be placed near enough to the suspected nodule to allow palpation, which usually allows accurate localization.—D.J. Sugarbaker, M.D.

*Reference*

1.  Mentzer SJ, et al: *Chest* 103(suppl):S415, 1993.

*Thoracoscopy of the Anterior, Middle, and Posterior Mediastinum*

**Thoracoscopic Resection of an Anterior Mediastinal Tumor**
Landreneau RJ, Dowling RD, Castillo WM, Ferson PF (Univ of Pittsburgh, Pittsburgh, Pa)
*Ann Thorac Surg* 54:142–144, 1992                    13–35

*Introduction.*—The role of thoracoscopy has been expanded to include the resection of apical bullae, pleura-based lesions, and selected pulmonary nodules.

*Case Report.*—Woman, 69, had coughed intermittently and nonproductively for 10 months and had a soft tissue density in the anterior mediastinum. Contrast CT confirmed a 5-cm mass without evident local invasion. A double-lumen endotracheal tube was placed to collapse the left lung, and a thoracoscope was introduced via an 11-mm trocar. Five trocar sites in all were required to introduce endoscopic instruments and dissect the mass from the pericardium and thymus. An encapsulated thymoma was discovered. The chest tube was removed on the following day, and the patient did well.

*Discussion.*—Thoracoscopic resection of thymic tumors may prove useful in selected patients and precludes the need for median sternotomy. Total thymectomy remains the standard approach to patients with myasthenia gravis or more advanced disease.

▶ The treatment and diagnosis of anterior mediastinal masses have traditionally posed a challenge to thoracic surgeons (1). Therapeutic resections have been confined principally to resection of cysts and thymic tumors or thymectomy in myasthenia gravis. Thoracoscopic resections in the mediastinum should be limited at this time to resection of benign disease, in which the extent of resection is assured and therapeutic efficacy maintained.

The case reported here indicates that a benign thymic tumor can be removed thoracoscopially (with 5 ports). The question is whether this is advisable in the good-risk patient. Thymomas do recur with some proclivity. Therefore, one needs to be careful in generalizing from what can be done thorascopically to what should be done as standard therapy. The other point to keep in mind is that assessment of the invasiveness of a thymoma is usually based on visual inspection and palpation. The ability to make these determinations thoracoscopically has not been established.—D.J. Sugarbaker, M.D.

*Reference*

1. Sugarbaker DJ: *Ann Thorac Surg* 1993. In press.

---

**Creation of a Pericardial Window Using Thoracoscopic Techniques**
Ozuner G, Davidson PG, Isenberg JS, McGinn JT Jr (Staten Island Univ Hosp, NY)
*Surg Gynecol Obstet* 175:69–71, 1992                                    13–36

---

*Introduction.*—The optimal treatment of pericardial effusions remains controversial. A technique was developed in which minimally invasive procedures are used to create a pericardial window.

*Technique.*—After intubation in the supine position, the patient is turned to the right lateral decubitus position so that the incision can be made. The pleura is carefully incised and the left lung allowed to collapse. A Goldberg mediastinoscope and laparoscopic instruments are used to perform the procedure through a small anterolateral thoracostomy. The phrenic nerve is identified and the pericardium incised anterior to it. With the aid of a flexible choledochoscope passed through the mediastinoscope, loculated pericardial effusions can be drained. A thoracic catheter is placed before reexpansion of the lung, after which the wound is closed.

*Discussion.*—Both pericardiocentesis and pericardiotomy fail to allow for continued drainage. By creation of a pericardial window, free and persistent communication exists between the pericardial and the pleural or peritoneal cavities. The technique described here requires a minimal incision, provides optimal visualization of the pericardium, and makes it possible to obtain a sufficient specimen for pathologic examination. Conditions such as loculated collections can be treated without a thoracotomy.

▶ This report is interesting because the technique described is not truly video assisted, but entails passing instruments and a choledohoscope via a mediastinoscope for drainage of pericardial effusions. The adequacy of the pericardial window remains in doubt via this technique, however, because the width of the exposed field is the width of the scope. The approach would not appear to represent an improvement over traditional transdiaphragmatic drainage.

The technique outlined by Mack et al. (1) describes a means of performing a pericardiectomy via the 3-cannula video assisted thoracic approach. The improved visualization and size of the pericardial resection capable via this technique, would appear to make it superior to the technique of Ozuner et al. For more information on this topic, the study by Sugimoto et al. (2) is recommended.—D.J. Sugarbaker, M.D.

*References*

1. Mack MJ, et al: *Ann Thorac Surg* 54:403, 1992.
2. Sugimoto JT, *Ann Thorac Surg* 50:442, 1990.

**Thoracoscopic Resection of a Posterior Mediastinal Neurogenic Tumor**

Landreneau RJ, Dowling RD, Ferson PF (Univ of Pittsburgh, Pittsburgh, Pa)
*Chest* 102:1288–1290, 1992                                    13–37

*Introduction.*—Posterior mediastinal masses are usually treated by surgical resection. Thoracoscopic resection of such a mass, found at pathologic evaluation to be a benign, encapsulated nerve sheath tumor, was successful in 1 patient.

*Case Report.*—Woman, 35, who underwent chest roentgenography because of possible exposure to tuberculosis, was found to have a soft tissue mass. A year previously she had received a renal transplant because of lupus nephritis. The patient was asymptomatic, and findings on a chest roentgenogram obtained 6 months earlier were normal. Computed tomography and MRI showed no evidence of local or spinal canal extension of the mass. When exploratory thoracoscopy revealed a localized lesion, thoracoscopic resection of the mass was performed. Endoscopic scissors and tissue forceps were introduced through trocars. Small vessels were controlled with electrocautery current delivered through the endoscopic scissors, and larger vessels were managed with an endoscopic clip applier. When the tumor was detached from the chest wall, it was placed into a surgical glove and removed through the midaxillary trocar site. The postoperative course was uneventful, and the patient was discharged from the hospital 5 days after surgery.

*Conclusion.*—With recent improvements in video optics and endoscopic surgical techniques, many thoracic problems may be treated with minimally invasive surgical techniques. Newer imaging techniques can identify those tumors with intraspinal extension that require an open, 1-stage approach. In selected patients, exploratory thoracoscopy followed by thoracoscopic resection offers an alternative to thoracotomy.

▶ This report describes the successful removal of a benign schwannoma of the posterior mediastinum using thoracoscopic techniques. Again, it is clear that the authors are well versed in the technique and are in fact, pioneers of this approach. That is sure to revolutionize thoracic surgery. However, as they point out, the decision as to the appropriate means of managing the tumors often depends on the intraoperative findings (1). About 10% of these lesions extend into the foramen, and if not appreciated by the surgeon could cause devastating complications. One must be prepared, and prepare the patient, for open thoracotomy should difficulty in intraoperative assessment or resection be encountered.—D.J. Sugarbaker, M.D.

*Reference*

1. Shields TW: Primary tumors and cysts of the mediastinum, in Shields TW (ed): *General Thoracic Surgery.* Philadelphia, Lea & Febiger, 1989, pp 1096–1123.

---

**Thoracoscopic Long Oesophageal Myotomy for Nutcracker Oesophagus: Initial Experience of a New Surgical Approach**
Shimi SM, Nathanson LK, Cuschieri A (Univ of Dundee, Dundee, Scotland)
*Br J Surg* 79:533–536, 1992                                          13–38

---

*Introduction.*—Noncardiac chest pain is usually associated with reflux disease or motility disorders. The results of drug treatment are uncertain and no better than placebo in relieving chest pain in patients with diffuse esophageal spasm and nutcracker esophagus. Surgical management in severe cases has consisted of long esophageal myotomy, a procedure requiring posterolateral thoracotomy and a long convalescence. An alternative thorascopic technique was developed.

*Patients.*—The technique was performed in 3 women aged 25, 42, and 38 years. All had angina-like pain unresponsive to medical therapy. One complained of pain on swallowing. Perfusion manometry suggested a diagnosis of nutcracker esophagus (high-amplitude esophageal peristalsis) in all 3 women.

*Technique.*—The procedure, performed with the patient under general anesthesia, is based on a multipuncture method and a left thoracoscopic approach. A flexible endoscope is inserted to identify and lift the esophagus. The myotomy begins in the lower esophagus. If normal, the lower esophageal spincter is left intact. If hypertensive, the myotomy is extended to the gastroesophageal junction. The duration of the operation has ranged from 90 minutes to 3 hours.

*Results.*—Postoperative pain was minimal, and all 3 patients were ambulatory within 24 hours. The only complication was a minor chest infection in 1 patient. Lung reinflation after the procedure was rapid and uncomplicated in each case. With a maximum follow-up of 12 months, all patients were free of chest pain and dysphagia.

*Conclusion.*—Nutcracker esophagus is a common cause of esophageal chest pain. Surgery is usually successful, but it is performed infrequently because of the need for an extensive thoracotomy. Thoracoscopic myotomy can be performed safely, with good results and rapid recovery. Pain relief has been obtained in 5 of 6 additional patients treated since this report was completed.

▶ The esophagus has only recently been the object of thoracoscopic procedures. The myotomy performed in this fashion took up to 3 hours of operative time. In addition, the dreaded complication of perforation, although it did not occur in this series, may be difficult to assess thoracoscopically. Caution will need to be the foundation of the extension of thoracoscopic surgery to the esophagus, because it is an unforgiving organ when inadvertently injured. Indeed, benign esophageal surgery for motility disorders is challenging for surgeons when performed in the traditional manner and will undoubtedly remain so regardless of operative technique (1).—D.J. Sugarbaker, M.D.

*Reference*

1. Sugarbaker DJ: *Surg Rounds* February:93, 1993.

---

**Thoracoscopic Enucleation of Leiomyoma of the Oesophagus**
Everitt NJ, Glinatsis M, McMahon MJ (General Infirmary, Leeds, England)
*Br J Surg* 79:643, 1992                                    13–39

---

*Introduction.*—Esophageal leiomyoma, an uncommon benign lesion, rarely becomes malignant. About 90% of the patients with this lesion, however, usually have it removed because of adverse symptoms. Thoracoscopic resection is preferred because it is less invasive. In a patient with a midesophageal leiomyoma, the lesion was removed by thoracoscopic enucleation.

*Case Report.*—Woman, 48, had experienced epigastric discomfort and heartburn for 3 years. She had a recent history of dysphagia and retrosternal pain on ingestion of solids. A barium study demonstrated the presence of a midesophageal leiomyoma. The 2-cm lesion was removed with the transthoracic endoscopic technique, after which the patient fully recovered. After induction of general anesthesia, the patient underwent endotracheal intubation. The tumor was located in the posterior esophageal wall, medial to the azygos vein, using a flexible endoscope. Dissecting forceps and a hook diathermy were inserted through the cannulas, after which the esophagus was rotated to allow performance of a longitudinal myotomy over the tumor with diathermy. The tumor was then totally enucleated and removed through a 20-mm cannula. Histologic analysis confirmed the diagnosis of leiomyoma.

*Discussion.*—Thoracoscopic resection is less invasive than open surgery. The technique avoids the problems associated with thoracotomy e.g., atelectasis and scarring. It also reduces the need for analgesia and the morbidity and mortality associated with the more involved general surgery.

*Conclusions.*—This technique is a less invasive means of removing an esophageal leiomyoma. It also allows for an open approach if the removal through the thoracoscope becomes impossible, or if hemorrhage follows a perforation.

▶ Resection of an esophageal leiomyoma is done when there are symptoms of obstruction. The clinical diagnosis of the lesion is not in and of itself a reason for removal. The case report is of interest because in this well-selected patient, thoracoscopic resection was easily accomplished and resulted in lowered morbidity.

We have performed several of these resections and find the use of the intraoperative endoscope of importance. It improves visibility and assures the surgeon that the mucosa is not torn or perforated during the resection. We have not found it necessary to close the longitudinal muscle after the resection.—D.J. Sugarbaker, M.D.

*Transthoracic Thoracoscopic Sympathectomy: Indications, Techniques, and Assessment of Outcome*

▶↓ The traditional approach to patients with hyperhidrosis and Raynaud's phenomenon, requiring surgical disruption of the sympathetic chain, has entailed limited transaxillary thoracotomy or limited posterolateral thoracotomy. Because the clinical results of this procedure are not always readily apparent, some surgeons use it only rarely. The following reports review new technical approaches to the procedure and new ways of assessing its clinical efficacy.—D.J. Sugarbaker, M.D.

### Endoscopic Transthoracic Sympathectomy: Experience in the South West of England

Adams DCR, Wood SJ, Tulloh BR, Baird RN, Poskitt KR (Cheltenham Gen Hosp, Cheltenham, England; Bristol Royal Infirmary, Bristol, England)
*Eur J Vasc Surg* 6:558–562, 1992
13–40

*Background.*—Surgical procedures for thoracic sympathectomy are intricate and may require several days of recovery in the hospital. The patients, predominantly females, may be left with sizeable scars. Because the supraclavicular approach entails a risk of Horner's syndrome, an endoscopic approach was used for 45 procedures in 26 patients. Follow-up data were available for 27 procedures carried out in patients with hyperhidrosis and for 10 others performed in management of Raynaud's phenomenon.

*Technique.*—General anesthesia is induced using a double-lumen endotracheal tube, and pneumothorax is produced. An end-viewing fiberoptic endoscope with video camera attached is passed. The pneumothorax is adjusted with carbon dioxide. A second incision is made over the same intercostal space to pass a 5-mm cannula for a diathermy probe, forceps, or scissors, as needed. Coagulation diathermy currently is applied to the second through the fourth ganglia and the intervening sympathetic chain, avoiding the stellate ganglion. Better exposure may be achieved by opening the parietal pleura over the sympathetic chain, minimizing the risk of damaging the stellate ganglion.

*Results.*—All patients with hyperhidrosis improved immediately, and all of those who were followed maintained a good or excellent outcome. All but 1 of the patients with Raynaud's phenomenon improved, but the effect appeared to decline over time. Four patients had asymptomatic pneumothorax that resolved rapidly with chest drainage. Two had a unilateral Horner's syndrome. The mean postoperative hospital stay was 3.5 days.

*Conclusion.*—Endoscopic thoracic sympathectomy now is the preferred approach. It is effective, safe, and well accepted by patients.

### Endoscopic Transthoracic Sympathectomy in the Treatment of Hyperhidrosis

Edmondson RA, Banerjee AK, Rennie JA (King's College Hosp, London, England)
*Ann Surg* 215:289–293, 1992
13–41

*Background.*—Axillary hyperhidrosis is managed by excising the eccrine glands, but if palmar involvement occurs, sympathectomy is the only option yielding lasting results. The results of 50 endoscopic transaxillary dorsal sympathectomies done in a 5-year period were assessed.

*Technique.*—An incision is made in the anterior axillary line over the third rib space, avoiding the long thoracic nerve. A Verres needle is inserted after clamping the appropriate side of the endotracheal tube, and the lung is slowly deflated by instilling carbon dioxide interpleurally. A laparoscope then is inserted to visualize the upper sympathetic chain. A second small incision is made over the fourth interspace to insert a diathermy probe, and the second through fourth ganglia with their interconnecting fibers are treated.

*Results.*—The procedure improved or eliminated symptoms of hyperhidrosis in most of the patients. All but 8% were very satisfied with the outcome. Three fourths of the patients experienced compensatory sweating, and 50% had gustatory sweating, but these effects were acceptable to the patients. No patient had a permanent Horner's syndrome.

*Conclusions.*—Endoscopic transaxillary dorsal sympathectomy is a simple, effective, and inexpensive surgical treatment for hyperhidrosis of the upper extremity. Only an overnight hospital stay is required.

▶ Care is taken to open the parietal pleura. This allows better visualization of the sympathetic chain and avoids damage to the stellate ganglion. The pleural dissection is facilitated by placement of a third port on the third cannula site. The 2 ports for dissection allow sectioning of the chain and the application of clips. We avoid the use of diathermy as it may lead to stellate ganglion disruption. It is important to resect 2 or 3 ganglia to assure complete nerve fiber transection (1).—D.J. Sugarbaker, M.D.

*Reference*

1. Mack M: *Ann Thorac Surg* 1993. In press.

---

**Transaxillary Endoscopic Laser Sympathectomy**
Austin JJ, Doobay B, Schatz SW (Hamilton Gen Hosp, Hamilton, Ont, Canada)
*Can J Surg* 35:414–416, 1992                          13–42

---

*Introduction.*—For half a century, surgeons have used thoratic sympathectomy and other procedures to treat a variety of vasomotor and neurologic disorders. These methods have produced serious complications, however, and lengthened hospital stays for some patients. The functional and cosmetic outcome of transaxillary endoscopic laser sympathectomy in treatment of hyperhidrosis was evaluated.

*Case Report.*—Woman, 20, had severe bilateral palmar hyperhidrosis that did not respond to medical treatment. Because the patient worked as a professional model and wanted to avoid a surgical scar, the transaxillary method was used in performance of laser sympathectomy. After general anesthesia induction, the patient underwent endotracheal intubation and was placed in the semilateral decubitus position. Her arm was elevated, and two 1-cm incisions were performed to insert the thoracoscopes into the third and fourth intercostal space. An air-cooled fiberoptic light guide in the endoscope was used to illuminate the operative area; the sympthetic chain was photocoagulated from the second to the third ganglion using the continuous-wave neodymium: yttrium/aluminum/garnet laser set at 1,064 nm. The patient left the hospital 2 days after surgery but returned 1 week later to receive a repeat procedure on the other side. The patient had a warm and dry hand immediately after the first surgery, whereas the untreated hand continued to perspire. Eighteen months of follow-up found the patient to have dry hands.

*Conclusions.*—Laser sympathectomy has been used successfully to treat causalgia, Raynaud's phenomenon, and reflex sympathetic dystrophy. A longer follow-up period is required, however, to assess possible relapse and return of symptoms. Currently, laser pulses have been increased to 15–18 W to prevent the possible regeneration of nerve fibers through the scar tissue.

▶ The combination of thoracoscopic techniques with laser coagulation will become more widespread in the future. The advantages of the laser here are the fact that ablation of tissue by thermal energy is not dependent on the flow of electricity, as it is with Bovie coagulation, making nerve damage much less likely.—D.J. Sugarbaker, M.D.

---

**Efficacy of Endoscopic Transthoracic Sympathectomy Assessed by Peroperative Palmar Temperature Measurement**
Chester JF, Jeddy TA, Taylor RS, Dormandy JA, Allt-Graham J (Taunton and Somerset Hosp, Taunton, England; St George's Hosp, London, England)
*Br J Surg* 79:752, 1992                                        13–43

---

*Introduction.*—Endoscopic transthoracic sympathectomy, first described in 1978, is the preferred treatment for palmar hyperhidrosis. Measurement of palmar temperature during endoscopic sympathectomy is useful in assessing the immediate efficacy of the procedure.

*Technique.*—The sympathetic chain under the parietal pleura running over the necks of the second, third, fourth, and fifth ribs is visible when the laparoscope is introduced through the fourth intercostal space in the anterior axillary line. If the chain is not visible, it may be palpable with the diathermy probe. Diathermy is used to coagulate the second, third, and fourth thoracic ganglia and the intervening chain, resulting in a characteristic charred appearance.

*Method and Outcome.*—Palmar temperature was measured during 6 sympathectomies with a disposable skin temperature sensor affixed to the patient's palm on the relevant side. All other factors, including anesthetic agents, were kept constant. A palmar temperature rise of 1.1–2.6°

C (mean, 1.6°C) was recorded on the relevant side within 3 minutes of coagulation of the sympathetic chain, whereas temperature on the side not operated on remained unchanged during contralateral sympathectomy. An average palmar temperature rise of 1.6°C predicted a good outcome, with abolition of palmar sweating for at least 6 months reported.

▶ This short report describes an easy method of assessing the neurogenic effect of the procedure in the operating room. The approach appears practical because it uses the contralateral palm as the control. Larger studies are needed to validate the technique.

Thoracoscopic surgery will provide a challenge to all surgeons. The need to provide appropriate, safe, and efficacious use of these new techniques will challenge the surgical community. Surgeons must keep in mind the clinical and biological behavior of the diseases they are treating as they devise new surgical therapy.—D.J. Sugarbaker, M.D.

# Subject Index

# G

Gallbladder
  sludge, 238
Gastrectomy
  in gastric carcinoma, pathology and
      prognosis in, 338
  partial, for benign conditions, long-term
      prognosis, 219
  smoking-related death after, 219
Gastric, 218
  acid production, effect of duodenal
      switch procedure in, 225
  bypass, long-limb, in superobesity, 222
  cancer, 333
    advanced, immunochemosurgery of,
        333
    FAMTX vs. etoposide, doxorubicin
        and cisplatin in, 340
    lymph node metastases in, endoscopic
        ultrasound of, 341
    staging, preoperative, endoscopic
        ultrasound vs. CT in, 342
    surgery, OK-432 after, 335
    surgery results, 333
  carcinoma
    pathology and prognosis after
        gastrectomy, 338
    resection, radical curative, 334
  duodenogastric reflux, 225
  emptying, effect of duodenal switch
      procedure on, 225
  replacement of esophagus, pyloroplasty
      vs. no drainage, 220
Gastroesophageal
  reflux, complicated, medical vs. surgical
      therapy, 209
Gastrointestinal, 207
  bleeding
    occult, surgical approach, 246
    upper, endoscopic injection treatment
        of, 224
  hormones, effect of duodenal switch
      procedure on, 225
Gel-filled
  breast prostheses, 385
Gene
  elastin, expression in skin fibroblasts,
      transforming growth factor beta
      up-regulating, 182
  epidermal growth factor receptor, in
      colonic anastomosis healing (in rat),
      188
  expression, down-regulation in CD8+
      T cells, 322

heat shock, expression after
    resuscitation from hemorrhagic
    shock, 47
p53 tumor suppressor, germline
    mutations in children and young
    adults with second cancer, 327
*ras*, mutations, in lung adenocarcinoma,
    as prognostic marker, 428
stress protein genes not transcribed
    simultaneously, 47
Glomerulosclerosis
  focal segmental, kidney transplant in, in
      children, 139
Glue
  fibrin, applications, 403
Glutamine
  enriched total parenteral nutrition,
      effect on tumor growth and host
      tissues, 197
  supplement of parenteral nutrition
      in marrow transplant, 198
      in sepsis of small bowel (in rat), 195
Gowns
  design needed to prevent nonsterile
      contact between surgeon and
      patient, 22
  surgical, in-use evaluation, 21
Graft
  arterial, infection, infrainguinal
      anastomotic, graft preservation in,
      125
  autograft for burns (*see* Burns,
      autografts for)
  Dacron, interstices, eradicating bacteria
      from, 126
  epidermis, cultured human, 399
  flap (*see* Flap)
  microskin, with pigskin xenograft
      overlay (in rabbit), 403
  pressure, in early reconstruction of facial
      burns, 66
  skin
    for burns (*see* Burns, skin grafts for)
    cultured, functional innervation of,
        399
  vein graft stenosis, balloon angioplasty
      limitations for, 373
  visceral grafts, composite, for intestinal
      transplant, 151
Growth
  factor
    beta 1, recombinant transforming, in
        ulcer healing, 184
    beta 1, transforming, in dermal
        wound healing, 183
    beta, transforming, in intestinal
        healing, steroid-impaired, 187

# U

# Author Index

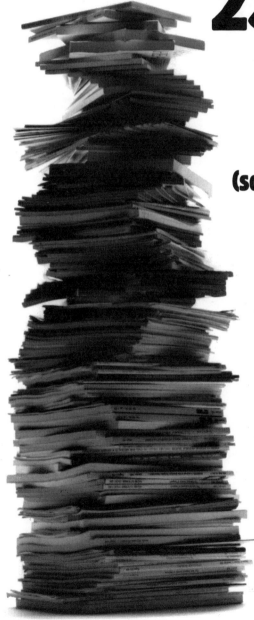

# We've read
# 236,287
# journal
# articles
## (so you don't have to).

# The Year Books–
# The best from 236,287 journal articles.

At Mosby, we subscribe to more than 950 medical and allied health journals from every corner of the globe. We read them all, tirelessly scanning for anything that relates to your field.

We send everything we find related to a given specialty to the distinguished editors of the **Year Book** in that area, and they pick out the best, the articles they feel every practitioner in that specialty should be aware of.

For the 1993 **Year Books** we surveyed a total of 236,287 articles and found hundreds of articles related to your field. Our expert editors reviewed these and chose the best, the developments you don't want to miss.

## The best articles–condensed and organized.

Not only do you get the past year's most important articles in your field, you get them in a format that makes them easy to use.

Every article that the editors pick is condensed into a concise, outlined abstract, a summary of the article's most important points highlighted with bold paragraph headings. So you can quickly scan for exactly what you need.

## Personal commentary from the experts.

If that was it, if all our editors did was identify the year's best articles, the **Year Book** would still be a great reference to have. (Can you think of an easier way to keep up with all the developments that are shaping your field?)

But following each article, the editors also write concise commentaries telling whether or not the study in question is a reliable one, whether a new technique is effective, or whether a particular trend you've heard about merits your immediate attention.

No other abstracting service offers this expert advice to help you decide how the year's advances will affect the way you practice.

## No matter how many journals you subscribe to, the Year Book can help.

When you subscribe to a **Year Book**, we'll also send you an automatic notice of future volumes about two months before they publish. If you do not want the **Year Book**, this convenient advance notice makes it easy for you to let us know. And if you elect to receive the new **Year Book**, you need do nothing. We will send it upon publication.

No worry. No wasted motion. And, of course, every **Year Book** is yours to examine FREE of charge for thirty days.